D0906189

DIGITAL RADIOGRAPHY:
A FOCUS ON CLINICAL UTILITY

DIGITAL RADIOGRAPHY: A FOCUS ON CLINICAL UTILITY

Editors

Ronald R. Price, Ph.D.
Director, Division of Radiological Sciences
Associate Professor of Radiology and Physics
Department of Radiology and Radiological Sciences
Vanderbilt University School of Medicine, Nashville, Tenn.

F. David Rollo, M.D., Ph.D.
Vice President, Medical Affairs
Humana Inc., Louisville, Kentucky
Professor of Radiology
Department of Radiology and Radiological Sciences
Vanderbilt University School of Medicine, Nashville, Tenn.

RC
78
.D494
1982

W. Gordon Monahan, Ph.D.
Product Director, Digital Radiography
Technicare Corporation
Cleveland, Ohio

A. Everette James, Jr., Sc.M., J.D., M.D.
Chairman, Department of Radiology and Radiological Sciences
Professor of Medical Administration
Lecturer in Legal Medicine
Senior Research Associate
Institute for Public Policy Studies
Vanderbilt University School of Medicine, Nashville, Tenn.

Grune & Stratton

A Subsidiary of Harcourt Brace Jovanovich, Publishers

New York   London
Paris   San Diego   São Paulo   San Francisco
Sydney   Tokyo   Toronto

© **1982 by Grune & Stratton, Inc.**

Grune & Stratton, Inc.
111 Fifth Avenue
New York, NY 10003

Distributed in the United Kingdom by
Academic Press Inc. (London) Ltd.
24/28 Oval Road, London NW 1

Library of Congress Catalog Number 82-083765
International Standard Book Number 0-8089-1544-4

Printed in the United States of America

6-14-84

CONTENTS

ACKNOWLEDGMENTS

We would like to acknowledge Humana Inc., Louisville, Kentucky, and the Technicare Corporation, Cleveland, Ohio, for their financial assistance in sponsoring the symposium on digital radiography that lead to this publication. We would also like to acknowledge the invaluable efforts of the editorial office staff of the Department of Radiology and Radiological Sciences at Vanderbilt University School of Medicine: Tom Ebers, Joann Fields, Ima Mosley, Terri Shaw, and Georgia Pilzak. We are most appreciative of the contributions by the authors of the individual chapters of this book, especially in light of their extensive and time-consuming clinical responsibilities in the development of this new diagnostic modality. Finally, the academic environment of our various institutions makes projects such as this one possible, for which we are most appreciative.

PREFACE

The digital imaging process affords far-reaching opportunities in diagnostic medicine. This methodology has significant implications for the acquisition, storage, manipulation, transmission or transfer, and display of data. This introductory text provides clinicians and scientists with the basic principles of digital radiography, relates early experiences in medical practice, and explores promising avenues of future application.

There are, of course, inherent limitations to any text about a methodology that is experiencing such dramatic and unpredictable growth. For this reason, we have purposely devoted a large portion of the text to basic principles and have discussed clinical experiences as generically as possible. Since this volume is primarily directed toward those persons responsible for using this exciting new technological advance in medical practice, the scope and content are clinically oriented, but background scientific information is provided as a basis for understanding present applications as well as future developments.

The first several chapters of *Digital Radiography* are devoted to the physical principles of digital imaging and the engineering technology that allows for clinical applications. Presenting the technology first allows the reader an enhanced appreciation of the virtues and limitations, as well as a realistic appraisal of the potential, of this method. From the initial clinical experiences with digital radiography, it appears that this method will achieve widespread use in the near future. Unlike pulsed Doppler, real-time ultrasound, or nuclear magnetic resonance imaging, digital imaging is in many ways similar to presently employed radiographic methods, which is a practical and important consideration in both physician and patient acceptance.

In other chapters financial aspects of digital radiography are explored and its health care implications compared with those of competing and complementary techniques. The remaining text is devoted to various applications of the technique, which range from cardiovascular assessment of children to the analysis of works of fine art. Finally, we have included a glossary of important terms used in this field. It has been our goal to produce a resource with which each reader can effectively assess the clinical utility of digital radiography.

CONTRIBUTORS

JOSEPH H. ALLEN, M.D. Section of Neuroradiology, Department of Radiology and Radiological Sciences, Vanderbilt University School of Medicine, Nashville, Tennessee

ALVIN N. BIRD, Jr., M.S. ADAC Laboratories, Sunnyvale, California

JAMES BLUMSTEIN, J.D. Vanderbilt University School of Law, Nashville, Tennessee

THOMAS B. BRUMBAUGH, Ph.D. Department of Fine Arts, Vanderbilt University, Nashville, Tennessee

EDWARD BUONOCORE, M.D. Department of Hospital Radiology, Cleveland Clinic Foundation, Cleveland, Ohio

M. PAUL CAPP, M.D. Department of Radiology, University of Arizona Medical School, Tucson, Arizona

JOHN C. CHAPMAN, M.D. Office of the Dean, Vanderbilt University School of Medicine, Nashville, Tennessee

JOSEPH DIGGS, M.D. Department of Radiology and Radiological Sciences, Vanderbilt University School of Medicine, Nashville, Tennessee

FRANK M. EGGERS, M.D. Section of Neuroradiology, Department of Radiology and Radiological Sciences, Vanderbilt University School of Medicine, Nashville, Tennessee

JON J. ERICKSON, Ph.D. Department of Radiology and Radiological Sciences, Vanderbilt University School of Medicine, Nashville, Tennessee

RONALD G. EVENS, M.D. Mallinckrodt Institute of Radiology, Washington University School of Medicine, St. Louis, Missouri

BARRY D. FLETCHER, M.D. Department of Radiology, Case Western Reserve University School of Medicine, Cleveland, Ohio

GERALD FREEDMAN, M.D.   Department of Radiology, Yale University, New Haven, Connecticut

JOE H. GALLAGHER, Ph.D.   Cleveland Clinic Foundation, Cleveland, Ohio

S. JULIAN GIBBS, D.D.S., Ph.D.   Department of Radiology and Radiological Sciences, Vanderbilt University School of Medicine, Nashville, Tennessee

ROBERT G. GOULD, Sc.D., Ph.D.   Department of Radiology, University of California, San Francisco, California

KEVIN GROGAN   Curator, Cheekwood Fine Arts Museum, Nashville, Tennessee

DONALD HALL, J.D.   Vanderbilt University School of Law, Nashville, Tennessee

RICHARD M. HELLER, Jr., M.D.   Departments of Radiology and Pediatrics, Vanderbilt University Medical Center, Nashville, Tennessee

EDWIN HILL   Technicare Corporation, Cleveland, Ohio

BRUCE J. HILLMAN, M.D.   Department of Radiology, University of Arizona Health Science Center, Tuscon, Arizona

WILLIAM HUNTER, Jr., M.D.   Technicare Corporation, Cleveland, Ohio

A. EVERETTE JAMES, Jr., Sc.M., J.D., M.D.   Chairman, Department of Radiology and Radiological Sciences, Professor of Medical Administration, Lecturer in Legal Medicine, and Senior Research Associate, Institute for Public Policy Studies, Vanderbilt University School of Medicine, Nashville, Tennessee

HOWARD JOLLES, M.D.   Department of Radiology and Radiological Sciences, Vanderbilt University School of Medicine, Nashville, Tennessee

CHIIMINY KAO   Technicare Corporation, Cleveland, Ohio

MARVIN W. KRONENBERG, M.D.   Departments of Radiology and Medicine, Vanderbilt University School of Medicine, Nashville, Tennessee

PETER L. LAMS, M.D.   Brompton Hospital, London, England

FREDERICK A. MANN, M.D.   Department of Radiology, University of Wisconsin Medical School, Madison, Wisconsin

THOMAS F. MEANEY, M.D. Department of Radiology, Cleveland Clinic Foundation, Cleveland, Ohio

CHARLES A. MISTRETTA, Ph.D. Medical Physics Section, University of Wisconsin, Madison, Wisconsin

MICHAEL T. MODIC, M.D. Department of Diagnostic Radiology, Cleveland Clinic Foundation, Cleveland, Ohio

W. GORDON MONAHAN, Ph.D. Digital Radiography, Technicare Corporation, Cleveland, Ohio

C. LEON PARTAIN, Ph.D., M.D. Department of Radiology and Radiological Sciences, Vanderbilt University School of Medicine, Nashville, Tennessee

HENRY P. PENDERGRASS, M.P.H., M.D. Department of Radiology and Radiological Sciences, Vanderbilt University School of Medicine, Nashville, Tennessee

JEFF POHLHAMMER Technicare Corporation, Cleveland, Ohio

ANN C. PRICE, M.D. Section of Neuroradiology, Department of Radiology and Radiological Sciences, Vanderbilt University School of Medicine, Nashville, Tennessee

RONALD R. PRICE, Ph.D. Department of Radiology and Radiological Sciences, Vanderbilt University School of Medicine, Nashville, Tennessee

ROSALYN REILLEY, M.D. Department of Radiology and Radiological Sciences, Vanderbilt University School of Medicine, Nashville, Tennessee

F. DAVID ROLLO, M.D., Ph.D. Humana Inc., Louisville, Kentucky, and Department of Radiology and Radiological Sciences, Vanderbilt University School of Medicine, Nashville, Tennessee

JOSEPH F. SACKETT, M.D. Department of Radiology, Center for Health Sciences, University of Wisconsin, Madison, Wisconsin

RONALD P. SCHWENKER, Ph.D. Photoproducts Department, E.I. DuPont de Nemours & Company, Wilmington, Delaware

MALCOLM SLOAN, R.T. Department of Radiology and Radiological Sciences, Vanderbilt University School of Medicine, Nashville, Tennessee

CLYDE W. SMITH, M.D. Department of Radiology and Radiological Sciences, Vanderbilt University School of Medicine, Nashville, Tennessee

CHARLES M. STROTHER, M.D. Department of Radiology, University of Wisconsin Medical School, Madison, Wisconsin

PATRICK A. TURSKI, M.D. Department of Radiology, University of Wisconsin Medical School, Madison, Wisconsin

R. E. WAYRYNEN, Ph.D. E.I. DuPont de Nemours & Company, Wilmington, Delaware

MEREDITH A. WEINSTEIN, M.D. Department of Diagnostic Radiology, Cleveland Clinic Foundation, Cleveland, Ohio

ALAN C. WINFIELD, M.D. Department of Radiology and Radiological Sciences, Vanderbilt University School of Medicine, Nashville, Tennessee

INTRODUCTION AND OVERVIEW

Ronald R. Price[1]
F. David Rollo[2]
W. Gordon Monahan[3]
A. Everette James, Jr.[1]

[1]Department of Radiology and Radiological Sciences
Vanderbilt University School of Medicine
Nashville, Tennessee

[2]Humana, Inc.
Louisville, Kentucky

[3] Technicare Corporation
Cleveland, Ohio

Arteriograms using intravenous injections of radiographic contrast media and conventional film-based systems were reported as early as 1939 (1). The development of catheterization techniques for the arterial administration of contrast media soon led to the replacement of the intravenous approach with the more invasive intra-arterial procedures. The morbidity associated with these invasive catheterization procedures was clearly outweighed by the improved resolution and contrast of the images relative to images obtained using intravenous procedures.

Digital Radiography is probably the most significant innovation in diagnostic radiology since the introduction of the CT scanner in 1972. The use of digital subtraction techniques and computer processing may now make it possible to return to intravenous angiography while maintaining good image contrast and acceptable resolution (Fig. 1). Other advantages of the digital technique include speed, flexibility and consistency.

Intravenous digital subtraction angiography using digitized video images from an image intensifier was pioneered

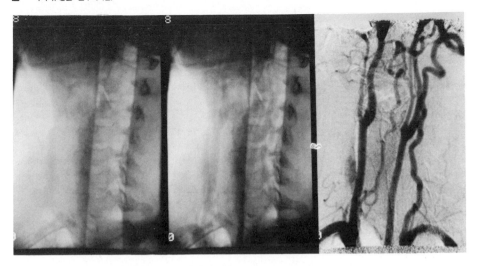

FIGURE 1. An example of intravenous digital subtraction
of the carotid arteries. (Left) Digitized pre-contrast or
"mask" image. (Center) Digitized image following intravenous
injection of 45 ml of contrast media. (Right) Image following
digital subtraction of the mask and computer enhancement.
Most of the vascular structures so clearly demonstrated in the
subtraction image can only be seen faintly in the image prior
to subtraction, illustrating the power of the digital
subtraction technique.

by several groups. Among those making significant
contributions were the University of Wisconsin (2-5) and the
University of Arizona (6-8). Since these early
investigations, essentially all of the major radiographic
equipment manufacturers now offer commercially available
digital radiographic systems (9). At the present time, it is
estimated that several hundred digital radiographic units have
already been sold and are in various stages of production,
delivery and installation.
      In this text, the editors have invited contributions from
individuals from all of the major groups who are currently
active in the development of digital radiography systems and
their clinical evaluation. Chapters have been continuously
added as advances have been made (10,11).
      As noted in the Preface, the text begins with a group of
four chapters (Price, Mistretta, Monahan, and Gould) to
develop a foundation of the basic physical principles,
intrumentation and terminology of digital radiography which
hopefully will aid in the understanding of the various

chapters presenting clinical experiences. Once the physical basis for digital radiography has been defined, the cost benefit ratio and legal aspects of both traditional and proposed procedures are considered. Three chapters (Freedman, Evens and James) are devoted to these important factors both from the private office setting and institutional practice points-of-view.

A chapter (Sackett) considering the important factor of injection techniques and contrast media has also been included prior to the group of eleven clinical chapters. The clinical topics include: head and neck angiography (Modic), cardiovascular (Smith), chest (Buonocore), pulmonary (Jolles), renal (Hillman), renal function (Meaney), peripheral vascular (Mistretta), pediatric applications (Fletcher and Heller), intra-arterial (Eggers) and a chapter on general topics (Bird). A chapter by Schwenker addresses the capabilities of analog film/screen systems for intravenous angiography, and the chapter by James explores the use of digital radiography in the analysis of art. The concluding chapter by Capp and others attempts to place digital radiography in its proper perspective in regard to other imaging modalities. These other modalities include ultrasound, both real-time and pulsed Doppler, nuclear medicine procedures, along with emission tomography and the other new and exciting imaging modality, nuclear magnetic resonance imaging.

The text concludes with a glossary of digital radiography terms which the authors hope will aid the reader in understanding this important new radiographic innovation.

During the course of compiling this document, significant advances in the implementation of this methodology came to our attention. Often we had to encourage individuals to commit their initial experiences to a public forum because of inherent risks involved in early publication. However, we believed these experiences to be promising and felt that they had significant future clinical implications.

We entertain the hope that this text will serve as a foundation to initiate a continuing experience in the digital imaging process. Digital Radiography II should keep pace with the developments and expanding clinical applications. Again, the general technique of digital radiology is advancing at such a pace that a text can only provide concepts which the practitioner may employ in order to be an informed participant.

REFERENCES

1. Robb, G.P., and Steinberg, I., Visualization of the chambers of the heart, the pulmonary circulation and the vessels in man: A practical method, AJR 41, 1 (1939).
2. Mistretta, C.A., and Crummy, A.B., Digital Fluoroscopy, in "Physical Basis of Medical Imaging" (C.M. Coulam, J.J. Erickson, F.D. Rollo, and A.E. James, Jr., eds.), p. 107, Appleton-Century-Crofts, New York, (1981).
3. Kruger, R., Mistretta, C., Houk, T., et al., Computerized fluoroscopy in real-time for noninvasive visualization of the cardiovascular system, Radiology 130, 49-57 (1979).
4. Kruger, R., Mistretta, C., Houk, T., et al., Computerized fluoroscopy techniques for intravenous study of cardiac chamber dynamics, Invest. Radiol. 14(4), 279-287 (1979).
5. Mistretta, C.A., Crummy, A.B., and Strother, C.M., Digital angiography: A perspective, Radiology 139, 273 (1981).
6. Nudelman, S., Capp, M.P., Fisher, H.D., et al., Photoelectronic imaging for diagnostic radiology and the digital computer, Proc. SPIE 164, 138 (1978).
7. Ovitt, T.W., Capp, M.P., Fisher, H.D., et al., The development of a digital video subtraction system for intravenous angiography, Proc. SPIE 167, 61 (1978).
8. Christenson, P.C., Ovitt, T.W., Fisher, H.D., et al., Intravenous angiography using digital subtraction: Intravenous cervicocerebrovascular angiography, AJR 135, 1145 (1980).
9. Couvillon, L.A., Jr., and Brenkus, L.M., The commercial systems for digital radiology, Diagnostic Imaging 4, 3 (1982).
10. Brody, W.R., Cassel, D.M., Somner, F.G., et al., Dual-energy projection radiography: Initial clinical experience, AJR 137, 201 (1981).
11. Price, R.R., Pickens, D.R., Smith, C.W., et al., Simultaneous bi-plane video-fluoroscopy, Radiology 143, 255 (1982).

2

BASIC PRINCIPLES AND INSTRUMENTATION
OF DIGITAL RADIOGRAPHY

Ronald R. Price
A. Everette James, Jr.

Department of Medical Imaging and Radiological Sciences
Vanderbilt University School of Medicine
Nashville, Tennessee

I. INTRODUCTION

The term "Digital Radiography" (DR) does not specify either a particular apparatus or a specific radiographic procedure (1,2). Digital radiography has come to imply a technique in which the traditional silver halide film/screen radiation receptor has been replaced by a photoelectronic receptor controlled by a computer. The advantages of digital over film-based systems include flexibility and the added facility for control and to manipulate image formation and presentation. The disadvantages of current digital systems include the relatively small field-of-view and reduced spatial resolution as compared to traditional film images (3).

Many of the system components and techniques used in the production of digital images are significantly different from conventional radiographic equipment. For this reason, a discussion of these components and the associated terminology will be presented in this communication. The authors felt this might be helpful prior to the presentation of the clinical experiences with the digital process. The components considered will include the computer system and peripherals, the video system and the analog-to-digital converter.

II. THE DIGITAL RADIOGRAPHY SYSTEM

Current digital radiographic (DR) systems can be divided into two broad categories. In our discussion, these will be termed digital video-fluoroscopy systems and scan projection radiographic (SPR) systems. The former is frequently referred to as digital fluoroscopy. The procedure most frequently performed using this system is called digital subtraction angiography (DSA). In SPR, collimated x-ray beams are used to scan the patient, either by moving the beam over the patient or by moving the patient through the beam. The detectors used in SPR systems are usually high efficiency scintillation crystals or high pressure xenon detectors. Scan projection radiography is used currently as an adjunct study by computed tomography to produce the survey images that are very helpful for determining the appropriate tomographic plane. Scan projection radiography is also produced commercially as a stand-alone device for low dose radiographic procedures, as will be discussed in the chapters by Jolles and Heller. This chapter will be devoted to the discussion of digital fluoroscopy.

Of the digital radiographic techniques in current use, DSA has received the most emphasis. DSA has provided, as a result of its increased contrast sensitivity, the ability to image arterial vascular structures by the injection of contrast media into the venous system. Visualization of the small density differences resulting from the intravenous injection has not, at this point in time, been possible with current film subtraction techniques. However, as shown in the chapter by Schwenker, this too may soon change.

The major components of a conventional radiography system (Fig. 1) include the source of x-rays (tube/generator), the image receptor (film/screen), the film processor/developer, and the film viewing station (light box). Analog film subtraction requires two additional steps between processing and viewing. These are to create the subtraction mask and the subtraction film. Of all of these components, only the x-ray source is common with the DR systems that are to be considered in this text.

In the digital video-fluoroscopic DR systems, an x-ray image intensifier replaces the film as the primary image receptor (Fig. 2). X-rays interacting with the image intensifier input phosphor are first converted to light photons within a scintillation screen. The light is, in turn, converted to electrons by a photocathode. The electron distribution closely mimics that of the x-ray distribution. This is because the scintillation screen thickness is kept

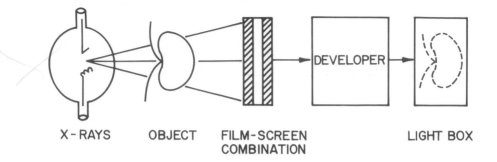

X-RAYS   OBJECT   FILM-SCREEN   LIGHT BOX
                      COMBINATION

CONVENTIONAL RADIOGRAPHY

FIGURE 1. The primary components of a conventional film-based radiography system are the source of x-rays (x-ray tube), the film/screen cassette, the film processor and viewbox. Of these components, only the x-ray source is common with digital fluoroscopy systems.

thin and photons do not migrate far from their point of production before being converted to electrons. The electrons are then accelerated and focused onto the image intensifier output phosphor. At the output phosphor, the increased energy of the electrons and the reduced size of the phosphor work together to produce an image with significantly enhanced brightness. The rather small image on the output phosphor (1-2 inches in diameter) is then viewed by a video camera (usually a lead-oxide vidicon).

Up to this point, the system for digital radiography is identical to a conventional video-fluoroscopic system. In a conventional fluoroscopic system, however, the images are viewed on a video monitor or recorded on a video tape or a video disk (analog storage devices). In the DR system, the video signals are converted to numbers and stored either in a computer memory or on a computer disk (digital storage devices). The part of the system which actually performs the task of converting the video signals to numbers is called an analog-to-digital- converter (ADC). The numbers corresponding to each part of the image are stored at high speed in special image memories and then transferred to either the digital disk or to a video device/disk, tape or monitor by way of a digital-to-analog- converter (DAC). The rates of this transfer are dictated by the specific storage device. The purpose of having the logarithmic amplifier placed between the video camera and the ADC is illustrated below. This will be amplified when the mathematics of the digital subtraction technique are discussed.

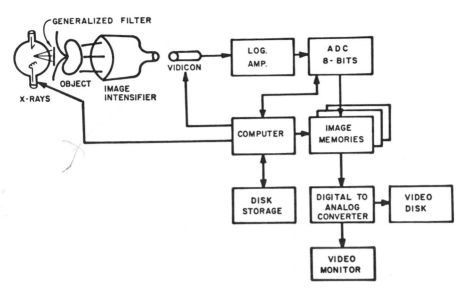

FIGURE 2. The primary components of a digital fluoroscopy system are the x-ray tube, image intensifier, a low noise video camera (lead-oxide vidicon), a logarithmic video amplifier, a high speed analog-to-digital converter (ADC), one or more image memories, a large digital disk for image storage, digital-to-analog converter (DAC) for displaying the digital images on a video monitor and a video disk or tape for rapid storage of subtracted images. For multiple energy procedures, energy spectrum shaping filters may be added.

The video camera which views the output phosphor image reproduces the image brightness distribution in a line-by-line fashion (Fig. 3). Each horizontal line of the image is represented as a voltage wave form, which varies in direct proportion to the brightness of the image at that point. The analog voltage signals are the input to the ADC (Fig. 4). The ADC then samples the continuously varying signal at prescribed time intervals and the sampling frequency determines the number of numbers that will be generated for each horizontal scan line. It is this feature of the ADC that determines the spatial resolution that can be achieved with a digital image. The range of magnitudes of the numbers generated by the ADC determines the contrast resolution or gray-scale resolution of the digital images. The images in Fig. 5 illustrate how the number of samples into which the image is divided and the number of shades of gray used to display the image affect the visual perception. Numerous image manipulation techniques

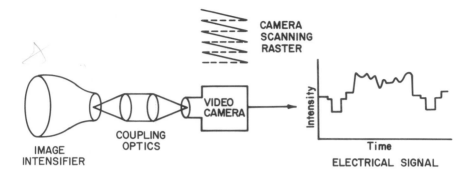

FIGURE 3. The video camera, through optical coupling, views the output phosphor of the image intensifier. The charge pattern on the light sensitive faceplate pick-up tube is read-out in a rectilinear scan pattern. A voltage signal corresponding to the light pattern is generated for each horizontal scan line.

have been developed which can affect the perception of an image without changing its information content. One such technique is interpolation (Fig. 6). The interpolation technique is usually applied to images which have small image matrices. Small matrices are often aesthetically displeasing

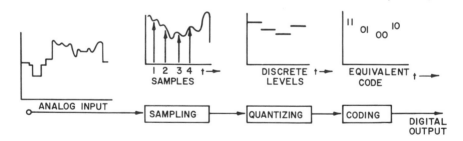

FIGURE 4. The analog voltage signal generated for each horizontal video line is the input for the analog-to-digital converter. The frequency at which the analog signal is sampled determines the spatial resolution of the digital image. The total number of samples across the horizontal line will equal the horizontal dimension of the digital matrix. The vertical dimension will equal the number of horizontal lines digitized. The quantizing phase of the ADC determines the number of shades of gray of the image. The coding phase assigns the binary number to each sample.

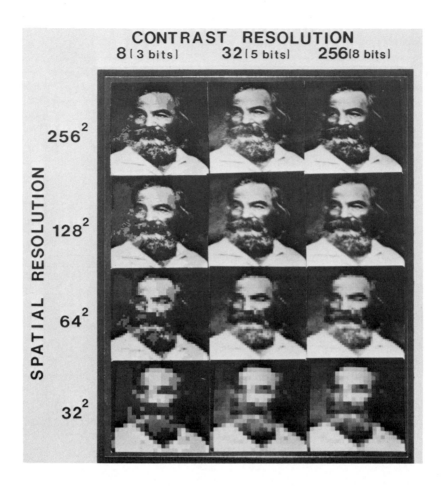

CONTRAST RESOLUTION

8 (3 bits)   32 (5 bits)   256 (8 bits)

SPATIAL RESOLUTION

256^2

128^2

64^2

32^2

FIGURE 5. The ADC parameters determine both the spatial and contrast resolution (shades of gray) of the digital image. An easily recognizable subject (Walt Whitman) illustrates how image perception changes as the shades of gray and spatial sampling vary.

because of the "blocky" appearance of the picture elements. By using a larger display matrix and "filling-in" between the actual picture elements one can improve the image presentation without actually altering the original image data.

Current DR systems digitize the video images in one of two ways. The two different techniques may be thought of in terms analogous to conventional filming and fluoroscopic procedures. One may thus refer to these as either the spot-film or "snap

F 4

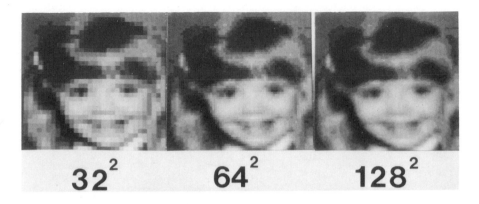

32^2 64^2 128^2

FIGURE 6. Interpolation can be used to improve the perception of a digital image without altering the image data. An image of the author's daughter was digitized originally into a 32 X 32 matrix with 16 shades of gray. By displaying the original data within larger matrices (64 X 64 and 128 X 128) and "filling-in" linearly between the original data, a more aesthetically pleasing image is obtained.

shot" technique or as a "continuous" technique (Fig. 7). In the snap-shot technique, the x-ray exposure is usually very short at high currents and the exposure is synchronized with the image digitization. The large number of x-rays and the short exposure time of the snap shot technique provide images of low statistical noise with minimal organ motion at the expense of low imaging rates. Currently, the systems operating in the snap-shot mode have maximum imaging rates of 1.5 to 3 images/second for a matrix size of 512 X 512 picture elements. Systems which operate in the continuous mode operate at relatively low fluoroscopic x-ray intensities but digitize the video images at the rate of 30 images per second; thus the temporal sampling with relatively low fluorscopic radiation dose rates at the expense of relatively noisy images.

Most systems operating in the continuous mode attempt to improve the noisy images by adding together a number of successive frames. The resulting image is less noisy. Due to the length of time over which the summation takes place, however, the image may suffer from motion artifacts. Since each video frame is created in 33 msec, each frame that is added increases the summation or integration time of the composite image by 33 msec, e.g., a three frame scan would correspond to a total time of approximately 100 msec. The

NON-INTERLACED
"spot film"

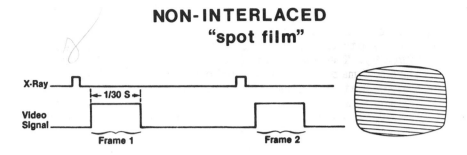

INTERLACE READOUT
(continuous)

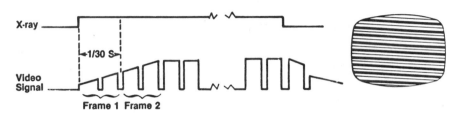

FIGURE 7. Two read-out techniques which are used in digital radiography are related to the manner in which the vidicon target is scanned and the x-ray beam is synchronized to this scanning. The pulsed or "spot film" technique delivers short pulses of x-rays at relatively high mA. The image "stored" on the vidicon faceplate is scanned line-by-line in a non-interlaced fashion. Another common technique utilizes standard 525 interlaced video read-out while x-rays are produced continuously at relatively low fluoroscopic mA. In the continuous mode, the first few images will not have useful data because the image is being read out at the same time as it is being created by the x-rays starting to fall upon the input phosphor.

distinction between the interlaced and non-interlaced read-out will be discussed further in the section of video principles.

III. IMAGE PROCESSING STEPS

The digital subtraction technique requires the capturing of a digitized mask image prior to the appearance of the contrast material. Subsequent images containing the dilutely opacified arteries are then also digitized and stored in an image memory or memories. The system is then employed to perform a subtraction of the mask and post-contrast images (Fig. 8). The steps in the creation of a DSA image are illustrated mathematically below. In addition, one can appreciate that the logarithmic rather than linear difference may be more useful. It is shown that the logarithmic difference is directly proportional to the amount of contrast material present and will be independent of the overlaying tissue thickness. This is not the case with linear subtraction. In most systems, a logarithmic amplifier is inserted in the imaging chain prior to computer storage. In this way, simple subtraction of the stored data will result in a logarithmic difference.

1. Acquire and store precontrast mask image--M(X,Y)

    M(X,Y) = number of x-ray photons detected by image receptor at location (X,Y)

2. Acquire and store images after contrast injection--I(X,Y). I(X,Y) is related to M(X,Y) by an attenuation factor $\exp[-\mu\rho\, T(X,Y)]$ resulting from the additional attenuation due to the presence of the contrast media.

    Mathematically, $I(X,Y) = M(X,Y)\, \exp[-\mu\rho\, T(X,Y)]$

    where

    μ = iodine attenuation coefficient (cm^2/G)

    ρ = iodine concentration (G/cm^3)

    T(X,Y) = the thickness of the opacified blood expressed in cm

3. The logarithmic difference image--D(X,Y) is directly proportional to the amount or thickness of contrast media T(X,Y) at each location

    $D(X,Y) = K\,[\ln M(X,Y) - \ln I(X,Y)]$

    and K is a constant.

The images presented in Figs. 9A and 9B illustrate the differences which are observed between images derived from linear and logarithmic subtractions. The object imaged in

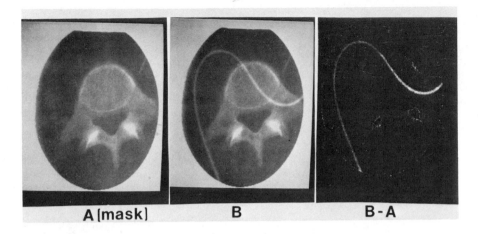

A (mask)   **B**   **B-A**

FIGURE 8. Digital video subtraction is illustrated by subtracting the mask image A from image B in which contrast media has been added to yield the difference image B-A of the contrast media alone.

Fig. 9 was a lucite stepwedge phantom on which two 1 mm plastic tubes had been taped. The lucite steps were 2 cm thick and ranged in thickness from 2 cm to 20 cm, with the thickest part of the phantom located at the bottom of the image. A mask image of the phantom was acquired first with the plastic tubes filled with saline. Repeat images were then made with the saline being replaced with iodine concentrations of 1 and 5 mg/ml for the left and right tubes, respectively. In each case, images were acquired both with and without the log amplification. The difference image with log amplification is shown in Fig. 9A. The difference image without the log amplification (linear) is shown in Fig. 9B.

Fig. 9B illustrates the point made previously that the amount of iodine (brightness) is a function of the total lucite thickness. The tube appears brightest at the top (small thickness) and quickly becomes imperceptible at large thicknesses (bottom). For the logarithmic difference image (Fig. 9A), however, this is not the case and the tubes are visualized with approximate equal brightness throughout their entire length. Fig. 10 illustrates the same point in a different manner and clearly demonstrates the advantage of using logarithmic processing when quantitative results are desired. The linear processing shows that the system produces unequal responses to equal increments of absorber thickness. The logarithmic processing, on the other hand, produces approximately equal system response to equal increments in absorber thickness.

IV. VIDEO PRINCIPLES

Video cameras may assume a variety of different sizes and shapes (4). They may be divided into two general groups: self-contained units in which one need only supply A/C power and a cable for routing the video signal to a monitor and two-unit systems in which the camera tube is driven by a

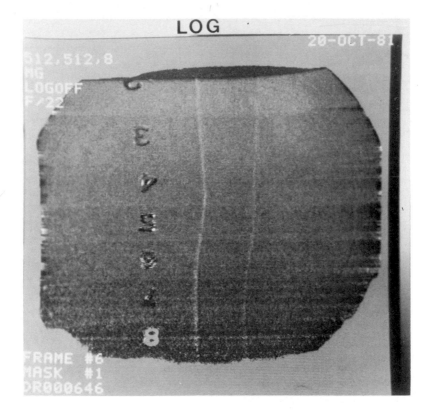

FIGURE 9A. A digital subtraction image of two 1 mm plastic tubes after having been filled with 5 mg/ml I (left) and 1 mg/ml I (right) of iodinated contrast media. The logarithmic difference shows the tubes to be of equal brightness regardless of the overlying thickness of lucite. Similarly, the tube with 5 mg/ml appears brighter than the tube with 1 mg/ml.

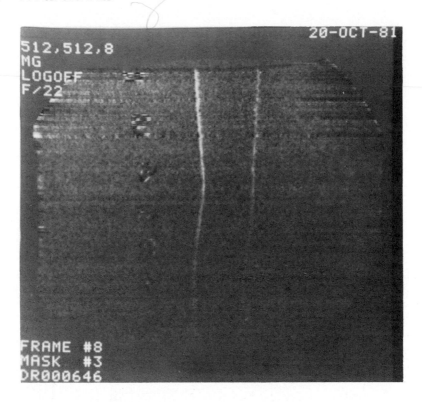

FIGURE 9B. Linear difference. The tubes are of unequal brightness with the brightness increasing with decreased overlying thickness of lucite.

remotely located camera control unit. The two-unit system is the design most frequently used for video-fluoroscopic applications. When the remote camera tube is used, it has the advantage of being smaller than a self-contained unit and also allows the major portion of the electronics to be isolated from heat, shock and vibration. In addition, since the camera tube itself usually requires few adjustments it can be kept in a relatively inaccessible location. The remote camera tube contains only the light-sensitive pickup tube, its associated scanning or deflection circuits and usually a video preamplifier.

Numerous types of light-sensitive video image tubes or pickup tubes have been developed to meet the needs of various applications. The differences in these tubes are primarily the composition of the photosensitive material on which the light pattern is focused and the method which is used to

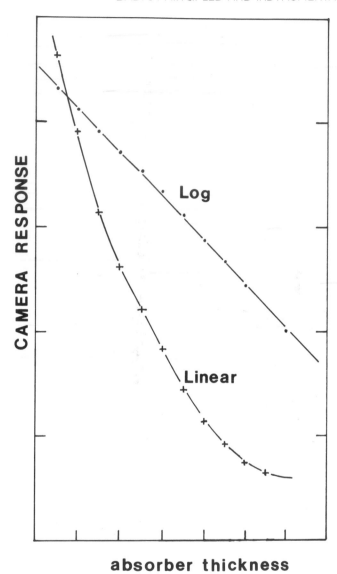

CAMERA RESPONSE

Log

Linear

absorber thickness

FIGURE 10. A plot of the DR numbers from a digital image of a stepwedge. DR numbers without log amplification of video show characteristic exponential dependence on stepwedge thickness. Plot after log amplification shows linear relationship with stepwedge thickness.

extract the electrical information produced by the light pattern. The vidicon pickup tube, or some variation of the vidicon using different types of photosensitive materials, are the majority of camera tubes in current use today.

The target or light-sensitive faceplate of the vidicon consists of a transparent conducting film on which a thin photoconductive layer has been deposited. Photoconductive material becomes a conductor when exposed to light. The target can be thought of as a large number of individual target elements consisting of a capacitor which will charge up in proportion to the amount of light falling on it when the conducting layer is connected to a positive voltage source. The charge pattern formed is thus proportional to the light pattern falling on the target. When no light falls on the target, the resistance of the photoconductor remains high and no charging should take place. Dark current, that is, current that is produced in absolute darkness, is an important feature of vidicon tubes. A large dark current is a very undesirable feature since dark current represents a primary source of image noise.

To transmit an image, it is necessary to convert the optical image focused upon the photosensitive surface of the pickup tube into a series of electrical signals. This is accomplished by scanning the target with a beam of low velocity electrons (5). The low energy electrons are deposited on the positively charged areas of the target causing a current flow which brings the target back to the negative potential of the beam. The magnitude of the developed current is proportional to the charge of the element being scanned. The magnitude of the charge is in turn proportional to the amount of light which fell on the target; thus, the output is an electrical rendition of the optical image. The electron beam is scanned over the target by being deflected in a raster pattern by magnetic fields which are generated by external coils. It is also possible to use electrostatic deflection techniques instead of magnetic deflection for scanning the electron beam (Fig. 11).

In scanning the target, if the beam intensity is too low, only those areas of the target which were not highly charged will be fully discharged. The result is that areas which have been exposed to a bright field may not be completely discharged during a single scan of the target. In this situation, the image of the bright pattern may continue to be seen for a long time after the illumination has been removed or, as is sometimes said, the high brightness areas tend to "stick". This phenomenon is commonly seen during video-fluoroscopic examinations when the image intensity is exposed to the direct unattenuated x-ray beam. This is also the phenomenon which produces the white tailing or smearing as

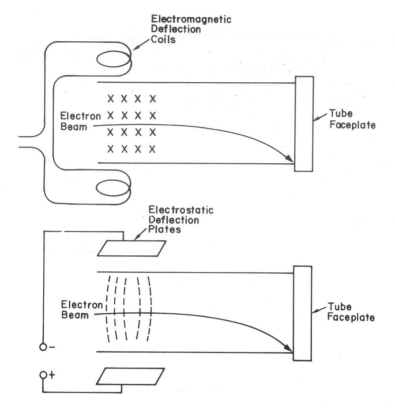

FIGURE 11. Schematic diagram showing how either deflection coils or deflection plates are used to scan the electron beam across the faceplate of a vidicon. The x's in the top figure represent magnetic field lines perpendicular to the electron beam. The curved broken lines in the lower diagram represent electric field lines.

a bright area is moved rapidly across the field-of-view. Vidicon targets can be permanently damaged by extended exposure to extremely bright scenes.

Although it is important to provide sufficient beam current, it must be realized that increasing beam intensity too much will increase the area of the scanning spot where the beam strikes the target and will thus cause a loss in resolution.

Another parameter of the vidcon which is also a function of the dark current is image "lag" or persistence. Lag is a measure of the decay in the output current after the illumination has been removed. Lag is manifested by the smearing of the edges of rapidly moving structures. A variation on the basic vidicon design has produced new types of tubes which utilize semi-conductor target materials. The advantage of these tubes is that they are fast (low lag) and exhibit extremely low dark currents, i.e., very low noise level. For these reasons, semi-conductor pickup tubes are the camera tubes currently used in most DSA applications. Specifically, most DSA systems employ lead-oxide vidicons - sometimes called plumbicons.

We have already described how an electron beam can be used to discharge a point on the target. In order to convert the entire scene, which has been optically focused on the target, into electrical signals, the beam must be scanned over the entire target area. All video systems use a rectilinear scanning raster. That is, the beam is scanned both horizontally and vertically with both motions being scanned at a constant velocity. Fig. 12 illustrates the motion of the beam over the pickup tube target. Since the beam is moving both horizontally and vertically simultaneously, the raster scan lines are at a slant rather than absolutely horizontal. The velocity of the horizontal is much faster than the vertical motion. It is the relative magnitude of these two scanning rates which will determine the number of horizontal lines that will be obtained during each scan of the target. A larger number of lines will discharge a greater portion of the target and will thus yield more information about the image. The dashed lines in the figure illustrate beam retrace. The retrace velocity is very rapid and the beam is turned off or deflected away from the target during this time so that no output will be generated during the retrace.

The vertical scanning frequency in the United States has been chosen as 60 per second. The vertical scanning frequency thus matches the frequency of the commercial A/C power supply. This is convenient since the A/C power line can be used as a synchronized source.

Standard broadcast video in the United States uses a horizontal scanning frequency of 15,750 lines per second. If one divides this by the vertical scan frequency of 60 per second, we see that one would achieve 262 1/2 horizontal scan lines during one vertical scan. The electrical signals produced during such a cycle is called a video field. The next video field will thus begin at a 1/2-line offset with respect to the previous field. Each alternate field scan is constructed so that the horizontal lines interleave, that is, the scan lines do not overlap exactly the same area on the target. The result is that the alternating fields actually contain different information and when alternate fields are combine, they yield an effective 525 horizontal lines. The two interlaced fields comprise one video frame whose frequency

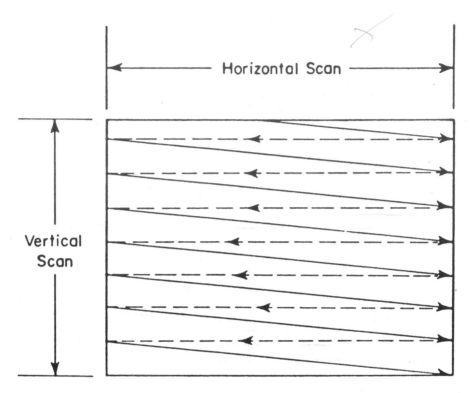

FIGURE 12. All video systems scan both the video pickup tubes and the video monitors in a rectilinear pattern. Since the electron beam is moving both horizontally and vertically at the same time, the horizontal scan line will be slightly tilted from the horizontal. The total number of horizontal scan lines will determine the vertical resolution.

is 30 images per second. In actual practice data from all 525 lines do not contain useful information since a number of horizontal lines are lost during vertical retrace. Similar to the horizontal retrace, the beam is turned off "blanked" and no output is generated. Typically, seven to eight per cent of the total horizontal lines may be lost during vertical retrace.

The standard 525 line interlaced scan is not the only possible way of scanning the tube target. There are DSA systems in use which utilize standard interlaced video and there are those who have chosen to use non-standard scanning rates. The advantages of using standard interlace systems include lower cost and the ability to use off-the-shelf video recording systems (disks or tapes). Non-standard systems are

being used which employ larger numbers of horizontal scan
lines as well as non-interlaced readouts. This arrangement is
sometimes referred to as progressive scanning. Higher line
density yields better spatial resolution and progressive
scanning in general yields more uniform images by avoiding the
intensity differences which sometimes occur between adjacent
fields in the interlaced mode.

V. VERTICAL RESOLUTION

The vertical resolution of a video system refers to its
ability to resolve horizontal lines. The more closely spaced
the horizontal scan lines are, the better the vertical
resolution will be. One would expect that the number of
horizontal lines should yield the same number of lines of
vertical resolution, but this is not generally the case.
Unlike radiographic film systems, where the resolution is
expressed in terms of line pairs, the resolution of a video
system is expressed in terms of the total number of lines. A
line pair in radiography (photography) is comprised of a
combined pair of radiopaque (black) and radiolucent (white)
strips of equal width. In video systems each strip or line is
counted individually regardless of whether it is black or
white. The difference is obviously a result of definition and
parameter chosen.
Fig. 13 illustrates the concept of vertical resolution and
the importance of the beam size on the target face relative to
the horizontal line spacing. If we assume that the image
focused on the target is a series of horizontal dark and light
lines and we also assume that the beam scanning path is
perfectly spaced and aligned with the lines in the scene, then
the vertical resolution would exactly equal the number of
actual horizontal scan lines. This will seldom be the case in
actual practice, so that the actual resolution will always be
somewhat less than the number of horizontal lines. At the
other extreme, if the beam paths were aligned so that the beam
spot was exactly half over the dark line and half over the
light line, there would be no evidence of the resolution
pattern on the output monitor at all. Since the output
current can obviously not simultaneously be both low and high,
the output is the sum of the two and the monitor image in this
case would be uniformly gray with no discernable structure.
In a standard 525 line system the vertical resolution is
usually about 350 lines. Fig. 14A illustrates vertical
resolution using a conventional x-ray phantom.

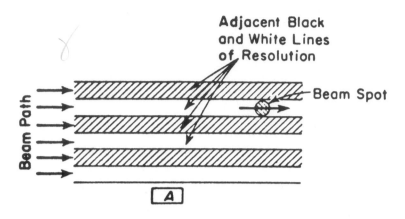

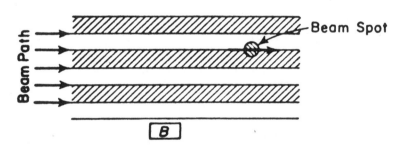

FIGURE 13. Vertical resolution. (A) If the beam path exactly matches the adjacent black and white lines with the beam scanning exactly over the center of a white line in one scan and then scanning exactly over the center of the adjacent black line with the next scan, the number of horizontal scan lines will exactly equal the vertical resolution. (B) In general, the vertical resolution will be less than the number of horizontal scan lines. This figure illustrates the extreme case where no lines will be resolved.

VI. HORIZONTAL RESOLUTION

In a manner similar to the definition of vertical resolution, horizontal resolution refers to the ability of the system to resolve vertical bars. However, in video systems all resolution measurements are defined in terms of the vertical image height. Thus, if a system is stated to have a

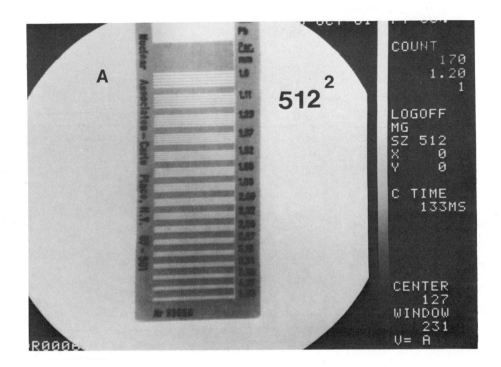

FIGURE 14A. Digital image of a resolution phantom (512 X 512). The slight misalignment of the phantom bars and the video scan lines reduces the vertical resolution to approximately 3-4 lines/mm (1.5-2 line pairs/mm). This image was taken in the 4.5 inch (114 mm) image intensifier mode. For 512 scan lines over a 114 mm field-of-view, this corresponds to a vertical sampling of about 4.5 lines/mm.

500 line horizontal resolution, this means that the 500 lines placed side by side would exactly fit the vertical dimension. Thus, in this way the fact that the horizontal and vertical dimension are different can be taken into account. In standard video systems the ratio of the horizontal dimension to the vertical dimensions is 4:3, with the horizontal dimension being greater.

The horizontal resolution of a video system is determined primarily by the system bandwidth or frequency response. The frequency response of a video system can be thought of in terms of its ability to respond to a black-white interface in a scene. Fig. 15 illustrates this concept. As the beam scans across the resolution lines, an output is generated. The sharp edge at the interface between each black/white line will be represented in the output as a square-wave with rounded edges. The higher the bandwidth the more accurate the representation of the sharp edge will be. At low bandwidth the edges become smoothed and adjacent lines tend to blur together until the lines can no longer be resolved (Fig. 14B). The bandwidth can be used to calculate the number of lines of horizontal resolution. A simple multiplication of the bandwidth frequency (usually expressed in megahertz, MHz) and the time that the beam spends in scanning the usable part of each horizontal line will yield the horizontal resolution

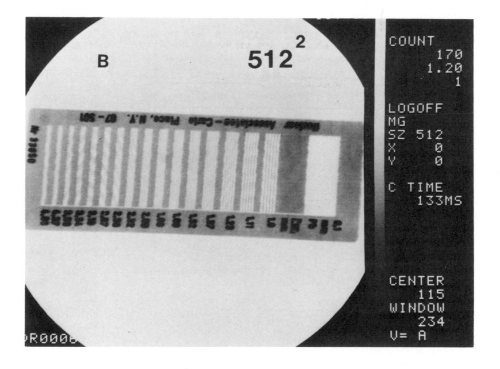

FIGURE 14B. Horizontal resolution. Digital image (512 X 512) of a resolution bar phantom. Resolution is seen to be less than 2 line pairs/mm. Moire patterns are seen in the high spatial frequency bars due to the interaction between the frequency of the bars and the sampling frequency.

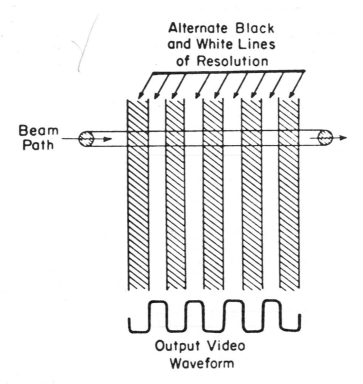

FIGURE 15. Horizontal resolution is illustrated as the response of the system as the electron beam scans across vertical bars. As the system response smooths out the edges of the resolution lines, the lines will smear together and can not be discerned (see Fig. 14B).

capability in terms of line pairs. This number is doubled to conform to the convention of line resolution rather than line pairs. For example, in a standard 525 line system the usable horizontal scan time (taking into account the 4:3 aspect ratio) is about 40 microseconds. Forty microseconds times 4 megahertz (the bandwidth of broadcast video in the United States) yields 160 line pairs or 320 lines of horizontal resolution. Using a 10 MHz bandwidth increases the number of lines to 800.

The above examples illustrate the fact that the amount of time available for scanning each horizontal line is directly related to the horizontal resolution. This fact should be considered when video systems with higher line densities are discussed. Since the vertical frequency is kept constant, it follows that there is less usable time for each horizontal scan line. If the bandwidth is kept constant, then the horizontal resolution would actually be decreased. For example, in a 1000-line system, to achieve 800 lines of horizontal resolution would require a 20 MHz bandwidth. Even though it would seem that all systems should be designed with extremely high bandwidths, this is not necessarily the case, since excessive bandwidth tends to amplify noise.

VII. PRINCIPLES OF DIGITAL SYSTEMS (COMPUTERS)

Images from conventional radiographic and fluoroscopic systems are referred to as analog images. These are differentiated from computer augmented images, which are generated from an array of store numbers. The latter images are designated as digital images and the process of generating the array of numbers is called image digitization. The primary distinction between analog and digital is that analog images exhibit a continuous spectrum of shades of gray, and digital images will be represented with a well defined discrete number of gray shades (6). If a digital system possessed a very large number of shades of gray, it would be impossible for the human eye to distinguish a digital image from its analog counterpart. There have been numerous experiments conducted that have attempted to determine the exact number of shades of gray that the human eye can detect. The number would appear to be somewhere between 8 and 64 but depends upon ambient light levels available in the viewing arrangement and also upon the scene surrounding the picture element that is being inspected (7,8).

The first bits of jargon one usually encounters in a discussion of computer systems are the terms hardware and software. Hardware refers to the physical components that we see and touch: the cabinets, the electronic circuits, lights, wires, power supplies and memory. Hardware also refers to the peripheral devices such as magnetic disk and tape drives, image display devices and operator terminals. Software, on the other hand, is the set of instructions that determine what functions are performed by the hardware and in what order they will be done. A set of instructions for a particular task is usually called a program. There are several categories of programs: system programs, utility programs and user application programs. The systems and utility programs are general programs that facilitate the handling of other programs. They are usually supplied by the computer vendor.

VIII. CENTRAL PROCESSING UNIT

The central processing unit or CPU is the brain of the system. The CPU transfers the stored program from memory, decodes the program instructions and executes them. The video camera views the output phosphor of the image intensifier at a rate of 30 frames per second. To keep pace with this rate, dedicated hardware must be used for both digitization and storate of image data in memory. Both the image memory (or memories) and digitizing hardware are peripheral to the CPU. Each is initiated and controlled by the CPU; however, because of considerations of speed, the CPU does not directly perform either the digitizing or the storage.

IX. IMAGE STORAGE

Once an image has been acquired in the image memory, the CPU will initiate the transfer of the image data from the image memory to a larger storage capacity device, usually a digital disk. The disk, being an electromechanical device, does not have the data transfer capabilities of the purely electronic data storage of the image memories. The result is that image data stored in digital form on the digital disk will, in effect, be "snapshots", with time gaps between successive images. The length of the time gaps will depend primarily upon the speed of the disk. Current DR systems utilizing high speed disks of the Winchester design are capable of storing digital images of 512 x 512 picture elements, at rates of 1-4 images per second. It should be emphasized that the digital images are created at video rates and that it is the digital recording of images that brings about the loss of time between stored images. This restriction on imaging rates, however, has presented a problem clinically only for cardiac applications. It should be mentioned, however, that there are several very high speed disks that are being advertised whose specifications indicate that they will be able to record digital images of 512 X 512 matrix elements at rates up to 30 frames/sec for time periods greater than 20 seconds.
      Since it is the total number of picture elements per image that dictates the image storage rate, one can easily realize

an increased digital framing rate of a factor of 4 by reducing the image matrix to 256 x 256. As will be seen later, a reduction of the image matrix size may compromise spatial resolution.

An alternate approach to image storage is to perform that digital processing required within the image memory (for most cases this is simple subtraction) and then to store the processed images in analog form rather than digital. Analog image storage devices (video tapes or video disks) can record images at video rates and in this mode will not result in time gaps between successive frames. With current technology the analog storage approach may be the technique of choice for cardiac applications where the ability to rapidly image is critical. The disadvantage of analog storage is that further image processing is somewhat hindered because analog storage will generally increase image noise, and images digitized for the second time will have a larger noise component, which in turn compromises image quality. As will be shown in later chapters in this text, however, this compromise has been accepted by several groups in specific clinical circumstances.

X. MEMORY

We have mentioned previously both computer memory and image memory. This distinction came not from physical differences but rather from the memory function. Memory whether used for program storage or image data storage can be thought of as a series of bins into which information can be placed for subsequent retrieval and manipulation. With an appropriate coding scheme, this stored information can represent numbers, letters or symbols. A memory is specified by not only the total number of storage bins or locations but also by the size of each bin, which determines the amount of information that can be stored at each location. In the particular case of the storage of a digital image, there is a one-to-one correspondance between each picture element in the image and a memory storage location. Thus, there is a direct relationship between the size of the image matrix and the amount of memory required to store it. For example a 512 x 512 image would require 261,144 memory locations for storage. Similarily, a 256 x 256 image would require 65,536. In computer jargon, the requirements are 256K and 64K, respectively, where 1K=1024. Each memory location is designated as a word. In some cases, a picture element may not require all of the storage capacity of a full computer word; a smaller memory unit called a byte may be used. A byte is usually equal to "one half of a word". In the following section on analog-to-digital converters we will see that the number of picture elements affects the spatial resolution of the image.

The size or storage capacity of a word of memory determines the magnitude of the number that can be stored. Information is stored in the computer memory as binary numbers. That is a series of 1's and 0's. In the decimal or base 10 number system, with which we are all familiar, there are nine digits, 0 through 9. In the binary system or base 2 there are only two digits 0 and 1. As with the decimal system, any size number can be constructed by using additional digits. The same is true in the binary system. Table I illustrates how the first 10 numbers can be represented in both the decimal and binary number systems. The choice of the binary number system for computer data storage was not by chance. It comes from the simple fact that, at some point, abstract numbers must be converted into a physical state if they are to be stored. In nature, it is easy to construct physical devices which will take on two distinct physical states, e.g., a switch is either off or on, a light bulb is lit or not, current is either flowing through a wire or it is not. Conversely, it is difficult to find physical devices which can take on 10 distinct states, as would be required by a decimal computer. Although decimal computing devices have been produced, it has been shown that binary devices are much more efficient for data storage and manipulation and require less hardware.

TABLE I. *Comparison of Decimal and Binary Numbers*

Decimal	Binary
0	0
1	1
2	10
3	11
4	100
5	101
6	110
7	111
8	1000
9	1001
10	1010

The smallest memory element thus becomes the physical representation of a single binary digit or "BIT". A bit thus can take on the values of 0 or 1. A combination of two bits can take on 4 values: 0, 1, 2, 3. By adding more and more bits, larger numbers can be formed. The maximum number that can be created from a combination of N bits is equal to 2^N-1. The -1 results from the fact that we always count zero as a number. The number of bits in a word of memory is a function of the specific computer. The most common size used in most DSA systems is the 16-bit word. The byte, probably the most frequently used storage unit, is equal to one half of a word or 8 bits. Using the above relationship between the number of bytes and the size of the number that can be stored, we see that numbers from 0-255 can be stored in a single 8-bit byte. If byte mode storage is used to represent the relative x-ray intensities falling upon the input phosphor of an image-intensifying tube, then each element of our digital image would be represented as one of 255 levels of gray. It might be noted, however, that the 8-bit grouping is not universally recognized as a byte. One may, on rare occasions, encounter 7-bit or 6-bit bytes. A 4-bit grouping is sometimes referred to as a "nibble".

XI. MEMORY TYPES

The implementation of computer memory usually takes one of two common forms. The oldest is the magnetic core memory, which is now being replaced in modern computers by solid state memory. Magnetic core memory consists of small ferrite rings arranged in arrays (Fig. 16). The arrays of the ferrite rings are organized to form bytes and words of the computer memory, with each ferrite ring being the physical manifestation of a single bit. The arrays of the ferrite rings are strung together by wires passing through the rings. The wires are strung in two directions, allowing a two dimensional representation to be formed. When a pulse of current is passed through the wires, the rings will be magnetized and the direction of the magnetization will depend upon the direction of the current. If pulses are simultaneously passed through the two wires intersecting a single ring, only that ring will have a unique magnetization. the rings also have a third wire passing through them. This third wire is referred to as a sense wire and is used to detect the direction of the magnetization. The direction of magnetization is defined as the storage of a binary one or zero. The ferrite ring memory has the compelling advantage that the current does not have

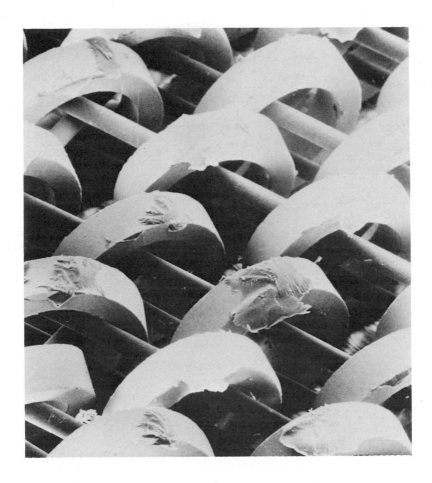

FIGURE 16. Electron microscope image of a portion of a core memory plane. The ferrite rings are magnetized and "read-out" by wires passing through the center of the rings. Wires running at right angles to each other generate two-dimensional (x,y) addressing.

to be continuously present for the magnetic ring to maintain its magnetization (memory). Therefore, this type of memory is referred to as permanent memory, meaning that if the computer itself is turned off, the memory will retain the information that has been stored. Magnetic core memory is becoming less common because of the expense involved in its construction and the large physical size required to accommodate large amounts of storage. The fact that the ferrite rings are referred to as magnetic cores accounts for the fact that frequently any

computer memory may be referred to as core. Solid state
memory consists of integrated circuits which mimic the
operation of the magnetic core. Solid state memory,
frequently referred to as semi-conductor memory, has made it
economically possible for many laboratory computers to have
relatively large storage capacities. Solid state memory is
sometimes referred to as volatile memory, meaning that if the
computer is turned off, the information stored within the
memory is lost. There have been modifications to computers
having solid state memories which cause the memory to be
powered by a battery when the computer is turned off, so that
the stored information may be retained. The primary
advantages of the solid state memory (MOS, metal oxide
sapphire), in addition to expense, are reduced space
requirements, reduced power requirements and, consequently
lower heat production. The almost unbelievable speed required
to convert a complete video image into digital numbers and to
store them in real-time is, in large part, made possible
through the very rapid access times of the computer memories.
Modern computer memories have access time on the order of 100
to 1,000 nano seconds (1 nano sec = 10^{-9} sec). There are
a number of new memory technologies which are becoming
popular. Probably the most frequently recognized potential
candidate for replacing solid state memories is referred to as
bubble memory which utilizes small magnetic domains for
storage.

XII. MAGNETIC STORAGE DEVICES

     As indicated above, magnetic memories are very fast and
can be made relatively large; however, the enormous amount of
data that is generated during a digital radiographic study
cannot be accommodated by reasonable memory sizes. The cost
is simply prohibitive; thus, an answer to the need for
peripheral storage is the magnetic disk. Magnetic disks are
available in a number of different sizes (i.e., storage
capacities). Disks are written in a manner similar to
long-playing phonograph records. That is, data are written in
concentric tracks at a density of 100 to 200 tracks per inch.
The position or address of any track is defined by the design
and construction of the particular disk system. The address
layout of the disk is further specified by sectors within the
tracks. Information then can be addressed to a particular
track for storage and retrieved. Data formats of disks are
not consistent among manufacturers. This results in some
incompatability and often means that one cannot store

information on a magnetic disk by one manufacturer and expect to retrieve information using another manufacturer's machine. Disks are characterized by both their total data storage capacity and their data transfer speed. Disks range in size from several thousands up to many hundreds of millions of words of storage.

Disk storage of data is slower than storage into magnetic memory. This limitation can be recognized fairly intuitively by recognizing that the data are being stored on a device which is not only electronic but mechanical. The mechanical motion comes from the fact that the disk is physically rotated; thus, in this type of data transfer we have left the electronic domain and gone to the physical domain, which results in a reduction in speed of storage. The reduction in the speed of storage is the primary reason why the images acquired in the digital radiographic study cannot, using current technology, be stored in digital form in real-time. However, disk technology is being improved, so that soon, through the use of multiple recording heads and other technological advances, it will be possible to record digital images in real-time. The limiting factor at present is the cost of manufacturing such a device.

Magnetic tape is similar to the magnetic disk in that the magnetic media are physically moved across a recording head. Similar to the disk, magnetic tape, because of its physical motion, is a relatively slow storage medium. Tape generally is written and specified in terms of its recording speed, density and number of tracks. Recording densities of current systems in common use in the medical environment range from 800 bits per inch (BPI) to 1600 BPI with nine tracks. There are magnetic tapes, however, up to 6050 BPI. Information is written on tape in blocks of pre-determined lengths. These blocks are usually separated by short sections of blank tape called inter-record gaps. There is no standard block length; however, most systems utilize blocks that are 256 words long. The magnetic tape's primary advantage is that the magnetic tape itself is relatively inexpensive and is thus used as a back-up or a permanent storage record of information which has been written on magnetic disk. The magnetic disk is used each day to store the image data as it is acquired, taking advantage of its relatively rapid storage rate. At the time the disk becomes full, one must either erase the disk by storing new data or copy the contents of the disk onto a magnetic tape for permanent archival. This is the typical method for archiving DR images. The amount of data that can be stored on a magnetic tape can be calculated knowing the writing density of the tape in terms of bytes per inch and the length of the tape. Tapes are sold in common lengths of 600,

1,200 and 2,400 feet long. Typically, a magnetic tape can easily accommodate over several million bytes of information.

XIII. THE ANALOG-TO-DIGITAL CONVERTER

The central feature of all digital imaging systems is the analog-to-digital converter (ADC) (6). The parameters of the ADC significantly affect the spatial resolution, the contrast resolution (the number of intensity levels in the image) and, in extreme cases, the image rate. The analog-to-digital converter accepts as input the analog video image. The analog video image is sampled by the ADC at specified temporal intervals. These intervals can be directly related to the spatial resolution of the image (Fig. 4). The sampling frequency of each horizontal video line determines the spatial resolution in the horizontal direction. The analog to digital-converter thus determines the number of picture elements into which an image is divided and this in turn determines the spatial resolution of the system. Not only does the characeristics of the analog-to-digital converter specify the spatial resolution, it also specifies the intensity resolution. Each sample is also digitized in regard to its analog voltage level. The higher the sensed voltage level, the larger the digital number generated. The magnitude of the digitized number represents the intensity level or shade of gray of the picture element and its relative location within the complete series of generated numbers determines its position within the image.

The characteristics of an ADC are specified in terms of the following parameters. The first parameter of the ADC is referred to as the ADC conversion time. Conversion time specifies the time that it takes for the ADC (which links the image intensifier video camera output to the computer) to convert the analog signals to digital numbers. The ADC used in digital radiography systems are sometimes called flash converters and are capable of converting 261,144 samples in each 1/30th of a second. That corresponds to an image matrix size of 512 X 512 elements being digitized within a single video frame of length of 1/30th of a second. As mentioned earlier, the conversion time of ADC's in current use are completely adequate to accommodate the imaging rates provided to us by the video camera. The limiting factor of the imaging rate, as stated earlier, is the magnetic storage on the digital disk. The second parameter frequently used to specify the ADC is the intensity resolution. The intensity resolution refers to the specification of the maximum number of bits into which the analog signal is converted for each picture element. The systems in current use utilize 8 bits, which corresponds to 256 shades of gray. The conversion time will also be a function of the number of bits.

The noise inherent within the video image in part dictates the number of shades of gray required to represent the image. As the noise level of the video camera is reduced, a more closely defined intensity range, with more bits in the ADC, will be needed. The third common term used to specify the ADC is the spatial resolution. The spatial resolution is the number of digital points into which the video image is converted. As indicated earlier, the video image is converted one horizontal line at a time; so the horizontal resolution is equal to the number of times that the horizontal scan line is sampled. Common matrix sizes are 512 X 512; that is, the horizontal line is sampled 512 times and there are 512 horizontal lines that are being sampled. Other commonly used matrices are powers of 2 below; that is, 256 X 256 and 128 X 128. The number of points within the vertical direction corresponds to the number of the video scan lines. Another parameter of the system is the dynamic range. The range of the analog video signals which are presented as input to the ADC must be matched to the characteristics of the ADC. Typically, the video signals will range from approximately 0 volts up to a maximum of somewhat less than 1 volt. The 0 volt level corresponds to the dark part of the image intensifier field; that is where no light is being produced, since very few x-rays have interacted with the input phosphor. The larger video voltage level corresponds to the greater light level areas of the field-of-view. The ADC must be matched to the video camera output in such a manner that all of the levels within the unsaturated dynamic range of the camera are contained within the dynamic range of the ADC. An eight bit ADC corresponds to 256 levels of gray. Therefore, the ADC must be matched so that zero voltage will correspond to the digital number zero and at the other extreme, one volt would produce the digital number 255.

As mentioned previously, in order to assure that the response of the system is linear in regard to the amount of iodinated contrast material that the system sees, one needs to compensate for the fact that the x-rays are being attenuated in a logarithmic fashion. Therefore, most systems utilize a logarithmic amplifier which is placed between the video camera and the analog-to-digital converter. The characteristic of the logarithmic amplifier is to enhance the lower voltage level, that is, to improve the detectability of the dark levels and to flatten out or to compress the brighter levels. The ADC must also be matched to the logarithmic output and the

video image that has been logarithmic amplified must also be
matched to the characteristics of the ADC. Some systems have
been designed which digitize the video signal without
logarithmic amplification, using the linear response, and then
take the logarithm after digitization. In these systems, in
order to maintain the information in the dark levels of the
image, it is important that one utilize ADCs with larger
number of bits, i.e., greater dynamic range. The information
thus is divided into smaller divisions in order that the lower
intensity regions can be recorded without loss. Thus we can
appreciate the importance of the ADC to the entire system and
to the digital process.

XIV. SPATIAL RESOLUTION

We have discussed in some detail how the spatial
resolution of the digital image is dictated in large part by
the spatial sampling of the ADC (see chapter by Monahan). We
assume that the reader is familiar with the more traditional
characteristics of x-ray systems and will not discuss in
detail the effect of these characteristics on the spatial
resolution. For reference, those characteristics which do
affect resolution are the x-ray focal spot size, the image
intensifier resolution and the video system resolution. The
effect of spatial sampling on spatial resolution is most
easily communicated by repeating a fundamental theorem of
information theory. This theorem states that no digital image
can reproduce a structure within an image that has spatial
frequencies higher than one-half the sampling frequency. The
sampling frequency is determined by the number of picture
elements into which the image is divided. The equation which
relates this limited frequency (L) in terms of line pairs per
millimeter to the number of picture elements is shown below:

$$L = \frac{\text{Number of picture elements in one direction}}{2 \times \text{field size}}$$

This limiting frequency can be seen to be directly
proportional to the number of picture elements (Fig. 17).
That is, the larger the number of picture elements into which
an image is divided, the larger will be this frequency and,
therefore, the smaller the structures which can be resolved.
Fig. 18 shows the plot of limiting frequency as a function of
image intensifier field size for a sampling of 512 samples
across the horizontal line. It can be seen that the
theoretical upper limit of resolution would be just slightly

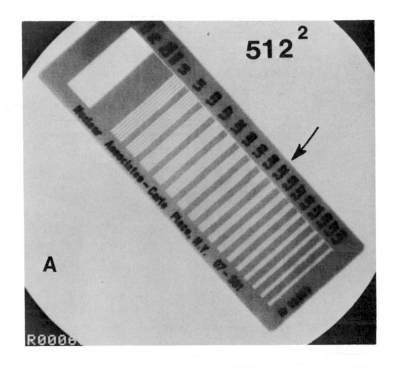

FIGURE 17A. Digital image (512 X 512) of a resolution bar phantom demonstrating approximately 2.32 lp/mm.

greater than 2 line pairs per millimeter for the smallest field-of-view in common use (4 inches). For the image intensifier field of 9 inches, we see that the upper limit is less than 1 line pair per millimeter. The implication of this is that the theoretical upper limit of resolution, for a 9 inch field-of-view using a 512 X 512 matrix, is approximately 1 millimeter for a maximally opacified structure. Note that this is an upper limit since other factors will degrade the response in most systems. It should be pointed out that the limiting frequencies shown in this figure are specified for opaque structures and most vessels are never completely opacified. Thus, the actual resolution will be somewhat degraded from the theoretical limits of resolution. Another phenomenon characteristic of digital imaging, called "aliasing", results when high spatial frequency structures are inadequately sampled. This is illustrated in Fig. 19 by the irregular patterns in the images.

Much interest has been expressed in increasing the
field-of-view of the image intensifier to allow a larger
portion of the anatomy to be imaged at the same time. It must
be recognized that there are limitations forced on the system
by the digital sampling resolution. If the graph in Fig. 18
were continued to a 16 inch field-of-view, we would see that
the spatial resolution would be greatly degraded. Thus, one
should emphasize that for larger image intensifier systems,
one must compensate by increasing the digital matrix size in
order to maintain adequate resolution. Another difficulty,
which can be recalled from earlier discussions, is that the
larger matrix sizes will have an associated increased data
density which will require longer storage times, therefore a
decrease in the imaging rate.

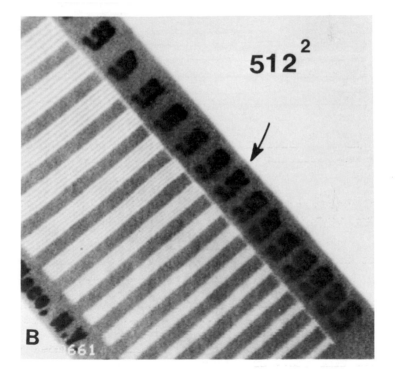

FIGURE 17B.   *Same digital image as shown in part A but
with zoom display for ease of viewing.*

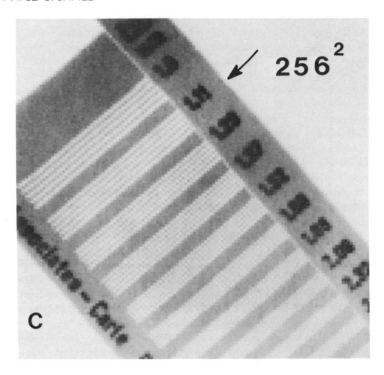

FIGURE 17C. Bar phantom imaged as 256 X 256 demonstrates how spatial resolution has been reduced relative to the 512 X 512 matrix image to approximately 1.11 lp/mm before significant aliasing errors (diagonal stripes) are seen.

XV. NOISE

Noise within the digital radiography image has a number of different sources. One common and easily recognizable component is quantum noise which results from the random absorption of x-rays within both the patient and the image intensifier input phosphor. Quantum noise can be minimized by increasing the number of x-rays, thereby increasing the total number of absorbed x-rays. Thus, this source of noise can be controlled at the expense of increased radiation exposure. Since the subtraction process tends to amplify image noise, it is essential that the images be acquired with as little x-ray quantum noise as possible. The relative noise of a picture element is inversely proportional to the square root of the total number of x-rays which have been absorbed at a particular picture element location. Thus, the uncertainty

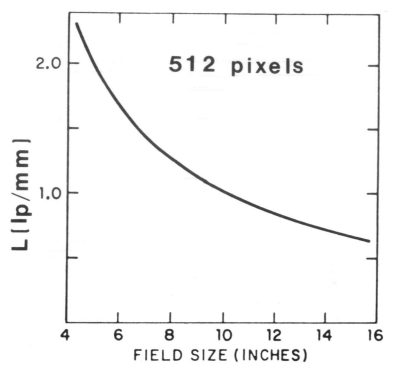

FIGURE 18. A plot of the limiting spatial frequency (line pairs/mm) as a function of the image field-of-view that can be resolved using a 512 X 512 matrix. Typical video-fluoroscopic image intensifiers range in size from 4.5 to 9 inches in diameter.

decreases as the number of detected x-rays increase. This implies that the areas of the image where small amounts of light are produced will have relatively higher noise levels or uncertainty than the bright areas. The difference image will tend to amplify this uncertainty. This phenomenon is called propagation of error, causing the low light (small number of detected x-rays) areas of the image to appear "grainy". Fig. 20 illustrates this point with an aortic arch study where the area over the vertebral column is underpenetrated and the overlying carotid artery poorly visualized.

A second source of image noise is commonly referred to as system noise and corresponds to the noise which is generated by the image intensifier video camera chain. In general, it has been found that the noise of the image intensifier system is smaller than the noise of the video camera system. Therefore, system noise generally is the result of the video noise. In order to minimize this source of noise, video camera systems which have extremely low noise levels are used in DR systems. In general, systems attempt to maintain high signal levels while decreasing noise levels. The noise level of a video system is generally defined as the video output level when the camera is in complete darkness. That level of noise is related to the maximum output of the video camera to yield the signal-to-noise ratio. The signal-to-noise ratio must be maintained as large as possible in order to decrease the effect of the video noise on the difference image. Current video cameras operate with signal-to-noise ratios within the range of 500 to 1,000. At the expense of motion artifact creation, the signal-to-noise ratio can be significantly increased by summing several frames together. Summation minimizes random noise components while enhancing the signal. The summation technique is commonly used by systems which operate in the continuous fluoroscopic mode (see chapter by Gould).

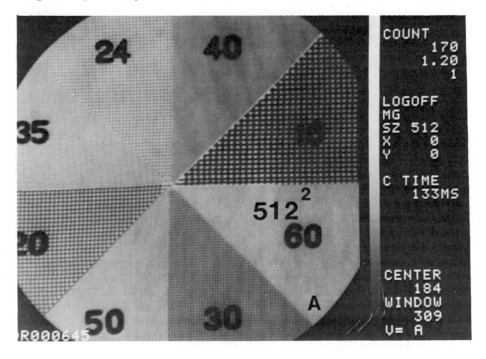

FIGURE 19A. Resolution phantom digitized at a 512 X 512 matrix with 4.5 inch field-of-view. Mesh size is identified by the numbers in terms of line pairs/inch. In the 512 matrix, the system can be resolved at least 40 lp/inch.

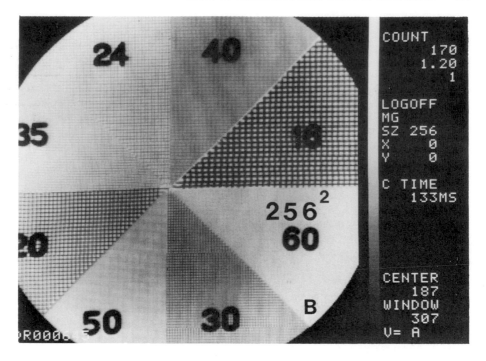

FIGURE 19B. Resolution wire mesh phantom at 256 X 256 matrix (4.5 inch field-of-view). Aliasing can be recognized as low as 24 lp/inch by the irregular intensity of the lines. More severe aliasing artifacts are seen at 35 lp/inch; however, the image of the 40 lp/inch mesh demonstrates a more subtle pattern which might be mistaken as true resolution rather than as artifactual.

An important feature of the video camera is the video gain. Increased gain will amplify very small signals, but camera noise will also be amplified. For this reason, the gain of the camera should be kept low in order to minimize the amplification of the video noise. If the gain is kept low, however, one must compensate by maintaining a relatively large amount of input light. This approach dictates that the system be operated at relatively high radiographic x-ray intensities rather than at fluoroscopic levels. An alternate approach would be to operate the camera at fluoroscopic intensities and then to sum together a number of video images to yield the same effect as an increased number of x-rays. It should be recalled that image noise is proportional to the total number of x-rays detected at a region and does not depend upon the time over which they were detected. Therefore, the mode at

which the data are acquired, whether in continuous
fluoroscopic mode at low x-ray currents or at pulsed
radiographic intensities, will result in the same noise level
as long as the total number of detected x-rays is the same.

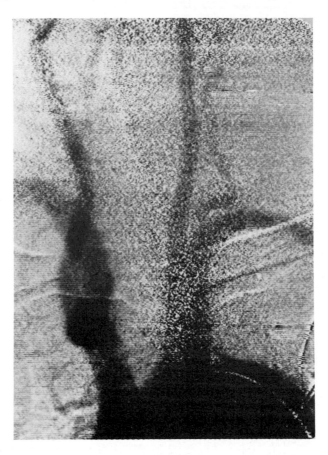

FIGURE 20. IV-DSA image of carotid arteries and aortic
arch demonstrating poor radiographic technique.
Underpenetrated areas over the vertebral column result in a
small number of x-rays detected by the image-intensifier.
Once the difference between the mask and contrast image has
been taken, the noise mottle, due to random variations in the
detected x-rays, becomes much more apparent. Image quality
may be improved by summing several images (both mask and
contrast images) together (at the expense of motion artifacts)
before subtraction or by increasing the radiographic factors
to higher currents, longer exposure time or higher KVp.

The x-ray quantum noise depends only upon the total number of x-rays and not whether the x-rays are absorbed within a short time period or absorbed over a relatively extended time period and then added together. An advantage to the pulsed system is that with short exposures the amount of the patient motion will be minimized.

XVI. ARTIFACTS

There are a number of artifacts resulting from the process and technology of digital subtraction imaging. The most common ones result from patient motion. If there is substantial motion between the mask image and the contrast images, then there will be artifacts produced in the difference image. Even very subtle motion on the order of a few picture elements can result in significant image degradation. Fig. 21 illustrates a carotid artery examination in which minimal motion has taken place (note cervical spine). Small vessels become completely obscured when the image is shifted, as little as one picture element (Fig. 22). In the head and neck images, the primary motion artifact is the result of swallowing (Fig. 23). Motion artifacts are generally easy to recognize. Motion resulting from a uniform shift can be corrected for by shifting the image a few picture elements in the direction of the motion. Motion which is non-uniform, in particular rotational motion, is a much more difficult problem. There are techniques under development which attempt to distort the image to take rotation into account. To date, however, these have not been extremely successful as will be necessary for routine clinical use.

Another common artifact results from the mismatching of the x-ray intensity with the dynamic range of the video camera and analog-to-digital converter. That is, if the light output of the image intensifier is too large, then it will saturate the video camera and those areas will all be represented at the maximum output level of the camera. Saturation results in a constant digital level with no information content. The term "saturation" is frequently used to identify those areas where the light level has reached the maximum operating level of the video camera. In those areas the difference will always be zero, because the digital number that has been stored in the computer would correspond to the maximum video level of 255 in each case. A similar effect can occur at low levels if the x-ray absorption in the patient is high and the light level produced in the image intensified is so low that it is below the analog-to-digital converter range. In this

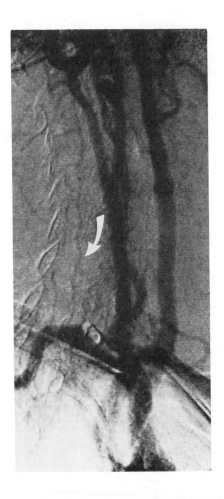

FIGURE 21.   IV-DSA carotid artery examination illustrating relatively little motion between mask and contrast image. Arrow points to small vessel which can be identified.

case, the values that are produced are a constant zero and when they are subtracted, the result will also be zero. Quantum mottle resulting from inadequate x-ray penetration over certain sections of the image is also a frequent problem and it is also a problem associated with the dynamic range of the system (see Fig. 20). Within the body, there are frequently regions of interest which include air interfaces close to dense bone interfaces. These present an extremely large range of x-ray intensities across the field of vision that must be accommodated by the image receptor. This range

of x-ray intensities is often too large for the recording
system and the result is image saturation. There are a number
of different techniques which are used to compensate for this
problem. The use of compensating wedges is the most common.
In this approach, the dynamic range is reduced by attenuating
x-rays in the "thinner" portions of the field-of-view so that
the x-ray intensity range will match the dynamic range
capability of the system. The dynamic range problem is well
illustrated by the aortic arch studies in Fig. 20, where the
lung field represents a very "thin" region and the base of the
skull represents a very "thick" region. Without compensating

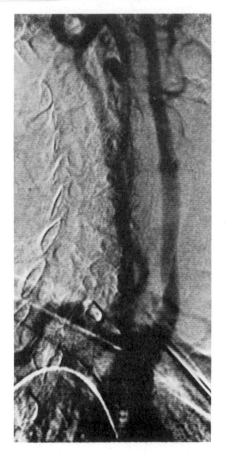

FIGURE 22. IV-DSA carotid artery image shown in Fig. 21
in which the mask image has been shifted 1 picture element;
the result being to obscure the small vessel shown in Fig. 21
as well as obscuring the carotid artery boundary.

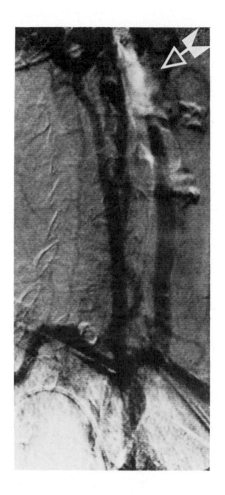

FIGURE 23. IV-DSA image of the same carotid artery examination shown in Fig. 21. This difference image was formed using a post-contrast image in which the patient swallowed. The swallowing artifact (white arrow) obscures the upper portion of carotid artery which can be clearly seen in Fig. 21, where a more appropriate post-contrast image frame had been chosen.

filters, it would be very difficult to form a single image which could contain both regions without saturation.

XVII. <u>SUMMARY</u>

Many of the difficulties in understanding digital imaging systems and computers in general stem from the "jargon" of the industry. This chapter is intended to amplify some of these terms and phrases and to assist in understanding what they imply in reference to medical digital imaging. Another goal of this communication is to give the reader some basic knowledge of the various system components and their characteristic parameters so that system purchases can be made in which the medical need and system capabilities are matched (9). For a more succinct presentation of the digital radiography terms and phrases the reader is referred to the Glossary of terms which has been included to aid in understanding this text.

<u>REFERENCES</u>

1. Mistretta, C.A., Digital videoangiography, <u>Diagnostic Imaging</u> 3:14, 1981.
2. Mistretta, C.A., and Crummy, A.B., Digital Fluoroscopy, in "Physical Basis of Medical Imaging" (C.M. Coulam, J.J. Erickson, F.D. Rollo, and A.E. James, Jr., eds.), p. 107. Appleton-Century-Crofts, New York, (1981).
3. Arnold, B., Eisenberg, H., and Borger, D., Digital videoangiography system evaluation, <u>Applied Radiology</u> 10(6), 81-90 (1981).
4. Hansen, G., "Solid-State Television Camera Tubes," pp. 63-80, Prentice-Hall, New Jersey, (1969).
5. Hansen, G., Solid-State Television System, Color and Black & White, in "Scanning Systems," pp. 83-102, Prentice-Hall, New Jersey, (1969).
6. Erickson, J.J., Price, R.R., Rollo, F.D., Pendergrass, H.P., Gerlock, J., Partain, C.L., and James, A.E., Jr., A digital radiographic analysis system, <u>RadioGraphics</u> 1, 49-60, 1981.
7. James, A.E., Jr., Goddard, J., Price, R.R., Jones, T., and Powis, R., Advances in instrument design and image recording. <u>Radiologic Clinics of North America</u> 18, 3-20, 1980.

8. Gibbs, S.J., Price, R.R., and James, A.E., Image
    Perception, in "The Physical Basis of Medical Imaging"
    (C.M. Coulam, J.J. Erickson, F.D. Rollo, and A.E. James,
    Jr., eds.), p. 295, Appleton-Century-Crofts, New York,
    (1981).
9. Price, R.R., Pickens, D.R., Smith, C.W., Lagan, J.E., and
    James, A.E., Jr., Simultaneous bi-plane digital
    fluoroscopy, Radiology 143, 255-257, 1982.

3

TECHNOLOGIC CONSIDERATIONS—EQUIPMENT, IMAGING PROCESSING AND
SUBTRACTION TECHNIQUES

Charles A. Mistretta

Departments of Medical Physics and Radiology
The University of Wisconsin
Madison, Wisconsin

I. X-RAY GENERATOR

X-ray generator requirements for subtraction angiography
vary depending on the specific application. Probably the
largest division occurs when one decides upon equipment for
cardiac or noncardiac applications. For imaging coronary
vessels or coronary bypass grafts, significant motion is
involved and a generator capable of high exposure rates and
short exposure times is preferred. However, in view of the
fact that intravenous techniques have found their largest role
in the examination of noncardiac vascular structures, it is
our opinion that longer exposure times, up to 100 msec, such
as are used in conventional angiography, are sufficient for
good image quality. Typically, researchers at the University
of Wisconsin use exposure times of between 30 and 250 msec and
employ digital image integration to combine the transmission
information from multiple television frames. When this is
done, x-ray tube currents of between 100 and 500 mA may be
used. If it is desired to use shorter exposure times, on the
order of 10 to 20 msec, a generator of 1000 mA or greater is
required. For most of the intravenous angiography work
presently being discussed, such a high power generator is not
required.

The pulse to pulse stability of the x-ray generator is a
rather important consideration. In the subtraction modes a
series of images is generated by subtracting images after
contrast injection from those prior to contrast injection.
Any appreciable increase or decrease in the x-ray tube output

from pulse to pulse will add an overall brightness component to the subtraction image and may decrease the range of contrasts which can be accommodated.

X-ray generator flexibility is also an important consideration. For implementing the various subtraction algorithms presently used, it is necessary to alter the exposure sequence of the generator. For maximum flexibility it should be possible to do this rapidly. For example, in coronary bypass imaging it is desirable to use a low x-ray tube current for the right heart phase of the examination and then to be able to rapidly switch to a high exposure sequence during the opacification of the left heart structures. For energy subtraction work, which up until this point has not shown as much clinical promise as the time subtraction algorithms most commonly used, the flexibility of the x-ray generator becomes an even more important consideration. Here, depending on the algorithm, it may be necessary to rapidly switch the energy of the x-ray generator at rates up to 60 times per second.

II. IMAGE INTENSIFIER

Intravenous angiography can be adequately done with most modern cesium iodide image intensifiers. The overall spatial resolution of the images is typically limited by the television camera rather than the image intensifier. In fact, in most cases it would be desirable to place greater emphasis on the quantum detection efficiency of the image intensifier rather than on the end-point spatial resolution. For quantitative studies, such as the determination of iodine concentration or cardiac ejection fraction, the contrast ratio of the image intensifier is especially important. Many image intensifiers have considerable lateral communication of information. This permits image brightness in one portion of the x-ray field to communicate with the darker portions of each picture element. Thus for quantitative studies image intensifiers with improved contrast ratio, or equivalently diminished veiling glare, are especially attractive.

The image intensifier format is also an important consideration. The new, large format image intensifiers provide the greatest flexibility, in that the area covered during a single contrast injection can be maximized. Thus, with the large format image intensifiers both kidneys may be studied simultaneously rather than with a separate contrast injection. For examination of smaller areas, maximum utilization of the available digital picture elements can be achieved by using the electronic magnification modes typically incorporated in these intensifiers.

III. TELEVISION CAMERA

The television camera is an important element in the imaging chain in that it is one of the main sources of image noise and is often the determinant of spatial resolution. In most digital angiography systems discussed thus far two types of television cameras have been used. These are the standard 1 inch Plumbicon and the larger Frogshead Plumbicon. The signal-to-noise ratio of the standard Plumbicon unit is typically on the order of 200 to 1, whereas the Frogshead Plumbicon has a signal-to-noise ratio on the order of 800 to 1. The 200 to 1 signal-to-noise ratio is sufficient for a large fraction of the imaging applications encountered. The basic question regards the amount of tissue variation contained within the video field. In the brightest portions of the image, the 200 to 1 signal-to-noise ratio is good enough to ensure that the quantum statistics, rather than the television camera, limits the overall signal-to-noise ratio of the image. For images having large tissue variations, and in which it is desired to visualize low contrast structures in areas corresponding to thick patient sections, the camera noise can dominate the overall signal-to-noise ratio. In these situations the Frogshead Plumbicon will provide somewhat better performance. The choice between the two also depends on the spatial resolution required. The standard 1 inch Plumbicon has a somewhat lower spatial resolution than the larger tube. Whether or not the Plumbicon is the limiting factor may depend on the number of digital picture elements contained in the processor memory. For applications involving 512 X 512 picture elements or less, the standard 1 inch Plumbicon is probably not a significant limitation. For systems intended to display 1000 X 1000 picture elements or more, the higher resolution tube would be necessary. At the University of Wisconsin, we have used both cameras and have the subjective impression that, for most of our imaging applications, using a 512 X 512 image matrix, there is little difference in the quality of the images obtained using the two cameras for a large fraction of the imaging situations which occur.

IV. A TO D CONVERTER AND LOGARITHMIC PROCESSING

The television information must be logarithmically processed in order to compensate for the exponential attenuation of the x-rays in the patient. There are two ways presently used to do this. One method involves the use of an analog logarithmic amplifier to stretch the dark portions of the image relative to the bright portions of the image prior to analog to digital conversion. When this is done, an analog to digital converter using 8 digital bits is sufficient for most applications. Since the main source of electrical noise comes from the television camera and not the logarithmic amplifier, the use of an analog logarithmic amplifier is not an important limitation. For extremely high contrast objects, the limited gain-bandwidth product of the analog logarithmic amplifier may lead to lower contrast transfer than might be achieved with a purely digital system. Most of the contrasts involved in intravenous subtraction angiography, however, are rather low and the limited gain-bandwidth product of the logarithmic amplifier is not a serious limitation.

Another alternative is to digitize the data prior to a digital logarithmic processing function. When this is done the requirements for the A to D converter are greater than in the previous case. If logarithmic processing is not done prior to digitization, there must be at least 10 bits of information in order for there to be adequate numbers of gray shades in the dark portions of the image. Either of the above two schemes can lead to excellent images and the choice of one over the other is largely a matter of convenience. One potential advantage of the logarithmic digital processing is that additional beam hardening correction information could be incorporated into the digital look-up table which performs the logarithmic function. This would be helpful in quantitative studies.

V. MEMORY CONFIGURATION

Most of the commercially available systems for digital angiography incorporate dedicated, real-time memories which are capable of storing information at video rates. This is necessary so that subtraction can be done in real time rather than having to slow down the data to accommodate the low data transfer rates of computers. For most applications, memory configurations of 512 X 512 pixels provide excellent image quality. For intravenous examinations, where contrasts are low, it is often difficult to tell the difference between images obtained with 256 X 256 matrices and those obtained with 512 X 512 matrices. The advantages of the larger picture element array become rather striking in the case of direct arterial injections where the subtraction images contain small, high contrast structures. This will be further discussed later on in this chapter.

The number of image memories required depends on the specific algorithm being executed. Most systems contain from 1 to 3 separate image memories and these are sufficient to accomplish the most commonly used algorithms. Greater numbers of memories permit specialized applications and are useful for research investigations.

VI. COMPUTER

We consider the role of the computer to be one mostly of image management and quantitation. Because of the high data rates involved, use of the computer on a pixel by pixel basis is usually not appropriate. Instead, the computer, whether it be a mini-computer or micro-computer, is used to reconfigure dedicated hardware which can handle the rapid rates associated with digital video processing. When the desired subtraction images have been formed by the dedicated hardware and stored, the computer can be used to further process or analyze these images in a post-processing configuration.

The computer will play a particularly important role in the quantitative evaluation of videodensitometric data. Such quantitation requires more flexibility than can be easily incorporated in the form of hardware. The computer will, through software programming, permit the user to perform a variety of analytical studies in an attempt to derive physiological information. Of particular importance in these investigations will be the corrections for x-ray scatter and veiling glare in the image intensifier. Although these corrections have, in some instances, been incorporated into the hardware, operations such as image blurring through convolution are easily accomplished by a computer. In addition, the computer provides a flexible means of data formating and display.

VII. SUBTRACTION ALGORITHMS

A. Mask Mode Radiography

In mask mode radiography, a pre-opacification image is stored in memory and is subtracted from a series of post-opacification images at a rate typically between 1 and 2 per second. Whether the mask is taken before the injection or following the injection depends on the anatomical region being studied. In the region of the aortic arch or the heart, it is important to take the mask before the injection of contrast in order to prevent venous structures from appearing in the subsequent subtraction images. For sites which do not overlap the venous injection path, the pre-opacification mask may be taken following completion of the injection but prior to opacification of the vessels of interest.

The x-ray factors chosen for the examination depend on a number of variables. It is desirable to keep the x-ray spectrum rather close to the K-edge of iodine at 33 keV. In practice x-ray energies on the order of 40 keV are optimal from the standpoint of maintaining iodine contrast and achieving adequate x-ray transmission. In order to achieve this, kVp values between 60 kVp and 80 kVp are generally used, depending on the thickness of the patient. Often one has to make the choice between using a larger television aperture, which reduces the required exposure for optimal television performance, and increasing the kVp, which might permit the use of a small aperture but which may compromise iodine contrast. The availability of a high power x-ray generator does provide some flexibility in this regard. Adequate x-ray statistical information may also be achieved through integration in regions where significant arterial motion is not expected.

B. Mask Mode Fluoroscopy

Mask mode fluoroscopy, or continuous subtraction imaging, is often accomplished using a pre-injection mask which is integrated over a significant fraction of the cardiac cycle, in order to produce an average blurred mask. This mask suffices to cancel enough anatomical information that the iodine in the subtraction display can be enhanced by a factor of about eight. Because the mask does not correspond to all subsequent phases of the heart, some mis-registration artifacts are visible. The display, however, does provide greatly enhanced visualization of the iodinated structures.

This examination has been useful in the evaluation of left ventricular function and is also being studied in connection with the evaluation of the patency of coronary bypass grafts. Mask mode fluoroscopy, like mask mode radiography, requires that the patient suspend respiration for the duration of the examination. Because the examination is usually done to study the heart, it is important to take the mask prior to the injection of contrast material.

The x-ray exposures used in mask mode fluoroscopy may vary greatly depending on whether it is desired to study the left ventricular wall motion or to study the patency of bypass grafts. In the latter case, significantly higher x-ray exposure is desirable. For evaluation of the left ventricle, fluoroscopic level currents of a few mA are probably sufficient. For evaluation of bypass grafts, we have had our best success using a dual dose mode in which low current is used during the right heart phase and the current is used for 3 to 6 seconds during opacification of the left heart. Study of the short high dose portion of the examination is facilitated by storing the information on a video disk and then viewing the disk in a dynamic mode in which the disk is repetitively moved between an upper and lower track number, so that the observer has sufficient time to become oriented to the anatomy.

C. Time Interval Difference (TID) Imaging

TID was developed in an attempt to reduce the effects of respiratory motion. In TID, rather than displaying the entire iodine signal, only short term changes in the iodine signal are displayed. The characteristics of TID mode are white signals during increases of iodine such as occur during expansion of the left ventricle, and black signals during contraction. Areas of dyskinesis show up as anamalous gray shades, for example, a black area on a white border. Experiments with animals in which the left ventricular has been infarcted have confirmed that irregular motion shows up directly in this mode.

D. Other Modes

Several other imaging modes have been studied or are undergoing further study. Among these are the so-called functional imaging algorithms in which the time of arrival of the contrast or the time of maximal opacification is displayed as a gray scale. Such displays may be useful for detecting

abnormalities in organ perfusion, such as asymmetrical
perfusion of the right and left kidney.

Subtraction images have been formed by several
investigators using continuous x-ray exposure with integration
times considerably longer than those used in mask mode
radiography. These techniques, under favorable circumstances,
can provide a dynamic display of the iodine flow, and through
extensive integration, can provide static images with adequate
quantum statistics. Further research is necessary, however,
to see if such an imaging procedure will be able to deal with
the very real problem of patient motion. Another closely
related approach involves the use of two digital memories
which integrate information from the past in such a way that
the combination of the information from these two memories is
particularly sensitive to various temporal frequencies, and in
particular can be matched to the temporal frequencies which
characterize the passage of an intravenously administered
contrast bolus. Again the basic question which must be
researched in connection with such algorithms is their
sensitivity to various forms of patient motion.

VIII. SHORT TERM DATA STORAGE

The means of data storage used for digital angiography
applications can be roughly divided into two catagories:
analog and digital. The advantages of digital storage are
that once the data has been digitized no further degradation
of the image can occur during reprocessing operations. It
also provides a certain flexibility in that, unlike the case
of analog storage, it is not necessary to be able to
anticipate the degree of contrast enhancement which is optimal
for a particular imaging situation. With analog storage, if
too large a contrast enhancement factor is chosen, the data
may saturate in such a way that reprocessing is not possible.
With the digital storage, the enhancement factor can be chosen
during reprocessing. In clinical practice, however, the
variation in the desired contrast enhancment factor is
sufficiently small that one can use analog processing without
frequent problems.

One of the disadvantages of digital storage is that
devices of moderate price do not have sufficient speed to
record continuous subtraction fluoroscopic information and are
limited to frame rates on the order of 1 to 2 per second at
512 X 512 or about 6 per second at 256 X 256. The University
of Wisconsin has recently developed a real-time disk unit,
patterned after a similar development originally done by the

Ampex Corporation which permits us to write 30 images per second, having a picture element array of 512 X 512. However, the development cost for this device was on the order of $150,000. It is presently not clear that the cost of this device can be reduced to a point which would make it cost effective.

If digital pre-processing and enhancement of iodine information utilize digital processing, then analog storage devices can be used to store mask mode fluoroscopy data and, using data redigitization, permit reprocessing of data without significant addition of noise. The fundamental principle involved is that fully processed and enhanced iodine information leads to an iodine signal on the order of 10 times bigger than that present in the raw video data. Placement of such an enchanced iodine signal on the video disk has the same result as if the disk had a signal-to-noise ratio 10 times larger than it has under normal circumstances. The advantages of using analog disks for data storage are lower expense and the ability to store data at real-time frame rates. It is likely that economic considerations will dictate the use of analog storage devices on commercial systems, at least for the purposes of dynamic examinations. Digital disk storage is quite feasible in the case of serial mask mode radiograpic imaging, where the frame rates are modest.

IX. IMAGE REPROCESSING

The most severe limitation to time-dependent subtraction angiography is patient motion. Patient motion often occurs between the time of the pre-opacification mask and the images which are sequentially obtained after opacification of the arteries of interest. When motion occurs it is very often useful to try early (or late) images as alternate masks for the purpose of subtraction. In the case of digital storage it is possible to store all of the images in unsubtracted form. As mentioned above, however, since the contrast enhancement factors are generally predictable, it is perhaps more advantageous in our opinion to subtract images in real time, so that the image sequence can be displayed during the passage of the iodinated contrast material, and to store only subtracted image information on an analog disk. In order to reprocess images stored in this way it is only necessary to subtract a pair of subtraction images. Because each of these has the original mask, as a subtracted element, the further subtraction of these two images causes cancellation of the original image with the net result that the first of the image pair serves as a mask for the second. This can be done quickly and reliably and in most cases the reprocessed image does not appear to have a significant increase in noise relative to the original image. More importantly, the effects of motion are often eliminated in this way.

Many investigators are studying the possibility of moving images relative to each other in order to compensate for patient motion. This kind of correction can produce striking results in some situations. However, it has not been demonstrated yet that such a technique will be important in the majority of clinical situations. University of Wisconsin scientists early investigated this possibility but were limited to only horizontal and vertical motion of the images with respect to one another. Rotation is another possibility being incorporated in some present devices. It is not clear, however, that any two dimensional rotation or translation will be sufficient to compensate for the motion, which is in general a complicated three dimensional process. More complicated algorithms involving non-linear stretching of images are also being tried. The results of these investigations are awaited with considerable interest.

X. ARCHIVAL STORAGE

The two most common methods for archival storage of intravenous subtraction angiographic data are videotape and film. In the devices we have used clinically, the subtraction information, which is primarily stored on analog disk for short term storage and reprocessing, is also simultaneously transferred to a video tape cassette and eventually to film using a multiformat camera. Digital storage of information on digital tape is too bulky for practical purposes and conventional video disks are also unsuitable for archival information. Laser disks are under investigation by several companies and may provide a reasonable means of long term storage of angiographic data. These devices, if their writing speed can be increased economically, may also play a role for short term data storage.

XI. FUTURE DEVELOPMENTS

Although there will be improvements in presently available equipment, it is probably safe to say that improvements of image quality will not occur as rapidly as they did following the introduction of computerized tomography. The improvements in that case were closely related to the evolution of the detector system. In the case of videoangiography, the image intensifier and video systems are already very well developed because of their use in previous applications. Nevertheless, it is reasonable to expect that some improvements in present equipment will occur. I have the feeling that the evolution of the equipment will be reminiscent of the hi-fi stereo equipment market, where rather simple inexpensive equipment already provides much of the peformance needed for a large majority of situations. For the purposes of intravenous angiography, I think it is clear that presently available commercial systems already do an excellent job.

One area where new algorithms and improved equipment may make a difference is in the area of coronary vessel imaging. In this case, it would be preferable to store a whole series of EKG labeled pre-opacification images during the heart cycle. Removal of mis-registration artifacts would aid in the visualization of bypass grafts and coronary arteries. The use of cine pulsing and sequential scan television operation will also help to improve the motion blurring, which is probably an important limitation of the present system. EKG gated exposures at end-systole and end-diastole are already possible with present equipment. It is the impression of the University of Wisconsin investigators that dynamic displays throughout the cardiac cycle are helpful for assessing vessel information.

For most intravenous angiography work, a 512 X 512 matrix appears to be adequate for use, in connection with a 6 inch or 9 inch intensifier. Larger matrix sizes would be useful in connection with larger format image intensifiers. Even in this case, however, it is likely that a workable mode of operation would be to do a moderate resolution survey scan and then, on a subsequent injection, to use electronic magnification in order to gain higher resolution over a smaller portion of the clinically relevant region.

The use of higher resolution systems may not be justifiable in the case of intravenous angiography, where contrasts are relatively low. The use of digital subtraction in connection with arterial injections has recently become of interest, however. To the extent that one might be able to eliminate film angiography entirely, using digital imaging, it may be necessary to increase the spatial resolution of the digital system in order to more closely match that provided by the film. Applications in this area include neuroangiographic examinations using aortic arch injections and screening for coronary disease using aortic root injections.

Another area in which considerable development is anticipated is in the quantitation of iodine distribution and flow. Here all that is required is the analysis of the digital images, using a computer to process the information included in a region of interest, which can be designated by a lightpen or similar technique. In this area present equipment is either adequate or easily upgraded to provide this capability. Most of the developmental work, once the equipment is in place, will consist of development of appropriate software analysis programs. We would like to re-emphasize that the data obtained from image intensifier systems is not directly quantitative except in selected applications, where errors may cancel through the use of ratios or where specific corrections are made for the effects of scatter and image intensifier veiling glare.

REFERENCES

1. Mistretta, C.A., Digital videoangiography, Diagnostic Imaging 3(14) (1981).
2. Mistretta, C.A., Crummy A.B., and Strother, C.M., Digital angiography: A perspective, Radiology 139, 273-276 (1981).
3. Mistretta, C.A., Crummy A.B., Digital Fluoroscopy, in "Physical Basis of Medical Imaging" (C. Coulam, J. Erickson, F. Rollo, and E. James, eds.), p. 107, Appleton-Century-Crofts, New York, (1981).

4

POTENTIAL ASSESSMENT OF CARDIAC FUNCTION WITH DIGITAL RADIOGRAPHY

W. Gordon Monahan
Chiiminy Kao
Edwin Hill
Jeff Pohlhammer
William Hunter, Jr.

Technicare Corporation
Cleveland, Ohio

I. INTRODUCTION

Angiocardiography is the visual documentation and quantitative analysis of the changes in x-ray absorption, both temporal and structural, that result from contrast-filled cardiovascular structures. Typically, this technique is used to obtain diagnostic information which is required to determine and monitor patient management. Invasive catheterization procedures are not ideally suited, however, to be used as screening diagnostic tests or for serial follow-up examinations to monitor the course of a patient's medical process or treatment regimen.

The increased availability and reduced costs of high speed data acquisition and processing equipment, coupled with the development of improved electronic components, has so improved angiographic techniques that imaging of low contrast signals has become feasible. In addition, these developments have been instrumental in shifting the emphasis from opacified hollow organ measurements to quantitative analysis of the radiographic images. Credit for much of the basic investigation in this field should go to researchers at the Universities of Wisconsin and Arizona (1,2). Each of these groups has several chapters in this text.

The technology, known as Digital Radiography or DR, was initially applied .to cardiovascular studies because it provided for the clinician a less invasive technique. This technology is being researched as a method for contrast ventriculography because of its millisecond framing rates and good spatial resolution. Although still in their infancy, digitial radiography cardiac techniques will be presented in this chapter to illuminate the facile aspects of a DR system and its potential for providing the physician with cost and efficacy advances in the routine assessment of cardiac function.

II. EQUIPMENT CONSIDERATIONS

Although the fundamentals of this process have been treated in many other chapters and in detail by Price as well as Mistretta, we will mention the basic principles in a summary fashion for the reader's orientation. A digital radiography system will usually include standard fluoroscopic x-ray equipment, plus the addition of a computer-based imaging chain. The primary difference between a digital imaging chain and a standard x-ray imaging chain is the conversion of the television signal from analog to digital form. The resultant digital signal is temporarily stored in computer memory where it can be processed and then returned to analog form for display. If post-processing is desired, the same image may be redigitized, re-processed and transferred to permanent storage on a digital disk. The digitization process allows great opportunities for the clinical user of this equipment.

Nuclear cardiology has successfully applied digital processing techniques to the quantitative assessment of cardiac pathophysiology. Several recent review articles have described this facility (3-6). The computer performance necessary for acquiring and processing gamma camera data, however, is approximately a factor of four times less than that needed for digital radiography. The digital radiographic process demands high speed (on the order of 1/30th sec.), large volume data handling (the number of data bits is calculated by taking 512^2 x 12 x number of frames), which has been a challenge only recently met by computer capabilities.

To describe cardiac motion with DR, at least 20 frames of data should be obtained during a single cardiac cycle. A complete examination of the cardiac function also requires measurements to be made at rest and immediately following exercise, resulting in heart rates from 60 to 180 beats-per-minute. To meet these sampling requirements, an imaging device would then have to acquire data at a rate of

60 frames/sec. Standard video framing rates are 60 fields/sec., or 30 frames/sec. since two fields are interlaced to produce one complete video frame.

Images can be acquired at 30 frames/sec. up to the total capacity of the memory. Due to the expense of memory components, the size is usually restricted to 2-8 image planes. If the image resolution is decreased by a factor of two in both dimensions, the image total can then be multiplied by four. Therefore, from 8-32 images can be acquired with a 256^2 resolution or, in like manner, from 32-128 images can be acquired with a 128^2 resolution.

This capacity has been found adequate for most studies. If more frames are required, then the images must be transferred to a storage device, such as a magnetic disk. If only qualitative results are desired, the data can be converted to analog form and stored on video tape or played out onto a video disk recorder. However, if the images are to be used in post-processing algorithms, then a digitized form of the data must be preserved. Current technology in magnetic disk subsystems limits data transfer rates to approximately 1.5 frames/sec., with each frame consisting of 512 x 512 pixels and each pixel being 16 bits deep. The corresponding recording rates for 256^2 and 128^2 matrices are 6 and 24 frames/sec., respectively.

III. TECHNICAL CONSIDERATIONS

Digital radiography has introduced important changes in the manner in which angiography is practiced. Yet, if this new modality is to reach its fullest potential as a diagnostic method for cardiac evaluation and many other low-contrast studies, several factors related to the image quality must be more completely understood.

If good x-ray beam collimation is used to reduce scatter, the major factors which affect system performance, in terms of radiation dose and image quality, are: 1) the x-ray tube focal spot size; 2) blur at the image intensifier caused by the scintillator screen's thickness; 3) the TV camera data sampling aperture and the output matrix size; and 4) the finite number of x-ray photons available, relative to the number of x-ray photons detected.

An effective aperture for an image intensifier television system approximately corresponds to the unsharpness at the edge of an output image produced by a sharp-edged object. The aperture is calculated from (7):

$$\text{Aperture} = [2 \int \text{MTF}^2(f)df]^{-1}$$

where the MTF (modulation transfer function) is the calculated response function of the system to a sinusoidal bar pattern. When several components of a complete system contribute to image quality, their respective apertures add in quadrature. By using the measured line spread function for an image intensifier, its contribution to system aperture can be calculated. Also, the largest matrix size currently available for most digital radiography systems is 512 X 512, and thus the magnitude of the pixel size component of each system aperture can be similarly determined. By treating geometric magnification and focal spot size as variables, the system aperture functions were calculated over the usable range for the device.

It is evident from an inspection of the curves (Figs. 1,2,3) that significant improvements in image quality will not be obtained by using radiographic magnification without increasing the data acquisition matrix size. In addition, for magnifications less than 2 X's, more than twice the improvement in system aperture is gained by changing the matrix size rather than the focal spot size; while the 0.6 and 0.3 mm focal spot curves show that the system aperture size remains relatively constant across the increases in magnifications.

With respect to photon detection, Albert Rose (8) has significantly contributed to our understanding of human and electronic vision. During 35 years of research in television systems, he developed an extremely simple and useful criteria for the number of photons required to detect an object with a given level of contrast. This number is:

$$N = \frac{25}{C^2 d^2}$$

where C is the object's contrast with respect to its surroundings, d is the object's size, and N is the number of photons per unit area detected for that object. This expression forms the ultimate limit for the performance of an imaging device. Fig. 4 compares the contrast-diameter performance of a specific digital radiographic system (Technicare DR-960) with an ideal imaging device, according to the Rose criterion. The deviation of the curves from an ideal imaging device is due to the finite resolution of the individual components in the system.

Objects smaller than the pixel size are observable in the limit of 100% contrast. These objects would not be produced

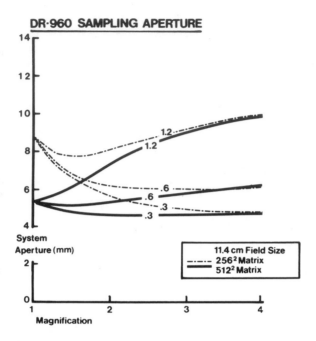

FIGURE 1. Plot of system aperture functions assuming the variables of geometric magnification (horizontal axis) and focal spot size (on lines) for a 11.4 cm (4.5 inches) field-of-view and 512 X 512 and 256 X 256 image matrices. The sampling aperture is calculated from the contributions to system MTF due to focal spot size, image intensifier blur, pixel size and both geometric and electronic image magnification.

at their correct size or contrast due to each pixel having a uniform gray shade in the output.

In order to use the Rose data to advantage in determining the likely performance of a digital radiography device in a clinical setting, the following experiment was performed (9). A patient being evaluated for carotid artery disease was given a peripheral venous injection of 40cc Renographin-76 followed by a 20 cc push of 5% Dextrose. A series of images was obtained of the neck region with a 1.0 mR exposure at the face of the image intensifier and at one-second intervals, to record the passage of the contrast bolus. After completion of the study, representative image frames were selected and subtracted for evaluation of contrast perfusion.

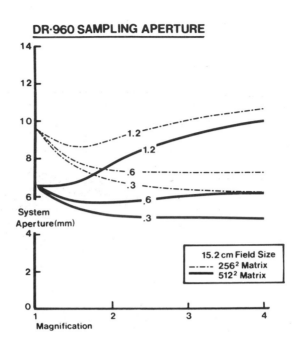

FIGURE 2. System aperture function as a function of geometric magnification and focal spot size for a 15.2 cm (6 inch) image intensifier field-of-view.

A second study was collected identical to the first but with only a 0.1 mR exposure measured at the level of the image intensifier. These images are shown in Fig. 4.

By calculating the object contrast for various sizes of vessels, the curve of presented object size versus object diameter was estimated (Fig. 5). The superposition of this curve on the contrast-diameter curve for 1.0 mR points out the useful operating range of a digital radiography device for intravenous angiography.

The machine's performance is the physical limit, and the calculated vessel contrast for an intravenous injection versus the vessel's diameter is the physiologic limit for this type of study. By plotting the performance curve for a typical film-screen system along with these other curves, the superior detection capability of a digital radiography device for imaging low contrast objects is indicated. This is accomplished by the preservation of detected photons using the gain of the image intensifier. Fig. 6 demonstrates a comparison of the photon gain through a digital radiography system to the photon gain of a film/screen system.

IV. CARDIAC MEASUREMENTS

In digital radiographic cardiac studies, the patient, in a supine position, receives a 40 cc intravenous injection of contrast material followed by a 20 cc 5% dextrose bolus to assist in maintaining the concentrated nature of the contrast media. The heart is imaged in either the LAO, RAO, or AP projection, and image frames are acquired at a rate of from 6-15/sec., depending upon the size of the digital matrix. The bolus of contrast material is injected at a rate of from 10-15 cc/sec. which results in a 6-to-8 sec. imaging time to demonstrate the left ventricle. In this "first pass" study, there are usually at least five cardiac contractions that

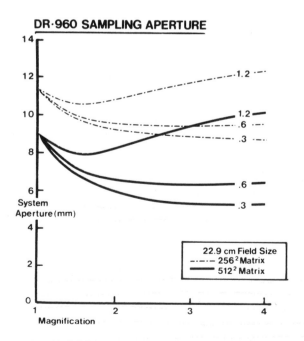

FIGURE 3. *System aperture functions as a function of geometric magnification and focal spot size for a 22.9 cm (9 inch) image intensifier field-of-view.*

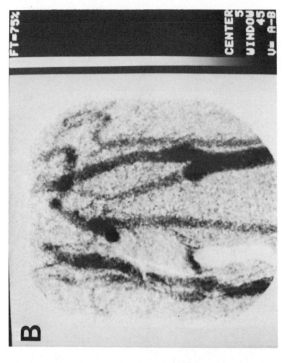

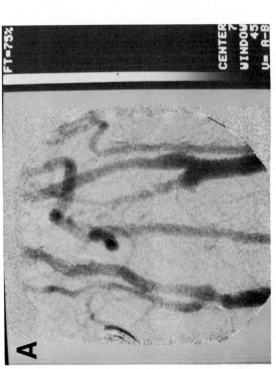

FIGURE 4. The carotid artery image (A) was performed with 1.0 mR exposure at the level of the image intensifier; image (B) is a repeat of the study, but with only 0.1 mR at the intensifier. Clearly, smaller vessels are visible in the higher exposure study, thus illustrating the Rose criterion more practically.

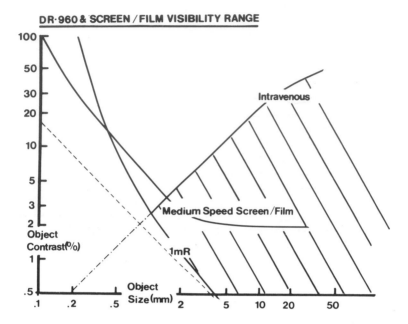

FIGURE 5. Ideal visibility curves using the Rose criterion for a film/screen system and Technicare DR-960 Digital Radiographic System. The measured values are typical for a digital radiography system performance for a 1.0 mR exposure at the face of the image intensifier. The physiologic limit was determined from measurements made on carotid artery examination images. The film/screen curve was generated from a medium speed system's response.

share maximum contrast material concentration. The following techniques are in developmental stages and should only be considered as potential DR applications.

V. EJECTION FRACTION

A left ventricular ejection fraction measurement can be made with an electrocardiographic gate to assure that good systolic and diastolic image frames are obtained. After the injection of a contrast media in a peripheral vein, an anteroposterior projection is viewed fluoroscopically to determine when the bolus has reached the left ventricle.

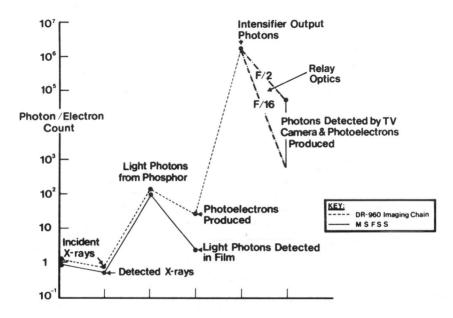

FIGURE 6. Comparison of photon conversion efficiencies for a specific digital radiography system and a film/screen system.

Since it takes from three to four cardiac cycles for maximum contrast concentration to arrive, the operator delays the initiation of the image recording sequence until the left ventricle is visibly observed. Data acquisition commences on the next R wave peak of the cardiac cycle. Using a 15-cm mode image intensifier magnification, and a 256^2 matrix, good spatial resolution is obtained. Images are stored in computer memory at 30 frames/sec. until the memory's capacity is reached (Fig. 7). Depending on the heart rate (at least one R-R interval in most patients), this method results in up to 32 data frames. The process can be repeated with frames allocated to digital disk storage sequentially as acquisition and storage overlap.

At the completion of data acquisition, images are reviewed in a "cine" format so that regions of interest can be selected for computation of time-density curves. Frames representing end-systole and end-diastole are used to calculate ejection fractions by either the area-length or the DR number methods,

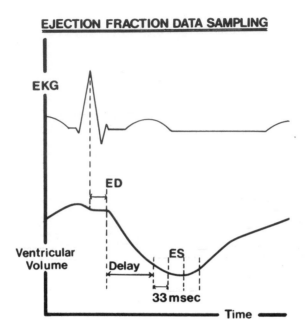

EJECTION FRACTION DATA SAMPLING

FIGURE 7. *EKG gate enables accurate determination of end-diastole. Rapid burst mode data acquisition is used to sample data at end-systole (33 msec intervals).*

as demonstrated in Fig. 8.   When DR numbers are properly corrected for scattered radiation from the patient, and veiling glare at the level of the image intensifier, these numbers accurately measure the product of the average absorption coefficient times the patient thickness, on a pixel-by-pixel basis. Therefore, a ventricular volume can be calculated which will be inaccurate by only a multiplicative constant.   By sampling the data at uniform intervals, a ventricular volume vs. time curve, similar to Fig. 9, can be obtained.

VI. REGIONAL WALL MOTION

Regional wall motion data can be collected in a fashion similar to the digital radiographic ejection fraction and ventricular volume determinations described above.   An alternative method is to use a constant rate and to then collect data continuously during the passage of the contrast medium bolus. For example, if 15 frames/sec. are recorded with a 128^2 matrix, wall motion can be viewed immediately following the study by replaying the acquired data from digital disk in a "cine" fashion.

For quantitative results, these same frames are used to calculate the average time to reach systole on a pixel-by-pixel basis. These data are then scaled and displayed on a gray scale image which is referred to as a "parametric" image (Fig. 10). Regions exhibiting rapid contraction appear at the black end of the scale, while the more slowly contracting regions are displayed in shades of gray. This type of display can be used to highlight explicit areas of akinesis.

To better define areas of dyskinesis, a phase analysis, with corresponding parametric image, should be performed. This involves fitting Fourier coefficients and phase angles to the pixel-value-vs-time data. Areas which are moving in synchrony will have the same phase and, therefore, will be displayed with identical gray scale values. The converse will obtain for those areas with dyskinesis.

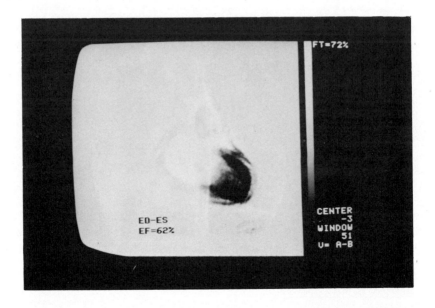

FIGURE 8. Cardiac ejection fraction image (end-diastole image minus the end-systole image). The ejection fraction image is calculated from the integrated DR numbers. Regional wall motion is apparent by inspection of the subtracted image data. This example represents an ejection fraction of 62%.

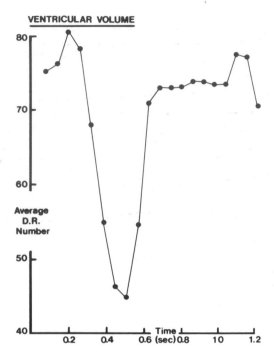

FIGURE 9. Ventricular volume curves are obtained from an area of interest chosen to encompass the left ventricle. The curve was obtained from a study in which images were acquired at 15 frames/sec.

VII. REGIONAL MYOCARDIAL PERFUSION

During the "cine" review of data for a first pass study, the observer will notice that myocardial wall thickness becomes quite visible, especially if a mask frame is taken from a point near the end of the study, where the contrast agent has entered the muscle's capillary phase (Fig. 11). These data suggest that a number proportional to regional myocardial perfusion might be obtained by integrating areas containing myocardium. To perform this calculation in a reproducible way, pie-shaped areas are centered on the left ventricle. A square area is positioned and sized to include all visible cardiac muscle. The particular algorithm used determines the range of the data in the square, and, while a threshold or lower level discriminator is applied (to avoid the inclusion of the contrast-filled left ventricle), it integrates the pie-shaped areas (Fig. 12).

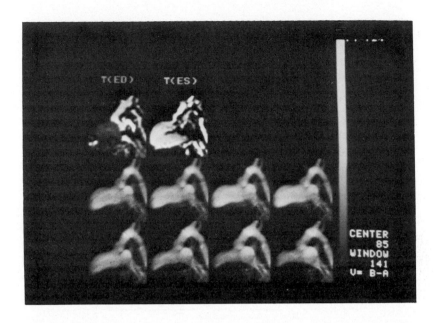

FIGURE 10. *Using DR number versus time data, time-to-maximum is determined on a pixel-by-pixel basis. These data can be used as a measure of regional myocardial wall motion. Upper left: end-diastole; upper right: end-systole. The eight images (left-to-right) move sequentially from end-diastole to end-systole.*

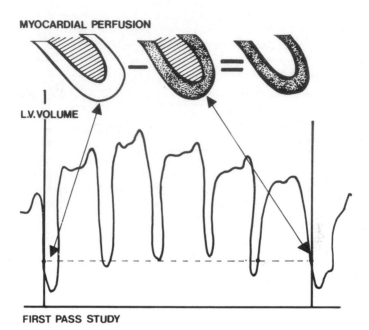

FIGURE 11. Illustration of the technique for using DR to assess myocardial perfusion. Prior to the first ejection of contrast material from the left ventricle, the myocardium contains no contrast agent. If a subsequent frame acquired at the same phase of the cardiac cycle and with the same amount of contrast in the left ventricle is subtracted, the result represents the residual amount of contrast material in the myocardium.

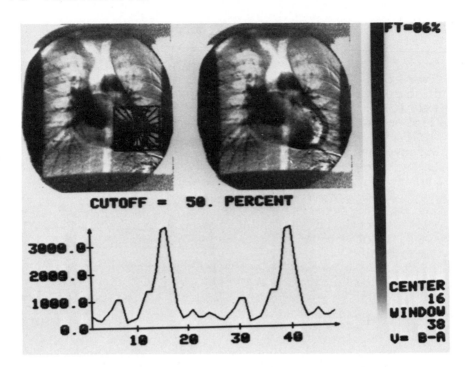

FIGURE 12. The integrated DR numbers are proportional to regional myocardial perfusion in the pie-shaped areas. Upper left image demonstrates the definition of the pie-shaped region-of-interest used to create the density versus angular position plot shown at the bottom.

VIII. SUMMARY

Digital radiography has the potential to be a valuable clinical method for evaluating left ventricular contraction, for detecting the presence and severity of regional asynergy, and for eliciting ejection fraction abnormalities at rest and during exercise stress. One would predict that as general clinical experience is gained, the value of this system to our cardiovascular diagnostic armamentarium will increase. Application of present and future biomedical engineering advances to this area should increase our facility in this evaluation process.

REFERENCES

1. Kruger, R.A., Mistretta, C.A., et al., Computerized fluoroscopy in real time for non-invasive visualization of the cardiovascular system. Radiology 130, 49-57 (1979).
2. Roehrig, H., Nudelman, S., et al., X-ray image intensifier video system for diagnostic radiology. SPIE 127, 216-225 (1977).
3. Bodenheimer, M.M., et al., Nuclear cardiology. I. Radionuclide angiographic assessment of left ventricular contraction: Uses, limitations and future directions, Am. J. Cardiology 45, 661 (1980).
4. Bodenheimer, M.M., et al., Nuclear cardiology. II. The role of myocardial perfusion imaging using Thallium-201 in diagnosis of coronary heart disease, Am. J. Cardiology 45, 674 (1980).
5. Berger, H.J., and Zaret, B.L., Nuclear cardiology (Part 1), NJM 305(14), 799 (1981).
6. Berger, H.J., and Zaret, B.L., Nuclear cardiology (Part 2), NJM 305(15), 855 (1981).
7. Schade, O.A., Image Quality - A Comparison of Photographic and Television Systems, RCA Publication, RCA Lab, Princeton, NJ (1975).
8. Rose, A., Vision Human and Electronic, RCA Lab, Princeton, NJ (1974).
9. Meaney, T., et al., Digital subtraction angiography of the human cardiovascular system, SPIE 233 (1980).

5

A DIGITAL FLUOROSCOPIC SYSTEM
USING TANDEM VIDEO PROCESSING UNITS

Robert G. Gould

Department of Radiology
University of California
San Francisco, California

I. INTRODUCTION

Recognition of the potential clinical impact of digital fluoroscopy has resulted in relatively recent, yet almost overwhelming interest by the radiologic community in this technology. Virtually all major x-ray manufacturers have marketed or plan to market a digital fluoroscopic imaging system. The early development work on digital fluoroscopy was done in academic centers, notably the Universities of Wisconsin and Arizona (1,2). The process, however, will predictably spread to other facilities for health care delivery.

Much of the excitement regarding digital fluoroscopy stems from the possibility of its application for intravenous (IV) angiography. This procedure presents a particularly difficult imaging task because subject contrast, defined as the change in x-ray attenuation along a projection through a vessel due to the presence of iodinated contrast medium, is quite low. While contrast medium injection factors (rate, bolus volume, initial iodine concentration) can affect subject contrast, significant dilution of the iodine occurs as it flows from the site of injection in the venous circulation, through the heart and lungs and, finally, to the arterial vessels of interest. Digital fluoroscopic systems are able to image low contrast vessels by subtraction, which cancels high contrast structures out of the image, and by image contrast amplification, which increases vessel visibility. These principles will be the focus of this chapter.

Because of the low subject contrast, the exposure to the image intensifier per image must be relatively large to overcome limitations imposed by quantum statistics. Typically, this exposure is between 0.25 and 1 mR for a satisfactory image (3). (For comparison, serial photospot images using 100–110 mm cameras are taken with 0.1–0.2 mR.) Different digital fluoroscopic systems deliver this radiation in different ways. Most systems presently available pulse the x-ray equipment several times per second at high current levels, usually 100 mA or greater.

Investigators at the University of California at San Francisco are investigating an alternative approach wherein a large number of video frames, produced while the x-ray equipment is operated at fluoroscopic levels (~5 mA), are averaged together to form an image (4,5). The averaging system has several advantages over pulsed systems, including:

1) It does not require an interface to the x-ray generator, connecting only to the video line from the TV camera on the image intensifier.

2) It does not require the low noise, high dynamic range television camera that is necessary with pulsed systems to reduce electronic noise. The frame averaging system reduces electronic noise as well as quantum noise by compiling frames.

3) Because of the advantages detailed in 1 and 2, the averaging system can use any reasonable quality, video equipped fluoroscopic system as it exists in nearly all radiology departments. This has significant financial implications (see chapters by Freedman and Evens).

4) It produces and stores a continuous subtraction sequence which can either be viewed in real-time or frozen at any point to create a hardcopy record for subsequent analysis and archiving.

5) The x-ray beam operates during the passage of the contrast medium through the vessels and is sampled continuously, thereby making better use of the available signal created by the transient presence of iodine. The signal is not constant, changing as the iodine concentration in the vessels of interest changes.

II. METHODS

A block diagram of the frame averaging digital subtraction fluoroscopic system is shown in Fig. 1. Video data from the camera on the image intensifier is recorded on a wideband VTR (Recortec) and also passed though a log amplifier to the digital hardware. This equipment consists of two video processors, made by Quantex Corporation (Sunnyvale, California), that operate in tandem.

The first processor operates simultaneously in an averaging and differencing mode. Its function is to: digitize an incoming video frame, subtract from it the exponentially weighted average of preceding frames, thereby creating a difference image, amplify the contrast in this difference image, average the incoming frame used to create the difference image into memory, and convert the difference image back to analog form. These operations are done at the standard video rate (30 frames per second). Note that the averaging process is continuous so that after the memory is subtracted from a frame, that frame is averaged into memory.

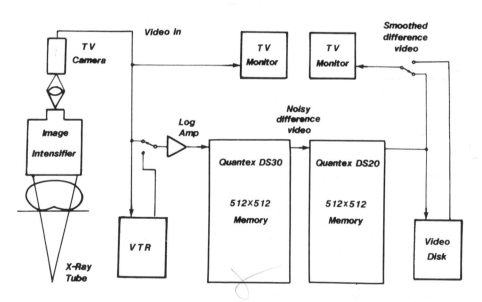

FIGURE 1. Schematic diagram of our frame averaging digital subtraction fluoroscopic system. Each processor has an 8 bit A/D converter with a 9.6 MHz sampling rate and can digitize a 525 line composite video frame into a 512 X 512 pixel matrix at a rate of 30 frames per second. Both processors have a memory depth of 12 bits.

The difference image produced by the first processor is noisy because of noise present in the images used in its formation. While the image in memory is relatively noise free (because it is the average of many frames), each incoming video frame has significant quantum and electronic noise. The function of the second processor is to average the noisy difference frames. A noise-reduced, real-time difference image is output from the second processor, recorded on either a videotape or disk recorder, and viewed on a standard TV monitor.

The number of frames averaged by a processor is determined by an averaging parameter: N, where N is a power of 2 between 0 and 7. It is set by the system operator. Clearly, the more frames averaged together (the larger N), the greater will be the noise reduction in the viewed image. The particular averaging algorithm used by the processors reduces noise in a stationary image by a factor that approaches $1/\sqrt{2N-1}$.

The number of frames that must be averaged to achieve adequate noise reduction in an intravenous angiographic subtraction image depends on the x-ray exposure rate to the image intensifier. We normally operate our equipment at 10-20 μR per video frame and average 32 or 64 frames (i.e., 1 or 2 seconds of video data).

Hardcopy can be obtained by freezing an image in memory of the second processor and transmitting this image to a multiformat camera. This action is usually performed after the patient procedure is completed by playing processed data from the video disk (tape) back into the second processor (Fig. 1), which is used to grab and store the desired image.

III. SUBTRACTION TECHNIQUES

An intravenous subtraction sequence is produced by the averaging system when a bolus of contrast medium is injected into the venous circulation. The x-ray equipment is activated several seconds before contrast medium is expected to arrive in the field of view and the fluoroscopic exposure is continued until the iodine has passed through this field. After initial adjustments of the processors, no intervention by the system operator is needed.

An interesting effect of this subtraction method is that the initial image contrast, produced when contrast medium arrives in the field of view, gradually diminishes as the bolus passes through the field. This fading occurs because video frames containing contrast medium are averaged into the memory of the initial processor. After the contrast medium has passed from the field of view and the image in memory contains contrast (but the incoming frames do not), a "reversal image" is observed. This reversal image can be useful in obtaining a diagnostic image if the patient motion occurs when the contrast medium reaches the field.

An alternative subtraction method is to freeze the contents in the memory of the first processor prior to the arrival of contrast medium in the field of view. This action results in a subtraction sequence during which image contrast does not fade as the bolus passes through the field. No reversal image would be produced in this mode.

The above subtraction methods work well if the arteries of interest remain stationary throughout the injection sequence. However, it is also possible to use the averaging system for subtraction imaging of the heart chambers. In this subtraction mode, the image in the first processor is frozen, as in the above subtraction method. Similar to the other methods, this image is formed by averaging a second or more of video data. During this period the heart moves and, consequently, this image is blurred (unsharp). It is formed prior to contrast medium injection. When the bolus is injected, the frozen image is subtracted from each incoming frame but the second processor uses a small averaging parameter of only 2 or 4 frames. This technique outlines the border of the heart chambers as the bolus flows through them. The real-time image seen by the system operator is noisy because the second processor averages together only a few of the incoming noisy difference frames. However, as the heart is a relatively thick object, subject contrast is higher than it would be in the arteries. Consequently, not as much noise reduction is needed to observe the desired detail.

IV. RESULTS

Typical intravenous images produced by the averaging fluoroscopic system are shown in Figs. 2-4. For patient studies, the catheter tip is positioned either in the inferior or superior vena cava and a bolus of 30 to 40 ml of contrast medium is injected at about 15 ml per second. All of the images are taken using a 9 inch diameter image intensifier.

A criticism of this system is that it might be more sensitive to misregistration problems caused by patient motion than are pulsed digital fluoroscopic units. Indeed, if the patient moves within the interval during which frames are

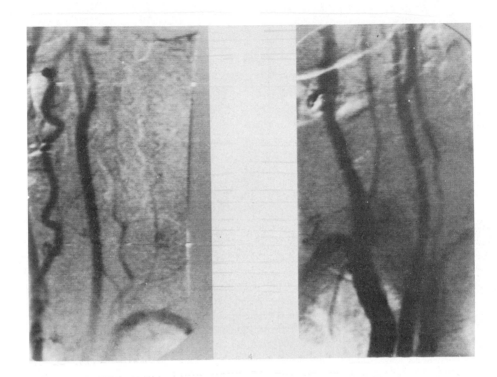

FIGURE 2. *Example images of carotid arteries made with the frame averaging digital fluoroscopic system. Both images were made by injecting a 35 ml bolus of contrast medium (Conray 400) into the inferior vena cava and operating the x-ray equipment at 68 kVp and 5 mA. The averaging parameter of both processors was set at 32.*

averaged, motion artifacts are produced. More motion artifacts are observed, larger averaging parameters are set on the processors. The 32 or 64 frame settings appear to be the best compromise between motion problems and noise reduction. These settings correspond to a time interval of 2 to 4 seconds. This is typically the same length of time as that between the formation by pulsed digital systems of the mask and the post-injection image. Consequently, it seems that the frame averaging technique is no more sensitive to patient motion than are pulsed techniques.

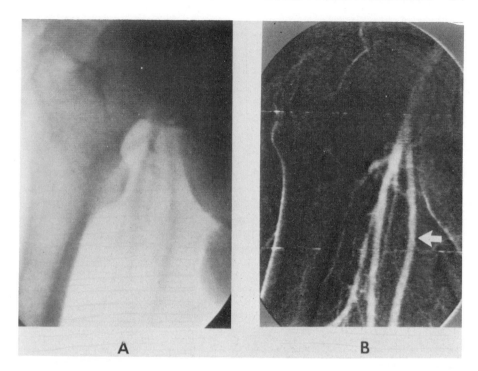

A   B

FIGURE 3. Image of the femoral artery, made with 35 ml
injection of contrast medium (Conray 400) into the inferior
vena cava. A patent femoral-popliteal graft (arrow) is seen
in the reversal subtraction image (Fig. 3B). Fig. 3A is the
image prior to subtraction. The averaging parameters of both
processors was set at 64.

V. CONCLUSIONS

Frame averaging techniques can be used to reduce noise in
digital fluroscopic subtraction imaging. It has the advantage
of easing the x-ray equipment performance requirements,
including those of the video camera, compared to pulsed
systems. Digital fluroscopic systems using frame averaging
need not interface with the x-ray generator but connect to the
x-ray unit only by the video line. These systems are flexible
and relatively inexpensive and have considerable potential in
clinical radiology.

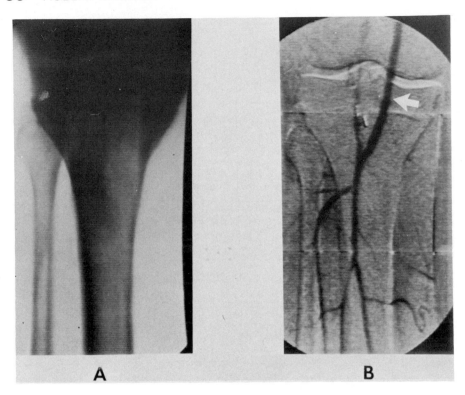

FIGURE 4. *Image of the trifurcation of the popliteal artery made with a 30 ml injection of contrast medium (Conray 400) into the inferior vena cava. A patent femoral-popliteal graft is indicated by the arrow (Fig. 4B). Fig. 4A is the post-injection image prior to subtraction and Fig. 4B is the subtracted image. The averaging parameter of both processes was set at 64.*

ACKNOWLEDGMENTS

The help of Paul Mengers of Quantex Corporation and of Dr. Martin Lipton of the University of California, San Francisco, in the investigation of our digital system is acknowledged gratefully.

This work was partially supported with grants from the Academic Senate and the Radiology Research and Education Foundation of the University of California, San Francisco.

REFERENCES

1. Kruger, R.A., Mistretta, C.A., Lancaster, J., et al., A digital video image processor for real-time x-ray subtraction imaging, Optical Eng. 17, 652-654 (1978).

2. Ovitt, T.W., Christensen, P.C., Fisher, H.D., et al., Intravenous angiography using digital video subraction: X-ray imaging system, AJR 135, 1151-1154 (1980).

3. Kruger, R.A., Mistretta, C.A., Riederer, S.J., Physical and technical considerations of computerized fluoroscopy difference imaging, IEEE Trans. Nucl. Sci. NS-28 (1981).

4. Gould, R.G., Lipton, M.J., Mengers, P., Dahlberg, P., A digital subtraction fluoroscopic system with tandem video processing units, SPIE 273, 125-131 (1981).

5. Gould, R.G., Lipton, M.J., Mengers, P., Dahlberg, P., Investigation of a video frame averaging digital fluoroscopic system. To be published. Proc. SPIE 314, 184-190 (1981).

6

COMPARISON OF OUTPATIENT DIGITAL ANGIOGRAPHY
AND INPATIENT ARTERIOGRAPHY: SOME FINANCIAL IMPLICATIONS

Gerald S. Freedman

Temple Medical Center
and
Department of Radiology
Yale Medical School
New Haven, Connecticut

A. Everette James, Jr.

Department of Radiology and Radiological Sciences
Department of Medical Administration
Institute for Public Policy Studies
Vanderbilt University
Nashville, Tennessee

with the assistance of

W. Hoyt Stephens

Department of Radiology & Radiological Sciences
Vanderbilt University
Nashville, Tennessee

I. INTRODUCTION

The application of biomedical technology, with the computer as a fundamental component, has found a significant application in diagnostic imaging. Digital radiography, when applied as contrast subtraction angiography, converts arteriography from what can be characterized as inpatient service with significant cost implications to a less expensive, safer technique that will most often be performed on an outpatient basis. These features of the digital technology will significantly alter the current clinical criteria for a large volume of angiographic studies. The advances in this type of medical imaging will quite likely lead to more widespread application of angiography as a diagnostic screening test in the evaluation of many disease processes. This chapter will consider the types of equipment currently used for hospital-based angiography and the financial implications of equipment currently being employed in an office practice as well as in inpatient or outpatient facility to perform digital angiography.

In this chapter, the cost-effectiveness of the outpatient diagnostic carotid examination will be analyzed. The total cost for evaluation of carotid artery disease is considered with regard to the larger population that may be expected to be studied by the safer and less expensive digital technique. A break-even analysis for various angiographic rooms will be developed graphically for a more universal application. This exercise will be coupled with a cost-effective analysis for the evaluation of carotid artery disease. The authors accept the circumstance that these evaluations are, at best, preliminary and represent extrapolation from historical precedent. However, we hope to provide a framework and potential template for future analysis, when the data base will become larger and more predictable with the rapidly expanding experience. For purposes of future calculations of reimbursement and cost as well as resource allocation, the reader should be aware that the anticipated experience and activity should improve the accuracy of these determinations.

II. EQUIPMENT ANALYSIS

At present, all the major medical imaging manufacturers and a number of for-profit companies new to the field are either offering or developing digital radiographic systems. As noted, a number of companies in related fields of medical imaging, such as computer sciences, information transfer, and signal detection, are developing independent systems of their own. Within such a short period of time as a year, the medical consumer will probably have more than a dozen image processors to consider. This will involve communication with groups and firms previously unfamiliar to the user. Therefore, general guidelines become increasingly important.

It appears that the price of a digital processor, which would be added to the existing x-ray system, should range from a "bare-bones" minimum of $150,000 to approximately $300,000 for a complete (full-blown) system with continuous real-time recording capability. The decision of which to choose should be based on the individual circumstances. For best results, the digital radiographic equipment should be used in conjunction with a "state-of-the-art" image fluoroscopic system. One can, however, modify an existing fluoroscopic room with newer components to optimize the room for digital radiography. Table I lists the x-ray components that should be available in an optimized fluoroscopic room, improved or equipped to effectively add a digital capability. These components will most likely include an x-ray tube with high heat capacity, a cesium iodide-image intensifier, preferably larger than 9 inches, a specialized television camera with an excellent signal-to-noise ratio, and a power injector for contrast media delivery. These general requirements may be modified as the available instrumentation advances and the clinical potentials become more apparent. The identification of these components of a digital facility as new capital expenditures is a philosophical one but has important and extensive implications.

III. FIXED AND VARIABLE COSTS FOR DIGITAL RADIOLOGY FACILITIES

Table II lists the spectrum of costs that one might anticipate to comprise the value of a radiographic room fully equipped for digital angiography. The values here range from a low of $300,000, which assumes the acquisition of a computer for $150,000 and modification of an existing radiographic room whose initial value is assumed to be $150,000. More realistically, if one were to purchase an x-ray room for this purpose, it is likely that an expenditure of at least $300,000 would be required for new equipment; if, in fact, the room is to be designed to perform conventional angiography as well,

TABLE I. *X-ray Components*

X-ray Tube and Housing	$15,000
Cesium I - Intensifier 9"/14"	30,000/75,000
TV - Camera	20,000
Power Injector	10,000
	$75,000/115,000

TABLE II.

X-ray room	Computer	Equipment total	Annual cost[a] true lease	Annual cost[b] installment
$150,000	$150,000	$300,000	$ 85,500	$100,000
200,000	200,000	400,000	114,000	134,000
250,000	250,000	500,000	142,680	168,000
350,000	250,000	600,000	171,000	200,000
450,000	250,000	700,000	199,500	234,000
500,000	300,000	800,000	228,000	268,000

[a]True lease - 5 years at 15% (10/81).
[b]Installment contract at 22% interest (9/81) - 5 years.

more than $500,000 will be required to make this improvement.
Column 3 in Table II lists the total value of equipment in the
the room under consideration; this valuation encompasses a
range from $300,000 as a minimum assignment to $800,000 as a
maximum. To determine the operating costs for this equipment,
one could value the equipment using either a true-lease or an
installment contract method. The values listed for these
calculations are based on current interest rates. (Note that
the finance charge for carrying such a room at this time is
approximately $100,000 to $200,000 a year.) This particular
calculation represents the main component of the fixed cost,
to which rent and a number of other costs must be added.

To the total annual cost for the operation of the digital
radiology room should be added additional costs: servicing
the equipment, the cost of personnel, administration,
insurance, remodeling, utility, etc. (Table III). The main
component of variable cost is supplies, which is approximately
$100 a case for a central catheterization and approximately
$50 a case for exams performed with a peripheral intravenous
injection. The final columns total the annual cost based on
either the assumption of 1,000 cases per year (4 per day), or
2,000 cases per year (8 per day). With peripheral injections,
significant reductions in room time can be achieved and some
institutions are reporting 16 or more cases per 10-hour day
(see chapter by Modic). However, it would appear that with
present staffing patterns and available instrumentation, a
figure of 6-8 per day would be realistic.

IV. FIXED COSTS FOR OUTPATIENT DIGITAL ANGIOGRAPHY

Substantial savings in capital investment for the digital
radiographic procedures and needed resources can be realized
if an existing fluoroscopic room has characteristic features
that can be adapted for digital angiography or other digital
procedures. For the calculation, one can assume that there is
unused time in that particular room. If modifications similar
to those described in Table II, which include the acquisition
of a new video system, as well as a new image intensifier tube
and possibly a new x-ray tube, which were assumed to require
an allocation of $100,000, were added to a room whose
depreciated value is assumed to be $100,000, one would assume
that the capital cost following purchase of a $200,000 digital
process would then be $400,000. If this expenditure is
compared to the cost of an angiographic suite, which usually
will require an allocation in excess of $500,000, there is
often a significant capital cost savings. Furthermore, if

TABLE III.

Equipment[a] annual cost	Service annual cost	Personnel[b]	Misc.[c]	Supplies[d]	Annual[e] total	Annual[f] total
$100,000	$30,000	$50,000	$50,000	$100,000	$330,000	$430,000
134,000	40,000	50,000	50,000	100,000	374,000	474,000
168,000	50,000	50,000	50,000	100,000	418,000	518,000
200,000	60,000	50,000	50,000	100,000	460,000	560,000
234,000	70,000	50,000	50,000	100,000	504,000	604,000

[a]Installment contract at 22% interest (9/81) – 5 years.
[b]Assumes 2.5 people.
[c]Space, administration, insurance, remodeling, utility.
[d]Supplies $100/case, 1,000 cases/year (Table IV).
[e]Assumes 1,000 cases/year.
[f]Assumes 2,000 cases/year.

digital equipment were added to a conventional angiographic suite, the typical capital expenditure for rooms of this type will usually be in excess of $700,000. (See chapter by Evens.) From Figure 1, one can interpolate that, on the assumption of 8 cases performed in a single day, a savings of perhaps $75 a case would result from the use of a digitally equipped fluoroscopic room rather than a digitally equipped angiographic suite. This is based upon the effect of difference in financing alone. These fixed costs may very well change with the effects of "economics of scale". As our clinical experience is expanded, we may decide more, or even fewer, peripheral injections are appropriate. It may even develop that physicians will become convinced that technical personnel may monitor the injection procedure. From discussions in this text, it will become apparent that this

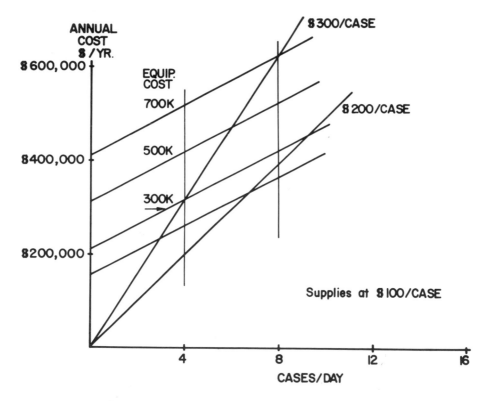

FIGURE 1. *Estimated arrival cost per year for a digital radiography system as a function of the number of patients examined per day. Cursors are plotted for initial equipment costs of $200K, $300K, $500, and $700K.*

decision has financial, legal, and health care implications. The practical aspects of the patient throughput are very important in determining the financial viability of any planned facility.

V. VARIABLE COST FOR OUTPATIENT OFFICE EXAM

Certain assumptions will be utilized here as if they were sacrosanct but it is recognized that these are subject to change. It is common practice at this time to perform digital subtraction angiography following the placement of an intravenous catheter in the superior vena cava or inferior vena cava. Table IV analyzes the supplies that are needed for such a central catheterization. In the office practice of the first author, these expenses approximate $100 per case; in some instances where difficulties with the catheterization are encountered, the cost can substantially exceed this figure. The actual cost saving potential of digital angiography can be much more easily achieved if peripheral injections are sufficient for purposes of contrast media delivery and patient safety. Several institutions, including the Cleveland Clinic as noted in the chapter by Meaney, routinely perform digital angiography following the placement of a short intracath in a vein in the antecubital fossa. Approximately a 50% reduction in variable costs could be realized if this technique proves to be satisfactory.

Anticipated improvements in contrast materials could provide the density needed, even with current technology, to deliver peripheral boluses with the same resulting contrast density in the artery. (See chapter by Sackett). This is an area of research being conducted by a number of institutions. One can anticipate that marked improvements will be made, especially in the use of non-ionic contrast media.

VI. COMPARISON WITH ANGIOGRAPHY BY ARTHERIAL CATHETERIZATION

In comparing digital radiography with arteriography, consideration must be given not only to the cost factors involved but also to risks of complication and the potential biological burden. The risks and implications from radiation are discussed elsewhere in this chapter and text. The cost factors are certainly related to other tests and treatment associated with the disease process. Arteriography generally requires hospitalization and the attendant "routine" laboratory tests. The hospitalization might include surgery or the treatment of a secondary diagnosis. In the circumstance in which no operation is required and the patient is to only have the diagnostic procedure, a more direct comparison can be made with digital intravenous angiography, which normally will not require the hospitalization. Thus, we would hope that in this text a comparison can be made based on costs of the implication from the procedures alone.

The Association of American Medical Colleges reports data from 24 teaching hospitals showing an average length of stay of 6.45 days with an average total charge of $1678 for diagnostic evaluation of symptoms of transient cerebral ischemia (1). This cost is calculated without surgery and absence of a significant secondary diagnosis. This might be compared to a $500 charge for digital angiography which would result in a saving of over $1100.

The relative costs can also be compared for the case of inpatient studies for both conventional and digital angiography. The costs of supplies for a bilateral carotid/cerebral arteriography are shown in Table IV-B. These costs are similar to those in Table IV-A, except for additional catheters, guide wires, and a very large increase in film utilization. The costs of the conventional angiography are detailed in Table IV-C and show a total cost of $1000 (excluding overnight hospitalization), which can be compared to the $500 cost for digital angiography. In this case, the savings in the outpatient population for each study might be as high as $700 per procedure. Further savings for carotid/cerebral angiography now done on an inpatient basis would increase by approximately $300/day. Regardless of whichever comparison one makes, the savings are significant; the financial implications are yet to be specifically determined.

VII. THE PARAMETERS OF JUSTIFICATION OF DIGITAL RADIOGRAPHY: "BREAK-EVEN ANALYSIS"

A more useful manner to approach certain aspects of this data may be to consider it graphically by means of a technique known as a break-even analysis (2,3). In this part of the communication, the previous assumptions will be utilized to evaluate the financial implications of digital radiography.

Figure 2 plots the fixed costs of $230,000 per year, to which the variable cost of $100 per case is added. Therefore, at 8 cases per day, the total annual cost for a 250-day year

will approach some $430,000. In order to determine the
break-even analysis, divide the total of $430,000 by 2,000
cases per year. In so doing, it is determined that $215 per
case would have to be charged in order to provide adequate
funds for fixed and variable expenses. Note that this assumes
100% payment for all the cases performed. Realistically,
receipts are more likely to be approximately 85-90% of billing
charges. These revenue shortfalls are a result of bad debt
and the acceptance of assignment. Therefore, by accounting
for these constraints, one would probably have to charge $250
per case in order to "break even".

Figure 1, again, is a more general illustration of the
break-even analysis; various equipment costs are considered.
The variables result in a family of parallel sloping lines in
which the variable costs (the slope) is the same but the fixed
costs vary as a result of the value assigned to the equipment
used in each hypothetical circumstance. This graph

TABLE IV-A. Digital Angiography Supplies

Items	Cost
1. *Syringes - Power Injector*	$ 8.50
2. *Floppy Disc*	10.00
3. *Poly-Line Towels*	.25
4. *Sterile Gown*	4.15
5. *Sterile Sheet*	2.24
6. *Absorbent Towel*	1.62
7. *Sterile Gloves*	2.35
8. *Contrast - 200cc*	19.12
9. *IV Admin. Set*	1.90
10. *Catheter*	11.50
11. *Vessel Dilator*	2.99
12. *Guide Wire*	9.19
13. *Connector*	2.00
14. *Jelco Needle*	3.16
15. *Steri-Drape*	2.16
16. *IV Solution*	7.53
17. *Syringes*	.48
18. *Scalpel*	.34
19. *Needle*	.79
20. *Local Anesthetic*	.70
21. *Film*	2.88
TOTAL	$93.85

TABLE IV-B.   *Arteriographic Supplies*

Items	Cost
1. Syringes - Power Injector	$ 8.50
2. Floppy Disc	10.00
3. Poly-Line Towels	.25
4. Sterile Gown	4.15
5. Sterile Sheet	2.24
6. Absorbent Towel	1.62
7. Sterile Gloves	2.35
8. Contrast - 200cc	19.12
9. IV Admin. Set	1.90
10. Catheters (2)	23.00
11. Vessel Dilator	2.99
12. Guide Wires (2)	18.38
13. Connector	2.00
14. Jelco Needle	3.16
15. Steri-Drape	2.16
16. IV Solution	7.53
17. Syringes	.48
18. Scalpel	.34
19. Needle	.79
20. Local Anesthetic	.70
21. Film [92 (14x14) @ 1.62 ea]	149.04
TOTAL	$260.70

encompasses the most likely range of equipment costs and patient charges. For example, if one were to evaluate a room whose equipment cost was $500,000, in which one expected a case load of 6 patients per day, then one would have to be compensated approximately $300 per case plus professional fees and bad debt for a total of $500/case (Table V). The reader will note that this calculation assumes 100% utilization of the room for digital radiography, which will not always be the case. However, the graph could also be used for rooms which will have a mixed patient load and more than a single function. For example, if a $500,000 room is only used 60% of the time for digital angiographic studies, then one should assign a value of $300,000 ($500,000 x 60%) with a resulting value for this purpose. Only 4 digital cases would be required at $300 per case for a break-even point of 60% utilization; the remaining 40% utilization would be expected

TABLE IV-C.   *Typical Costs of Carotid*
              Arteriographic Procedure

Time required: 2 to 2-1/2 hours

Salaries/fringes
(2 Techs for 2-1/2 hrs at $9.00/hr) $ 45.00

Supplies (Table IV-B)   260.70

Equipment
(Assume $450,000 - 5 yr basis
 annual costs - Table II = $199,500
 8 hr/day - 2080 hrs/yr or $95.91/hr.)   239.78
                                             545.48

Overhead
(Assume 25% admin. costs, rent, etc.)   136.37

Professional fee
(Assume $100/hr -
 3 hrs to complete report)   300.00
                                            $981.85

With a slight change in overhead or
professional fee, the cost approximates $1000.

---

to pay for itself on a similar analysis by performing other cases employing the space, personnel and equipment.

The costs of performing digital intravenous angiography have been explored in order to further evaluate this concept. This was chosen because substantial reductions in the cost of health care and savings of general resources can be achieved by utilizing this procedure rather than its alternatives. If for example, one were to consider the carotid angiogram, which will be the example used for the remainder of this communication, the charge for this radiographic study is at least in the $1,000 to $5,000 range. The relatively high cost of this procedure is due in part from the requirement that a carotid angiogram be performed as an inpatient hospital procedure necessitating several days hospitalization. The patient most often arrives for admission the day before the study and is discharged the day after the completion of the study. This hospitalization is required to properly monitor several aspects of this procedure, including the site of

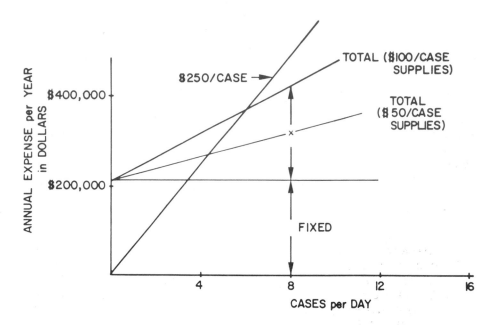

FIGURE 2. Plot of fixed costs of $230,000 per year to which variable costs are added.

puncture and catheterization through the arterial wall. The hazards of this type of procedure are eliminated in digital angiography since the catheter and contrast media are introduced on the venous side rather than the arterial. The

TABLE V. Proposed Charges - Digital Angiography

Hospital Charges[a]	*$300*
Professional Charges	*150*
(Surgical Fee	
& Interpretive Fee)	
	$450
Bad Debt (10% Approx.)	*50*
	$500

[a]*6 cases/day*
$500,000 equipment cost

lower pressures in the venous side do not require the same post-procedure monitoring. The change of monitoring, allowing one to perform the study as an outpatient, results in a $750–$900 savings by allowing one to perform the study as an outpatient. Moreover, the low patient risk associated with digital angiography now makes it possible to perform these studies not only more expeditiously on an inpatient basis but on an out-hospital basis. The first author has been performing outpatient digital angiography in a private office for the past 12 months, and the total charge for carotid angiography is approximately one-third the charge for carotid arteriography in the community hospitals in the geographic area.

VIII. REIMBURSEMENT

Medicare's position on reimbursement for the digital radiographic procedure has not been entirely clarified. This appears to be a quite reasonable circumstance in that our experience with this technology is in its infancy and is continually evolving. Some prognostication might be derived from a quote in Medical World News (4) in which Rowan of the Health Care Financing Administration (HICFA) states that Medicare will be reimbursed for these procedures but does not indicate the level of reimbursement. In Connecticut, where the the first author practices, the local Medicare representatives have not received instructions. Blue Cross/ Blue Shield, of course, operates on a more regional or local basis. As with computed tomography, which carried no Blue Shield obligation to its contracted subscribers, the Blue Shield fee schedule in Connecticut provides for significant professional benefit coverage for angiography of the various vessels (Table VI). Without significant modification of the coding of the fee schedule or change in total reimbursement, digital radiography might be substituted in place of conventional angiography. Refinement of existing fee schedules should ideally be undertaken on a local basis. This symposium has demonstrated that practices are quite varied and the cost and reimbursement implications quite profound.

IX. CERTAIN CLINICAL APPLICATIONS OF DIGITAL ANGIOGRAPHY

The major considerations of this text have been the basic science principles of the digital radiography process.

TABLE VI. *Fee Schedule for Blue Cross/Blue Shield in a Selected State*

Diagnostic Vascular Procedures

Aortography		
Abdominal, thoracic, terminal...............	*161*	*185*
Arteriography		
Renal, celiac, mesenteric, thoracic		
or any single *artery*....................	*159*	*188*
Combination of any two *studies or a*		
bilateral study........................	*242*	*260*
Combination of any three or more *studies*.....	*274*	*323*
Femoral, unilateral.........................	*117*	*132*
bilateral.........................	*217*	*217*
with terminal aortogram............	*190*	*206*
Aorto-iliac...................................	*120*	*142*
Splenoportogram..............................	*124*	*136*
Non-selective coronary.......................	*255*	*301*
Non-selective pulmonary......................	*178*	*196*
Angiocardiogram (Ventriculogram), unilateral.	*198*	*218*
bilateral..	*205*	*226*
Pulmonary angiogram, unilateral..............	*207*	*219*
bilateral..............	*207*	*244*
Selective bilateral carotid and vertebral		
(4 vessels)......	*308*	*363*
Selective bilateral carotid (2 vessels)......	*240*	*274*
Selective carotid and *vertebral (2 vessels)*..	*260*	*284*
Selective carotid or *vertebral (1 vessel)*....	*175*	*207*
Transfemoral selective catheterization,		
one vessel......	*231*	*273*
two vessels......	*296*	*318*
three vessels......	*396*	*398*
Arterial clot removal during catheter study..	*25*	*27.50*
subsequent to catheter study..............	*50*	*55*

However, clinical experience has been presented in detail. From the preliminary experience, it is clear that significant beneficial applications can be found in the visualization of the carotid vessels, the abdominal aorta, and renal artery evaluation, as well as digital studies of the peripheral vasculature. Probably future applications of this technology will be evaluation of cardiac performance, coronary bypass graft analysis, and, possibly, detailed studies of intracranial vessels. As a model for the application of this technology, the following discussion deals with an analysis of carotid digital radiography following the methods and techniques suggested by Detmer (5). The protocols chosen evaluate three levels of confidence as the outcome of digital radiography. In protocol 1, patients received conventional carotid arteriography only. In protocol 2, they are studied with digital angiography. Arteriography is performed only if the digital radiographic study is positive. In protocol 3, 50% of the positive digital studies require further arteriography prior to operation or decision. In protocol 4, it is assumed that only 5% of the positive digitial studies require arteriography prior to surgical intervention or decision. The remainder of the calculations are based upon these principles.

Table VII uses these four protocols in an analysis of a patient representing approximately 300,000 people and two major hospitals containing approximately 1200 acute beds. The 1977 cooperative study of transient ischemic attacks (TIA's) reported an average of 5.4 patients with definite diagnoses of this disorder per 100 acute beds at the participating hospitals (6). The highest reported patient diversity was 8.8 TIA's per 100 acute beds. This table assumes 8.5 exams per 100 beds and the calculations based upon that assumption result in an expected 100 angiograms per year. In protocol 1, assuming an average hospital charge for carotid angiography of $1,200 per case, this would result in an average per-lesion cost of $1,500, if 80% of the patients studied were abnormal. In protocol 2, the patients were initially studied by digital angiography at $420 per study and then the 80 positive cases were hospitalized to be studied with conventional arteriography; the total cost increased, averaging $1,720 per lesion. However, if only 50% of the positive cases were restudied with arteriography, as in protocol 3, the cost would be decreased to $1,120 per lesion. In protocol 4, in which 10% of the cases were positive studies, the cost per lesion was only $690. In this high risk group, an 80% yield for the studies has been assumed. It is likely that the low risk of digital angiography will increase the number of patients studied by this procedure. Presumably, the yield rate in this new population would then be reduced. Thus, Table VIII adds to the first population of 100 patients per year with a yield of 80%, a second population of 100 patients per year whose yield rate is assumed to be 40%.

In an analysis of protocol 3, it can be determined that twice as many patients (200) could be studied by digital radiography at a cost per lesion which is less than the cost

TABLE VII. Analysis of Four Protocols[a]

Protocol	# Angio[b]	# Digital	# Lesions	$ Billed[c]	$/Lesion	Approximate Rem/Lesion	Increased Risk # Complications
1	100	0	80	$120,000	$1,500	26	0.5
2 (100%)	80	100	80	138,000	1,720	22	0.4
3 (50%)	40	100	80	90,000	1,120	12	0.2
4 (10%)	8	100	80	55,000	690	2	0.04

[a]These analyses presume the accuracy of IVA to approximately that of arteriography for both stenotic and ulcerative lesions.
[b]Assuming population selection: 8.5 exams/100 beds @ yield = 80% (4).
[c]Assumes angiography @ $1,200/case and digital @ $420/case.

TABLE VIII. Analysis of Four Protocols[a]

Protocol	# Angio[b]	# Digital	# Lesions	$ Billed	$/Lesion	Approximate Rem/Lesion	Increased Risk # Complications
1	NOT APPLICABLE						
2 (100%)	120	200	120	$228,000	$1,900	22	0.6
3 (50%)	60	200	120	156,000	1,300	17	0.3
4 (10%)	12	200	120	96,000	800	2	0.06

[a]These analyses presume the accuracy of IVA to approximately that of arteriography for both stenotic and ulcerative lesions.
[b]Assuming initial population: 8.5 exams/100 beds @ yield = 80%
Plus new population: 8.5 exams/100 beds @ yield = 40%

which would result if 100 patients were studied by conventional arteriography. Moreover, if the accuracy of digital radiography approaches that of conventional arteriography and only 10% of the patients require conventional arteriography, then twice as many patients could be studied, at half the cost when compared to conventional arteriography.

Aside from the financial implications, digital radiography promises to reduce the radiation burden and the risk of complication to patients. Detmer, et al. estimate that the average arteriogram requires approximately 20 rem per exposure, whereas the average digital angiogram examination will require about 3.6 rem. Furthermore, the risk from the interventional nature of the procedure will be lower with digital radiography. While both procedures have the attendant risk associated with contrast media injection and reaction, the arteriogram carries further risk due to bleeding, clot formation, and thrombus propagation during and subsequent to the study. These conventional arteriographic procedures are assumed to have a 0.5 risk of permanent complications, as suggested by the literature (7).

The introduction of digital technology to a modern, high quality image-intensification fluoroscopic room will provide substantial improvements in the field of vascular and other forms of imaging. The procedure is extremely cost-effective. It has the potential of providing comparable data to conventional arteriography for approximately one-third the cost. The overall savings for the entire health care system are difficult to determine since the low risk nature of the procedure will result in the relaxation of the indications for the procedure and possibly result in many more studies. Based on this analysis, the introduction of digital radiography should have impact on the patterns of practice as well as the monetary cost-effectiveness of screening for surgical lesions. It may appear that twice as many people will benefit from the money expended.

The implications for complications as well as the biological burden appear favorable for this technology. Data acquisition, storage, retrieval, and transmission will be significantly changed by the process. The financial implications of these effects of the digital process have not been emphasized in this communication but we predict they will be significant. Digital radiographic techniques appear to represent a significant advance from a number of aspects, only several of which have been the subject of this chapter.

In Table IX are listed the major suppliers of digital radiography systems at this time. This, understandably, represents data which is sure to be obsolete almost

TABLE IX. Current Commercial Systems of Digital Radiography

Company	Digital fluoroscopy systems	Comments
ADAC Laboratories	DPS-4100 Digital Fluoroscopy Unit	Add-on to existing image intensifier. General purpose system operating in both pulsed and continuous mode.
American Edwards Laboratories (American Hospital Supply)	CarDIAC-1000 (Utilizes a Quantex Image Processor)	Add-on system designed primarily for cardiac application and operates in continuous mode.
CGR Compagnie General de Radiologies	DIVAS (Based on Univ. of Arizona System)	Add-on or complete system. General purpose pulsed or continuous system.
Diasonics Corporation	DF-100	Add-on general purpose system.
Fisher Imaging Corporation	ARIEL-9 and VANTAGE 12 (ADAC Image Processor)	Complete general purpose system. C or U arm configuration.
General Electric Corporation	Digital Fluoricon 3000	General purpose system.
Instrumentation Camera Inc.	ICI-CAMTEK 1000	Add-on general purpose unit.

TABLE IX. *Current Commercial Systems of Digital Radiography (continued)*

Company	Digital fluoroscopy systems	Comments
Machlett Laboratories	DI-2200 (ADAC Image Processor)	Add-on general purpose unit.
Medical Data Systems	Spectra System	Add-on general purpose unit. Based on MDS nuclear medicine computer system.
Philips Corporation	DVI (Digital Vascular Imaging System) (Based on Univ. of Wisconsin System)	Add-on or complete system. Operates in continuous fluoroscopy mode.
Picker Corporation	DAS-211 (ADAC Image Processor)	Add-on general purpose system.
Quantex Corporation	DS-20, -30, and -50	Add-on. Operates in continuous fluoroscopy mode.
Siemens Corporation	Digitron and Angiotron	Digitron--Digital general purpose add-on. Angiotron--Special purpose vascular system.

TABLE IX. *Current Commercial Systems of Digital Radiography (continued)*

Company	Digital fluoroscopy systems	Comments
Xonics Corporation	XIDIS	Add-on or complete general purpose system
	Special Area Detectors	
Kontron Corporation	ZIKON-100	No image intensifier system. Uses luminescent screen viewed by video camera. Add-on.
Fuji Corporation	Imaging plate with heavy metal halite salts	Not a real-time system. Plate is digitizing and stored for post-processing.
Interchange Manufacturing Corporation	Digitized Plain Films	Add-on to existing systems by digitizing films and post-processing.

TABLE IX. Current Commercial Systems of Digital Radiography (continued)

Company	Digital fluoroscopy systems	Comments
	Scan Projection Radiography	
AS & E American Science and Engineering Corporation	Micro-dose	Flying spot scanner for low dose radiography. Complete system.
Picker Corporation	Line-scanned chest unit	Vertical scanned array of detectors for low dose chest radiography.
General Electric Corporation	CT/T 8800 – Based System (Based on work of Stanford Univ.)	Dual energy subtraction system.

immediately; nevertheless, these data may be of some assistance to those who are considering the purchase of a digital system.

REFERENCES

1. Bentley, J.D., Butler, P.O., A technical report - DRG case mix of a sampling of teaching hospitals, Association of American Medical Colleges Report (December, 1981).
2. Freedman, G.S., CT: A financial and legislative reappraisal, Applied Radiology (November/December, 1978).
3. Evens, R.G., Jost, R.G., Economic analysis of body computed tomography units incluing data on utilization, Radiology 127 (1978).
4. Rowan, C., Low risk angiography. Medical World News, pp. 50-52 (August 7, 1981)
5. Detmer, D.E, Fryback, D.G., Strother, C.M., Preliminary cost-effectiveness analysis of intravenous video arteriography for screening of transient ischemic attacks, in "Digital Video Arteriography" (C.A. Mistretta, A.B. Crummy, D.M. Strother, J.F. Sackett, eds.), Yearbook Medical Publishers, Chicago.
6. Swanson, P.D., Calanchini, P.R., Dyken, M.L., et al., A cooperative study of hospital frequency and character of transient ischemic attacks. II. Performance of angiography among six centers, JAMA 237, 2202-2206 (1977).
7. Eisenberg, R.L., Cerebral angiography: Conflicting testimony, AJR 134, 615-617 (1980).

7

ECONOMIC EVALUATION OF A DIGITAL ANGIOGRAPHY UNIT IN 1982

Ronald G. Evens

Department of Radiology
Washington University School of Medicine
St. Louis, Missouri
and
Mallinckrodt Institute of Radiology
St. Louis, Missouri

Diagnostic radiology has always been a specialty with relatively high costs due to its dependence upon sophisticated equipment, highly trained personnel, and large space allocations. Economic considerations are increasingly important with the recent trend in the use of higher cost equipment (angiography, computed tomography, nuclear cardiology, and digital applications). The last several years have also been a time of increasing awareness of medical costs by the public--including patients, politicians, third-party payors and physicians. The introduction of new medical technology is only one of many factors increasing the cost of medical care; others of more importance include access to care, inflation, the aging population, and medical payment policies (1,2).

Digital imaging units will undoubtedly have impact on diagnostic radiology (the subject of this text), and an evaluation of its economic impact includes consideration of expenses, associated charges to patients, and its relationship to a department or hospital budget.

I. FINANCIAL DATA ON DIGITAL ANGIOGRAPHY IN 1982

Table I presents data on projected expenses required to operate a digital radiographic unit, primarily for vascular studies, at the Mallinckrodt Institute of Radiology in St. Louis. It is important to note that these expenses include both technical and professional costs, which are separated in many institutions between the hospital and radiology group. The largest single category is salaries for 1.5 technologists, 1.5 nurses, 1 technologist aide, 0.5 electronic engineer, and 1 full-time equivalent radiologist. While salary levels vary among institutions and geographic regions, they are in a medial position in St. Louis and should approximate the salaries for similar personnel through the United States.

The second largest single expense is depreciation of equipment. The digital unit in current operation at the Institute is a single plane C-arm angiographic room with 525 line, high resolution TV-image intensifier and a 3-phase generator. The cost of this room is $700,000 and its adaptation for digital vascular studies is an additional $250,000, for a total of $950,000. This capital expense is depreciated over a 5-year period by a straight-line method. Please note that no debt was required by lease or borrowing and equipment expense would be higher if financing was necessary. Equipment maintenance has been calculated at 6% of the original purchase price, a relatively common figure for most manufacturers. An alternative purchasing formula is contained in the chapter by Freedman, Stephens, and James.

TABLE I. Annual Expenses of Digital Angiography - 1982

Direct Expenses	
Salaries[a]	*$ 224,650*
Equipment Maintenance	*57,000*
Supplies[b]	*102,000*
Total Direct	*$ 383,650*
Indirect Expenses	
Depreciation[c]	*$ 190,000*
Overhead[d]	*191,825*
Total Indirect	*$ 381,825*
Total Annual Expenses	*$ 765,475*

[a]Salaries = 1.5 technologists, 1.5 nurses, 1 aide, 0.5 engineer, 1 radiologist.
[b]Supplies = about $68/procedure, assume 1,500 procedures/yr.
[c]$950,000 for unit; depreciated by SLM/5 yrs.
[d]Overhead is 50% of direct expenses.

Supplies include contrast material, venous catheters, angiographic tray, sterile drapes, floppy disks, x-ray film, computer tape, etc. These costs currently approximate $68 per procedure in our institution.

Overhead is calculated at 50% of direct costs, a conservative estimate in most radiology departments and in the Mallinckrodt Institute. While this may seem high, overhead rates of 50%-100% of direct costs are common in business activities that are "service" in nature (e.g., other health care activities, architectural firms, and attorneys). Overhead costs include a variety of expenses that are necessary to diagnostic radiology but cannot be directly accounted to a particular procedure or radiologic room. Overhead must provide for the expenses related to administration, space and space maintenance, security, parking, accounting services, personnel office, educational activities (including house staff and continuing education), and the fringe benefits of staff. Necessary services of transcription and record keeping, billing and accounting, and insurance are also included in the overhead expense.

We estimate that 1,500 digital angiographic procedures will be performed in 1982 and the "bottom line" in Table I projects that our total annual expenses will be $765,475.

II. REVENUE ANALYSIS OF DIGITAL ANGIOGRAPHY

A financially viable diagnostic procedure should generate a profit (in order to provide capital for cash flow, future equipment and development) or at least "break-even". To break-even, net income must equal total expenses. A break-even point analysis of the Mallinckrodt digital angiography unit in 1982 is shown in Table II. In order to cover expenses with 1,500 procedures per year, the average charge per procedure should be approximately $655. This charge will provide gross revenues of $992,500; but since the Institute only receives a net revenue of 78% of gross billings (our total revenue deduction is 22% due to third-party allowances, partial pay/bad debt, and charity), the net revenues will be $766,250 or a net annual income of $875—essentially a break-even position.

TABLE II. Break-Even-Point Analysis - Digital Angiography

Total Expenses	*$ 765,475*
Revenue:	
Procedures	*1,500*
Average charge/procedure	*655*
Gross revenue	*982,500*
Revenue deduction[a]	*216,150*
Net revenue	*766,350*
Net Income	*$ 875*

[a]*Revenue deduction of 22% for third-party allowances, partial pay/bad debt, charity.*

III. THE IMPORTANCE OF PATIENT VOLUME

Most radiology expenses are fixed (expenses do not change with changes in volume) because of our dependence on equipment, space, and personnel (3). This important accounting distinction is the case for digital angiography, where approximately 85% of the costs are fixed. Where most of the costs are unrelated to procedure activity, the charge required to break-even is highly dependent on patient procedure volume estimates, as shown for digital vascular procedures in Table III. At the Mallinckrodt Institute the charge to break-even would vary between $936 per procedure at 1,000 procedure per year to $370 at 3,000 procedures per year. There are approximately 250 standard working days each year (we have found it difficult to perform scheduled procedures on Christmas or New Year's Day) so 1,000 patient procedures annually is four per day and 3,000 per year is twelve per day.

IV. POSSIBLE ECONOMIC ALTERATIONS

Revenue to a radiology department is based on three factors—charge, volume, and the amount of revenue deductions. The charge of digital vascular procedures should be based on an individual department's analysis of ecomomic factors (similar to this chapter) and modified by billing factors in the local geographic area. Revenue deductions can be improved by sophisticated billing methods and will probably be similar to other radiologic procedures in a given institution.

TABLE III. Volume Effect on Digital Angiography

Procedures/year				
1,000	1,500	2,000	2,500	3,000
Expenses[a]				
$731,475	$765,475	$799,475	$833,475	$867,475
Break-even-point charge[b]				
$936	$655	$512	$428	$370

[a] $68 variable expense/exam
[b] 22% revenue deduction

A careful projection of patient volume will be the single most important consideration regarding patient revenues in most departments and is the major theme of this chapter. Volume is influenced by what the facility can do (this is projected to be approximately 1 patient per hour) and what our clinical colleagues believe should be done. The limiting factor in many institutions will be the number of procedures requested, not what the facility can perform.

Expenses can be reduced in any of the categories of Table I. Fewer individuals or less qualified personnel, adaptation of currently available angiographic or fluoroscopic equipment for digital instead of new angiographic facilities and multiple possibilites for reducing overhead can be considered (4). It is unlikely that significant reductions in equipment maintenance, supplies, or the cost of digital adaptation will be possible. Reduction of expenses in any of these catagories is possible but not easy, particularly in the radiology department that has evaluated costs recently. When considering expense reductions, the quality of the final product (in this case a satisfactory diagnosis) must be protected. Several factors related to the quality of a digital vascular procedure (frame rate, number of television lines, image intensifier resolution, digital versus analog storage, software capabilities) are under evaluation and certainly will be discussed further in this text. While costs and quality may not be directly related, they are related.

The reader is cautioned about reducing the expenses of overhead or its allocation to a new digital vascular procedure. Overhead expenses are necessary for the successful performance of any diagnostic radiology examination. Since digital vascular studies are highly likely to replace current diagnostic examinations, overhead expenses for the radiology department must be recovered by newly established procedures.

V. CONCLUSION

A digital angiographic diagnostic radiology facility will have relatively large expenses that will total between $700,000-$900,000 annually in 1982. These expenses are not new or unique to diagnostic radiology and relate to the current cost of professional staff, space, equipment, and overhead. Procedure volumes will be important to establish a break-even charge that will vary between $370-$950 per patient procedure when 4-12 procedures are performed in a standard workday. The appropriate charge for economic viability will be similar to current special procedure charges and considerably higher than current standard radiographic or fluoroscopic charges.

REFERENCES

1. Moloney, T.W., and Rogers, D.E., Medical Technology--A different view of the contentious debate over cost, N. Engl. J. Med. 301, 1413-1419 (1979).
2. Evens, R.G., The economics of computed tomography: comparison with other health care costs, Radiology 136, 509-510 (1980).
3. Evens, R.G., Cost accounting in radiology and nuclear medicine, CRC Crit. Rev. Clin. Radiol. Nucl. Med. 6, 67-79 (1975).
4. Evens, R.G., Economic implications of a new technology installation, A CT model, AJR 136, 673-677 (1981).

8

CERTAIN LEGAL CONSIDERATIONS OF DIGITAL RADIOLOGICAL IMAGING

A. Everette James, Jr.[1]
C. Leon Partain[1]
Henry P. Pendergrass[1]

with the assistance of

James Blumstein[2]
Alan C. Winfield[1]
Donald Hall[2]
Thomas Sherrard[2]
F. David Rollo[1]
Ronald R. Price[1]
John C. Chapman[3]

[1]Department of Medical Imaging and Radiological Sciences
Vanderbilt University School of Medicine
Nashville, Tennessee

[2]Vanderbilt University School of Law

[3]Office of the Dean
Vanderbilt University School of Medicine

The application of biomedical techniques developed in physics, engineering and computer sciences has been the subject of this digital radiography symposium. This chapter will discuss certain principles of agency and evidence law and how these might be applied to digital radiography. The resources necessary to acquire these digital imaging devices, and the accompanying information transmission technology and new methods of archiving this digital data, are of such magnitude, public policies will be enacted to assure both public access to and protection from inappropriate acquisition and distribution of this technology. This technology will consider the combined effects of these legal principles in relation to medical imaging, with special emphasis upon the digital process.

I. <u>AGENCY LAW APPLICATION</u>

An agency relationship exists in order to enable health care deliverers to utilize the services of others and thus to accomplish what they could not achieve alone. Today, many aspects of the practice of medical imaging, as well as many forms of complex enterprises and professional activities, are conducted by agents (1,2). Because of the widespread use of agents, courts have formulated rules dealing with the agency relationships and their impact upon third parties of all types.

The law of agency has traditionally been the province of the courts rather than legislatures (3). As a result, agency law has not achieved the same degree of uniformity as many other legal areas. The inconsistent use of terms and varied concepts considered by the courts in dealing with agency problems has led to confusion about this subject. Certain general propositions may be stated which can offer substantial guidance, however.

This discussion will initially emphasize the issues of agency relationship creation and the principal's liability for the misconduct of the agent. An agency relationship involves at least two parties (3,4) usually referred to as principal and agent in situations where the issue is contractual in nature, that is, the agent enters into a contract on behalf of the principal. In an act of tort or omission when the agent injures another while acting on behalf of the principal, this is referred to as "master and servant" or, more recently, "employer and employee" (4).

The use of these terms by the courts has significance. They embody legal conclusions regarding the relationship between parties. The terms employer and employee, while encompassing the traditional view of the employment relationship, may include other persons who are not commonly viewed as employees but who meet the legal definition of the term (3). In the use of this technology discussed, such as digital storage, transmission, and retrieval, even machines and devices may operationally be considered "agents".

An agency relationship exists when parties consent to enter into a relationship whereby one party acts under the control for the benefit of the controlling party who may be termed the principal, master or employer. The party controlled is referred to as the agent, servant or employee.

Agency is in this instance a consensual rather than a contractual relationship (4).

If consent is deemed present, an agency relationship is one in which a party must be acting on behalf of the other party. This arrangement is often designated in terms of benefit, that is, the agent's actions operate to benefit the principal (4). This benefit element will be difficult to locate or identify and will cause interpretive questions when dealing with such complex technology as digital radiography, especially regarding information acquisition, storage, retrieval and transfer.

In an agency relationship, there must exist a potential for control of the principal over the agent. This requirement is not that of absolute physical control over all the acts performed by the agent, nor does it imply that the agent must constantly look to the principal for direction. Instead, it means that the principal must potentially have a general power to control the agent's actions. The courts phrase it as "a right to control" (3). Thus, because a radiologist in charge of the procedure has the administrative control to order a technologist, computer programmer, or physicist to discontinue an activity or to alter a certain procedure during digital radiography, the right to control may be said to exist even though the physician may not be present when nonphysicians are performing their duties.

Because an agency relationship can be found to exist when there is consent, benefit and control, parties during any phase of the digital radiography process may create an agency relationship without realizing they have done so. As a practical matter, agency relationships are created constantly, and the law is clear that the intent of the parties specifically in relation to agency is not relevant in determining whether or not one exists. In an informal manner and without formal disclosure, agency relationships may be created. This is very likely in large departments of imaging during complex imaging procedures requiring a team such as digital radiography.

An unwitting agency relationship can also occur when an agent creates a sub-agency. For example, a technologist or computer scientist, acting clearly as an agent for the medical imaging physician, may, during a digital radiography procedure request an assistant or attendant to perform certain actions which ultimately are for the benefit of the radiologist. This act on the part of the technologist or computer scientist may constitute the creation of a sub-agency although the physician has not interacted directly with the sub-agent. The only requirement is that a sub-agency be implicitly or expressly authorized by the physician or scientist or that it be reasonably foreseeable that a sub-agency may be necessary in order to carry out the request mandated for the procedure. In the event a court finds a sub-agency to exist, the principal may be held responsible for the actions of the sub-agent (4).

It is often not difficult to find an unwitting agency relationship between physicians, especially in more traditional roles. An example that might apply to certain digital procedures is the case of Rockwell vs. Kaplan, 404 Pa. 574, 173 A2d 54 (1961). The plaintiff submitted to surgery for removal by Kaplan of a bursa from his right elbow. The anesthesiologist selected by Dr. Kaplan, who was chief of Anesthesiology, administered anesthesia by injection to Mr. Rockwell's left arm in such a manner as to obstruct blood flow to the extremity. The surgeon did not discover the error until the arm had been so damaged that amputation was required. The considerations in this text regarding intracath injections into the peripheral vein versus superior vena cava may have parallels to this case.

In the Rockwell vs. Kaplan litigation, the issue involved only the extent of the surgeon's liability. The court found that Dr. Kaplan had not been negligent but that the anesthesiologist had. The court, however, held that the anesthesiologist had been acting, during the course of the operation, as the "employee" or agent of the surgeon. Thus, Dr. Kaplan was held liable for the error of his "employee". One could imagine a similar series of circumstances in an image manipulation experiment or during a digital radiology examination.

In the case described above, the surgeon and anesthesiologist believed that they had not created an agency relationship but were acting as independent professionals. The court found the requisite elements of agency: consent, benefit, and the potential right to control. The court stated that the necessary right to control existed, although the surgeon would not ordinarily tell the anesthesiologist how to perfom the anesthetization, he could have discontinued the operation at any time. This control over the procedure during which the faulty injection was administered was held to be adequate evidence of control by the surgeon over the anesthesiologist. This decision, while not stating the universal rule, does indicate that some courts may be persuaded to find an agency relationship in complex medical circumstances, such as digital radiography exams, that they do not fully understand. This "master of the ship" logic for surgeons in operating theaters may also apply to specialists in medical imaging in digital angiography suites.

Once an agency relationship has been found to exist, the question then becomes to what extent and under what

circumstances the principal shall be held responsible for the
conduct of the agent. An agency relationship is said to exist
if there is the ability of the agent 1) to create contractual
rights in favor of the principal, and 2) to subject the
principal to personal liability. The significant question for
the physician is the power of the agent to make the principal
responsible for the acts or omissions of the agent. The law
generally refers to this as "respondeat superior" ("let the
master respond") or, in a phrase gaining wider acceptance,
"vicarious liability". Whatever the term employed, the law
contemplates that the principal shall be held liable
regardless of any personal fault on the part of the agent.

A doctrine of liability without fault is a significant
exception to general Anglo-American jurisprudence, which
generally tends to equate legal responsibility with fault.
Perhaps the primary reason to have liability without fault in
a agency circumstance is that the principal enjoys benefits
conferred upon him by the agent. The law has determined that,
in return for the privilege of employing agents, the principal
should be prepared to take responsibility for any harm
suffered by others as a result of the agent's actions (4).
The imposition of vicarious liability is not a promise or
inevitable consequence of an agency relationship. Many agency
relationships will permit the agent to bind the principal to a
contractual obligation, but by its arrangement will not
contain the elements necessary to create vicarious liability
for the agent's wrongful conduct. Assuming the existence of
an agency relationship, the first additional element that must
exist is the principal's right to control the details of the
agent's work. Would this mean specific knowledge of a
computer program for temporal subtraction edge enhancement?
If this right to control is found, the courts will term the
relationship to be one of "employer-employee" or
"master-servant".

Another element that affects the imposition of vicarious
liability is the determination that the employee's actionable
conduct took place "within the scope of employment". Both of
these factors must coexist before a court will find the
"employer" liable (4). In radiology, these are constantly
changing. Control for the purpose of finding an employment
relationship contemplates a different and stricter standard
than that necessary to find a mere agency. The right to
control must be more specific and more direct. The issue of
whether this right to control exists is an elusive one and
depends upon the facts and circumstances of the terms of the
employment relationship in each particular instance.

Courts have looked to certain factors which are outward
manifestations of a right to control the details of an

employee's activities. These factors may vary. The number of factors required before an employer–employee relationship can be found to exist is also rather unclear. They include: 1) The extent of control which, by agreement, the principal may exercise over the details of the agent's performance of duties. 2) Whether or not the employee is engaged in a distinct occupation or business. The relation to the general context of the digital process would be important. 3) The degree of skill required by the employee. This is a criteria very important for discussion of digital process. 4) Whether the employer supplies the technology, instrumentation, and specific working environment for the employee. In imaging departments, this factor is particularly germane. 5) The length of time for which the person is employed. 6) The method of payment, whether by time or by completion of a particular activity. 7) Whether or not the employer has the right to terminate the activity or to discharge the employee (3). Even though a court may find an agency relationship, and more than that, an employment relationship, an employer will not be held liable for the acts of employees unless it is also determined that employees caused the injury complained of while acting within the "scope of their employment".

Whether or not one is acting within the scope of this employment is also a question of fact and is perhaps as difficult to answer in a particular case as is the question of whether or not a right to control exists. As a general proposition, to be within the scope of employment, conduct by the employee must be of the same general nature as that authorized by the employer, or it must be incidental to, or a reasonable and foreseeable consequence of, the conduct authorized (4). As we extend the digital radiography process these circumstances will continue to grow.

Stated and "working" policies here may differ in medical imaging departments but it is generally the routine conduct of the department that is considered policy. An example is intravenous injection of contrast media for certain radiographic studies such as digital radiography. If it is the general conduct of the department to allow technologists or nurses to perform these injections, then it will be considered within the scope of their employment to do so, despite disclaimers to that effect in the formal instrument of their contract. It is important to note that the courts are willing to interpret scope of employment quite liberally, thus including a broad range of activities that arguably would fall outside the normal duties of an employee. The more complex the technology, the wider this interpretation.

In addition to vicarious liability for the wrongful acts of an employee, the formation of an agency relationship in

health care delivery may have other potential implications.
For example, if agents or employees become aware of certain
facts or, by virtue of their position, should be aware of
certain facts, that knowledge or notice may be imputed to the
person in charge. Liability may occur although the medical
imaging physician does not presumably have any reason to be
aware of the facts in question.

Agency law suggests that agents have a duty to disclose
relevant information acquired within the scope of their
employment to their employer (3). Thus, the disclosure by a
patient to a nurse, assistant, scientist, or technologist of
certain information important in making a diagnosis may be
imputed to the physician although the physician may never have
learned of that information from the nurse, the technician, or
the patient. As a result, an incorrect diagnosis may lead to
liability, since the physician would be on notice of the
information given to an employee. With the issue of contrast
media injections as discussed in the chapter by Sackett, this
becomes an important issue.

In departments as complex as those in medical imaging
today, the patient may have great difficulty distinguishing
the physician from the technological or nonphysician
professional staff. Disclosure of a significant medical fact
to any employee which should necessarily be transmitted to the
professional person in charge, can result in vicarious
liability. This obtains if it can be shown that the
assumption made by the patient was a reasonable and logical
one and that the employee should have been expected to
transmit the information to the physician because of the
nature of the employment relationship. An example that often
occurs is a clinical history of allergy to contrast media or
any other data suggesting a hypersensitivity state (5).

With the extension of health care delivery practices and
the formation of complex physician/scientist partnerships,
such as in digital radiography, the law of agency increases in
complexity. Generally, a medical partnership will be treated
by the courts just as any other business partnership.
Partnership law declares that each partner shall be held
responsible for the acts or omissions of the other partners.
Therefore, partners are mutual agents. If patients enter
medical imaging departments in which they may be seen by
different physicians who are part of that partnership, each
may be jointly and severally liable for the improper treatment
of patients by an employee of that partnership. Such
vicarious liability cannot be contracted away, although the
law does provide that any judgment against the partnership be
collected from the partnership assets first and subsequently
from the assets of the individual partners. Each partner has

a right of reimbursement from a partner whose wrongful conduct caused the injury, but this right will not be available if all the partners are blameless and the injury was due to the negligence of an employee (6).

When medical imaging physicians act as consultants, they will generally be considered to be "independent contractors". The finding of independent contractor status is the converse of finding an employment relationship. An independent contractor may, and, in most cases, will be, considered an agent. However, under agency law, by definition, independent contractors are not employees because they are not subject to a right to control over the details of work by the contracting party.

The court in Rockwell vs. Kaplan, however, found that the anesthesiologist was subject to a right of control by the surgeon and could be considered not an independent contractor, but an employee. This decision does not conform with the general rule for agency interpretations. There are cases where the injury to a patient can be attributed both to a primary care physician and to the medical imaging physician; both parties would be held jointly and severally liable. A third situation would occur where the primary care physician acts upon the performance and interpretation of study by the medical imaging physician. If such interpretation has been negligently made, thus causing harm to the patient, both physicians in such a situation will be held responsible. Under a Rockwell vs. Kaplan rationale, the primary care physician may also be held responsible, despite no fault on his own part. Where the Rockwell vs. Kaplan rationale is not recognized, the medical imaging physician would be deemed an independent contractor rather than an agent of the primary care physician. Therefore, the primary care physician would not be subjected to vicarious liability for any wrongful conduct by his colleague. Since the level of expertise would not be equal, it is generally held that the specialist in medical imaging is liable, as the physician ordering the study is in a secondary and dependent role. Early in new procedures such as digital angiography, this would be particulary important.

An area of concern to radiologists often arises in the consultative process when the conclusions of the consultant are at variance with those of his clinical colleague, who is primarily responsible for the patient's care. In complex circumstances, and with new imaging procedures, this variance may occur with regard to the most appropriate next study in a diagnostic evaluation. At times, the primary care physician can object to the recommendations of the consultant and continue to request an imaging study not recommended by the radiologist. Because consultants are independent physicians, they are at liberty to refuse to perform a study requested when their judgment so dictates.

The radiologist understandably could be held responsible for any damages to the patient due to a study not being performed. It is, therefore, a good practice to document the basis for refusal to perfom a certain study on a patient at the time such a refusal occurs (7). The professional obligation of the imaging consultant is to provide appropriate services to the patient. The legal obligation will be based upon the issue of causation—did the acts or omissions of the consultant or his employees cause the injury in question? The liability will be based upon the determination of the consultant's negligence in refusing the study. The most common decision, however, will be the choice of the imaging technology.

The law of agency is probably not one of primary professional interest to may scientists and physicians. However, with the increased demands upon the health care delivery system, it is inevitable that health care professionals will continue to depend upon large numbers of persons to perform many significant functions in the care of patients (8,9). Therefore, vicarious liability will continue to exist and grow, especially in conjunction with our expanding technology. Certain basic aspects must be appreciated. It is important to understand under what circumstances individuals will be acting as employees and in what situations one may have liability for their actions (8). Digital venous and arterial injection angiography are but the most prominent at present.

II. EVIDENCE

The digital radiography process and new forms of information acquisition, storage and display will make evidence law even more important. Evidence is anything which serves as a means to make facts clear to human understanding. The law of evidence is a set of rules which determines what may be shown to a "trier of fact". This law was originally decisional law but is becoming increasingly codified in statute and rules of court, such as in the recently enacted Federal Rules of evidence for United States courts. Medical images, as have been presented in this textbook, provide quite unique form of evidence both in format and display.

The first requisite for admissible evidence is that it be relevant to an issue in the trial. Evidence is determined to be relevant if its introduction would render some fact more probable. Evidence, however, is sometimes relevant only if certain other facts are also examined in the trial. Therefore, the fact or exhibit introduced, e.g., a digital study, may represent only one of many facts which may be required to substantiate a particular issue. With the images and archives discussed, the rules of evidence may prove difficult to apply in the usual manner.

Much of the evidence law reflects distrust of the reasoning powers of the jury. As an example, evidence is not admissible if it is more influential than seems reasonable. The judge determines when a jury can be trusted to understand the limitations of the evidence. Occasionally, evidence may be introduced which prompts the judge to warn against its limitations in his instructions to the jury. This sometimes applies to evidence which is highly technical, such as the complicated digital imaging studies discussed in this text.

The material used for illustration in medical malpractice trials must often be screened so that it will not be prejudicial or inflammatory. Photographs and other exhibits which tend to offend human senses are often ruled inadmissible as evidence because of the effect that they may have upon the jurors. Diagnostic images are not so likely to be understood by a lay jury, and are not usually objected to on this basis.

A form of evidence that is generally inadmissible is hearsay. This type of evidence (oral or written) is presented by someone other than the person who personally participated in the fact at issue. Hearsay evidence is not admissible as proof of fact in an assertion stated by a third person. One reason hearsay evidence is inadmissible is that it presents a belief held by someone who is not testifying and is thus not subject to cross-examination. This general principle is frequently violated in the evidentiary use of highly technical studies and tests, and there are numerous common law and statutory exemptions to hearsay evidence. With multiple and sequential viewing of images, what is direct and what is hearsay may be a very difficult determination. Storage of data on tapes, discs, and other forms of archiving is, predictably, going to change this process.

Hearsay evidence rules were originally based on the concept that there are peculiar dangers involved in perceiving, remembering, and recounting statements (written or oral) made by another person. Since the trier of fact has no direct way to determine the state of mind or the particular circumstances of the third person who actually was the creator of the evidence, "the philosophy of the optimum search for truth" is violated and the evidence is inadmissible.

Nonpermanent storage of images might well lead to problems in this area.

The hearsay rule is said to reflect the constitutional "confrontation" guarantee; the sixth and fourteenth amendments to the U.S. Constitution provide the right to confront accusers in federal and state criminal actions. The hearsay rule is concerned, in part, with insuring the fair presentation of evidence, which may diverge from what is deemed conducive to accuracy in fact finding. The hearsay rule encourages lawyers to search for more reliable bases of proving facts, and it may have beneficial effects on the long-term factual accuracy of the legal system. It will be interesting to see the evolution of decisions in this area.

One of the firmly established rules of evidence is that a lay witness is not permitted to give opinion regarding the existence or nonexistence of any fact involved in a legal proceeding. This opinion is the province of the judge or jury. The jurors initially form an opinion of the evidential facts, and from that, form other opinions regarding the ultimate facts. Determination of the existence or non-existence of all facts belongs to the jury. Witnesses furnish evidence and consequently present facts of which they have personal knowledge. The medical imaging physician most commonly appears in court as a witness providing opinion evidence; opinion evidence is only admissible when, in the judgment of the court, the opinion expressed will assist the jury in the search for truth.

A number of procedural rules of proper expert testimony are unfamiliar, difficult to comprehend, and do not appeal to the logic employed in the practice of medicine. Testimony of expert witnesses is different from that of ordinary witnesses regarding latitude of opinions, corroborative evidence, and techniques of substantiation. This will be even more difficult with images as they become more complex, not only in appearance but in storage, retrieval and presentation.

Expert opinion must be within the primary knowledge of the witness. With involvement of support personnel the physician may not be responsible for all. Deductions cannot be made by an expert witness if the jurors or judge could make those same deductions based upon their background and knowledge. Therefore, the specific expertise of the witness must be established, usually in court by the legal counsel who summoned the witness. The expert witness can be challenged (in at least a limited fashion) by the opposing attorney. With such specialized technology, the scientific background of the expert witness, and not exclusively clinical experience, may be of paramount importance.

The law does not require that an expert witness be better qualified than anyone else, but the witness should have sufficient expertise to assist the jury in a search for the truth. The level of expertise will determine the weight given to testimony by the judge or jury, but not the admissibility of that evidence. One need not be a member of the specialty of radiology or have specific credentials, such as computer or physics training, in order to qualify as an expert witness, but testimony by witnesses with this documented experience is usually given greater weight. We can probably expect to see more rigid, nationwide standards regarding the credentials of expert witnesses in the future. An expert witness cannot render an opinion without the accompanying facts on which the opinion is based. If the witnesses lacks primary knowledge, he may be questioned on a hypothetical statement of the facts.

The law assumes that cross-examination provides a fair mechanism for ascertaining the truth, e.g., treatises and medical textbooks are thus not admissible as evidence without corroboration. The philosophical basis of this rule is that a) the author of the text cannot be cross-examined or questioned by the opposing counsel or jury, and b) the medical literature often lags behind current medical knowledge. The data in this volume serves to emphasize the wisdom of this concept. Although we have attempted to publish this text in a very timely fashion, we recognize that digital radiography is continually adding to the data base. For this reason we have attempted to emphasize basic principles.

An attorney may use a medical text as an aid in framing questions, but it is not permissible to read from such texts to the jury. Textbooks may be used in most jurisdictions in the cross-examination of a witness for the purpose of contradicting testimony, if the expert witness believes they are authoritative works on the subject about which he has given an opinion.

Many cases hold that the cross-examiner may use only those passages from the literature which the expert witness has specifically cited as supporting his opinion. Other courts have held that when experts have relied generally or specifically upon other authorities, they may be confronted on the basis of yet another authority. One may refer to experimentation which exactly duplicates the facts at issue. In a field that is evolving with the rapidity of digital radiography, this determination will be exceedingly difficult. If experiments are utilized to refute the opinion of a medical expert witness, it must be shown that the experiments were made under essentially the same conditions as those that existed in the case on trial. With the complexity of this

technology, this similarity is difficult to establish and has
limited the use of experimental evidence in legal
proceedings.

The opinions of expert medical witnesses are frequently
contradictory. In recent years it has become easier to obtain
expert medical witnesses to testify for plaintiffs in
malpractice cases, and this trend has lessened the need to
utilize authoritative medical writings in cross-examination.
Medical expert witnesses are posed questions based upon
formulation of hypothetical situations, a technique which
allows great latitude in presenting the opinions of an expert
witness.

Hypothetical questions posed on direct examination are
required to be based on facts in evidence in the case on
trial. The Court must decide whether a hypothetical question
is based upon an adequate foundation for the expert opinion.
There are very few limitations with regard to hypothetical
questions when used on cross-examination. Counsel need not
stay within the facts that have been proven, and, in some
jurisdictions, is not bound by the scope of the subject matter
elicited upon direct examination.

For a proper perspective of digital images, a short
history of medical evidence from images may be useful.

Radiographs were first used as evidence in a case just
four months after Roentgen's discovery. An American actress
sustained an injury to her cuboid during a theatrical
performance in Nottingham, England, in September, 1895. The
radiographs made at University College Hospital revealed
displacement of the bone in her left foot. A quotation from
the transcript of the trial demonstrates the attitude of the
court: "The case is a distinct triumph of science and shows
how plain fact is now furnished with a novel and successful
means of vindicating itself with inerring certainty against
opponents of every class."

In December 1896, an x-ray was admitted as evidence for
the first time in a U.S. Court (10), a trial in which a number
of evidentiary precedents and rules of admissibility of
radiographs were established. The expert witness was
Dr. Buckwalter, a physician who had made the radiographs of
the plaintiff. View-boxes were placed in the courtroom to
demonstrate the patient's radiographs as well as to use
illustrative normals of the same area for comparison. A
Crooke's tube was used to demonstrate the methodology
employed. One might imagine the potentially elaborate
procedures associated with displaying digital images in court.
In the first case, the defense objected to the introduction of
the radiographs as evidence because the object at issue (a

fractured femur) could not be perceived by the unaided eye, therefore it could not be identified directly.

Judge Leferre's opinion regarding the radiographs as evidence was that they were only exhibits to be used in explanation of an opinion, and not primary but secondary evidence to make clear to the jury the testimony of the expert witness. The judge believed "x-ray photography" was a process known and acknowledged as a determinate science and admitted, over objection, the radiographs as evidence. One year later this opinion was cited and followed by the Supreme Court of Tennessee (11). In the Haynes murder trial of 1897 (12), an x-ray "plate" was offered to demonstrate that a foreign body lodged in the victim's neck was not a fragment, but the entire 32 caliber bullet.

Testimony in which the opinion of one expert witness is based upon that of another expert witness is considered incompetent and inadmissible. However, if certain standard tests and studies are shown to be accurate representations of the legal question at issue, they can be interpreted by the expert witness. The valid interpretations of an expert can occasionally be utilized by subsequent expert witnesses in forming the basis of medical opinions. An example is Hickey vs. Chicago Transit Authority (13). It was held that an attending physician may testify as to the pathology revealed by x-rays or similar tests, even though he did not perform the test and had sought the advice of a specialist in interpreting the results. However, the records must then be placed in evidence and the witness must be capable of at least interpreting the records. The need to rely upon the results from tests performed or interpreted by others has increased and probably will continue to do so as the degree of medical specialization increases (14). This would obviate the objection that in digital radiography a number of persons may be responsible for the study. With the complexity of medical images that have been presented in this test, many persons may be "responsible" for the production of the digital images.

Most authorities agree that before an "x-ray picture" is admitted as evidence, proof should be presented that it was taken by the method generally recognized in the specialty. With these new techniques, the courts will have a very difficult decision in this regard. Just as in the introduction of a number of other scientific and medical tests, accurate methodology must be shown (15). It must also be shown that it is an adequate representation of the object under investigation, although the science of radiography is so well-recognized as to render it no longer necessary for a witness to testify as to the reliability and trustworthiness of radiographs before admitting them as evidence (16-18). Will this also apply to digital radiography images?

It was initially believed that even lay persons could interpret radiographs because they were thought to represent an unusual form of photography. However, it is now generally held that radiographs as exhibits should not be presented to the jury unless the radiographs or other diagnostic images are interpreted and explained to the jury by a competent expert (19,20).

Although it has sometimes been allowed that a radiograph be interpreted by someone outside the field of medicine, this action has been considered poor legal practice. However, a scientist may be also necessary as a "co-expert" witness in the future. Most juries recognize that a person interpreting x-rays must be sufficiently familiar with both the medical and technical considerations; an expert in the field of radiography is preferred. In many cases involving osseous pathology, orthopedists and other specialists may testify with regard to the radiographs that bear upon their specialty. It has also been held that the average physician may be called upon to interpret a radiograph, although being a physician does not in itself qualify one as a competent interpreter of an x-ray picture (21). Technologists may testify as to the identification of radiographs and, in the future, the methodology used to properly create the digital study (22,23). The person interpreting the radiographs may refer to the opinion of others, but the report of the radiologist who is not in court cannot be used as testimony, as this type of evidence may be objected to on the hearsay principle previously discussed (24).

The courts have transferred to the field of radiography a number of the rules of admissibility applied to photographs (25). Objective evidence is that which the physician discovers by the use of his ordinary senses. Subjective evidence is that which the physician discovers from the expressions of the patient. Radiographs are regarded as objective rather than subjective evidence (26). Medical images of normal people (just as the normal values of any medical test) may be utilized to contrast with the radiographic images at issue in the litigation. We should experience this rather early as digital studies are first introduced into the courtroom. Copies of radiographs of data, such as thyroid function tests or the original report of any radiographic study, may be introduced, although in some ways they violate the best evidence rule. The best evidence rule, which states that any evidence introduced should be the original evidence. Copies of radiographs would then be subject to this rule of admissibility. With the complex and varied manner of digital recording, the "original" may be difficult to determine. It must then be shown that, through no fault of the person offering it as evidence, the original is not presented. However, with the storage and retrieval techniques as have been discussed, our concept of an "original" may lie somewhere in a computer memory, requiring a specific form of expertise to access.

The federal rules of evidence modify the best evidence rule and permit the use of duplicates, subject to some qualifications (27). In general practice with expert medical witnesses, physicians are allowed to testify about the findings of medical images that were obtained in their absence. The proper proof of their correctness and accuracy must first be established (28). The expert witness can render an opinion of what the medical image portrays after it has been properly authenticated. This opinion does not have to be substantiated by confirming data or other testimony, but can rest merely upon the belief of the medical imaging specialist.

The importance of the expert interpretation of medical imaging has been slowly recognized by the courts. Courts are willing to accept radiographs as accurate "pictures," but the specifics of what they represent have been considered of secondary importance (20). It has gradually become accepted that detailed explanations of the findings displayed by the images, as well as of their generation, are necessary for proper understanding by the jury. The most common method is to introduce the radiographs and to have the radiologist "read" them to the jury. As previously noted, reading the report of the radiologist who is not in the court is objectionable under the hearsay rule (24). Although improperly authenticated radiographs are occasionally admitted under the "shopbook" exception to the hearsay rule, medical reports are not generally admitted under a so-called "business entry" statute (29).

The development of special procedures and new imaging techniques has made the application of general evidence rules difficult because of the different format required for presentation of this data to the trier of fact. Angiograms have been used as courtroom evidence, although such techniques as ultrasonography, cine radiography, xeroradiography, and computed axial tomography have not yet been frequently introduced. Images from digital radiography, positron emission tomography, pulsed Doppler real-time ultrasound and nuclear magnetic resonance may await years before introduction.

The law is slow to accept new techniques, especially those which are scientific, until their validity has been firmly established; for example, handwriting identification tests, but not polygraph results, have been accepted as reliable scientific evidence. Knowledge of the rules of evidence may increase the understanding of radiologists during this evolutionary process and insure the proper application of these new techniques in the search for the truth.

III. CERTIFICATE OF NEED

This text addresses the acquisition of sophisticated and expensive technology (see chapters by Evens and Freedman). Resource allocation to assure access and distribution of computed tomography, angiography equipment, tele-therapy apparatus, and nuclear medicine laboratories has raised considerations that will certainly be "revisited" and probably reapplied to digital radiographic facilities.

A general consideration of the general legal principles would appear warranted. When Congress enacted certificate of need (CON) legislation, the intent was to regulate capital expenditures and distribution of the sophisticated and costly medical technology of that time. Section 1122 of the Social Security Act of 1972 had previously stated that facilities making capital expenditures without approval would be subject to loss of federal reimbursement for depreciation, interest, or return on equity in relation to these instruments.

The Planning Act of 1974 penalized any state that had failed by 1980 to designate agencies to perform certificate of need review. This penalty, if invoked, might include withholding federal funds for the development, support and expansion of health resources. The 1979 Planning Act Amendments introduced incentives for competition and gave rise to a number of exemptions from certificate of need requirements for health maintenance organizations. We propose that Congress by these legislative acts effectively made the decision that regulation and not the "free enterprise system" would govern the supply of institutional health services.

Many have felt that certificate of need concept was developed as a mechanism to control supply of health services by compelling the private sector to ration health resources. Historically, the health care industry has acquired excess capacity when allowed to operate in the marketplace without constraint. Excess hospital beds and expensive new medical technology can be significantly under-utilized, raising the cost per bed or procedure. Over-expansion of facilities should be tempered, insofar as possible, by projected need. The proponents of CON argue, in light of these circumstances, that regulation is potentially the most effective manner to achieve an appropriate balance between need and supply of new and sophisticated medical technology such as digital radiographic facilities.

In enacting the Planning Act of 1974, did Congress repeal the application of antitrust law to the activities of the health planning agencies? The language of the Planning Act does not state an exemption; if one is operative, the intent would be implied. Although the Planning Act may not have provided an exemption, there are at least two potential exemptions to antitrust enforcement. These are known as the Noerr-Pennington and the so-called "state action" doctrines (30,31). We will consider whether these exemptions should be operative in the health care regulation programs with a specific emphasis upon certificate of need for expensive medical technology. These, we believe, can be applied to the topic of digital radiography.

Should we choose regulation rather than the free market system for allocation of expenditures and resources applied to health care? Certain facets of present society may have characteristics that make the free enterprise system inappropriate in health care to assure public welfare and protection. The health care industry is an area in which this alternative line of reasoning has been traditionally applied. In this chapter, we will explore and evaluate the validity of these concepts.

If one views regulation and competition as mutually exclusive, then to consider certificate of need (CON) policies in an antitrust context may appear contradictory. Regulation permits and sometimes fosters a quasi-monopoly circumstance, whereas the Sherman Antitrust and the Clayton Acts tend to promote competition. The application of CON to act as an entry barrier for person and activities can also promote competition in some circumstances.

Often a single institutional provider (hospital) dominates the health care market to the extent that it can support the expansion and initiation of new services irrespective of the previous level of demand. Thus, with "high technology", the provider not only may create its own quasi-monopoly but also may control the sustaining and extension processes necessary for continued growth. If there are no competitive digital units in the area, it is possible for the institutional provider to operate in an uncontrolled fiduciary fashion (monopoly equivalent status).

Many contend that if the various health care judgments could be reduced to some common denominator such as costs in dollars or allocation of scarce resources, it might be possible for the consumer to become part of an effective decision process and act in a collective fashion.

Conceptually, if only the "best" medicine is acceptable, patients and physicians will invariably choose the more sophisticated alternative of care. This characteristic individual behavior, when placed in a general context, usually leads to the type of medicine we have considered in this text, which is technologically oriented. For these reasons, federal inquiry has been directed to many areas and procedures of medical imaging, including such methodologies as computed tomography, peripheral angiography and cardiac catheterization, nuclear medicine, and other technologically oriented procedures. Now digital radiography will also be considered.

The contribution of capital expenditures for these instruments to health care costs has been explored in such great detail that some now suggest that contributions of costs for the new technology have been overemphasized. Most would agree that other factors contributing significantly to health care costs have not been fully appreciated. Several will be explored in this chapter, but the major emphasis will be the legal considerations.

Antitrust principles often seem to be obviated by federal regulatory statutes, especially with regard to the health care industry. Usually, the formulators do not anticipate the implications of this control and from the wording of the legislation makes it difficult for one to determine if antitrust laws are repealed. Courts, in general, have not been disposed to imply legislative intent to nullify the control resulting from application of the Sherman and Clayton Acts. Only where cases of repugnancy between antitrust considerations and regulatory provision are believed to exist, do the courts appear to favor repeal of antitrust considerations. Even in this extreme case, antitrust laws are displaced only to the extent believed necessary to allow the regulatory provision to be effective.

A number of pronouncements and interpretations have demonstrated that Congress intended competition and regulation to act in a complementary fashion in supply allocation. Thus, antitrust laws were not to be abrogated by certificate of need legislation and implied immunity or repeal does not appear to prevail. The landmark decision in the state action doctrine is Parker vs. Brown (32). In this case, a producer attempted to enjoin the state government regulating the sale of an agricultural product in accord with a plan initiated by his competitors. The court declined to apply the Sherman Act because it believed that the Sherman Act should not prohibit economic restraints imposed by a state sovereign, as an act of government.

This concept of providing state policy supremacy over conflicting federal policy has proven problematical. If applied to CON regulatory activities in the medical technology area, Parker would protect an official agency decision made by the state as sovereign, pursuant to clearly defined federal and state economic regulatory policy. So long as the certificate of need considerations further the state's regulatory objectives, the state action doctrine should preclude antitrust liability (33). The Parker doctrine application is even more difficult when one considers that the CON considerations are a function of Health Systems Agencies (HSA); and HSA's are not solely governmental bodies but are often organized as private nonprofit corporations with participation of public as well as state government representatives. However, the state does have significant input into the CON process. State supervision of HSA guidelines, priorities and recommendations appears to compensate for state Parker exemption to HSA activities. Because the relation of the HSA/CON considerations to the state's sovereign activities is a variable one, Parker immunity is neither constant nor predictable. Although the circumstance may not provide a Parker exception, Noerr-Pennington immunity may obtain (34,35).

Under the Noerr-Pennington doctrine, concerted efforts to procure or influence government are, in general, exempt from applications of the Sherman and Clayton Acts even though these efforts may have an anti-competitive animus (36). Thus, providers (hospitals or physicians) may conspire to inundate and co-opt the recommendations of state agencies carrying forth CON legislation without antitrust liability. The single caveat to a general exemption appears to be that competitors must avoid providing known false information to the agencies if this data is critical to the decision process.

There are limitations to the conduct which is immunized by the Noerr-Pennington doctrine (36). If the intent of these activities can be shown not to influence government policy but rather to injure a competitor, the Noerr-Pennington doctrine does not apply. This doctrine appears to be based upon several basic principles, the first ammendment right to petition government, the need for the public to make its views known, and the resistance to use of antitrust legislation to regulate political activity. It has been emphasized that although Noerr-Pennington and Parker vs. Brown are ordinarily complementary, these are not correlative immunities. The origins of Noerr-Pennington are found in the Constitution, whereas in <u>Parker</u> they are found in congressional intent (35-37).

The <u>Noerr</u> immunity is much broader in scope than that provided by application of <u>Parker</u> principles. <u>Noerr-Pennington</u> is particularly important in those agencies that must administer certificate of need legislation (38,39). These agencies can usually be found to have sufficient governmental attributes under federal legislation to qualify for <u>Noerr</u> protection. This form of immunity offers providers significant protection when they seek to influence the certificate of need process. If a government official colludes with providers, the <u>Noerr-Pennington</u> immunity does not apply because it is felt that this behavior internally undermines the regulatory process. This rule is generally known as the co-conspirator exception (40).

Another exception which abrogates immunity is when the anticompetitive efforts of providers are addressed to agency officials acting in a commercial rather than a governmental capacity. To be applicable here this activity must occur when officials are administering CON legislation.

If a Health Systems Agency takes action inconsistent with the state health regulatory mechanism, this conduct will not be protected by either <u>Noerr-Pennington</u> or <u>Parker</u> doctrines. In analysis of certificate of need regulations, the legislators appear to have anticipated some of the antitrust problems that have occurred with implementation, but many were not even considered. The health planning process for digital radiography is sufficiently complex that intrusion of interest groups in the decision process is essentially mandatory. Government intervention into the health care market should not create a circumstance whereby providers can impede competitors by controlling the planning process.

Many believe that official co-conspiracy should be assumed when a provider evaluates the proposal of a direct competitor. A competitor should, in this context, be defined as an institution offering the same or similar health services. Since the Planning Act and antitrust laws allege to proscribe the same conduct, repeal of the antitrust laws should not be implied. Medical technology in the form of expensive instrumentation is assuming increasing importance. Decisions regarding certificate of need applications may be the primary determinant of the character of health care provided by any particular institution. Conduct of the decision process should be in such a manner as to minimize the opportunity for competing providers to have a significant judiciary role. The CON process is designed to protect appropriate provider involvement based upon the belief that these decisions are complex, and knowledge and appreciation of the technology are necessary to render an informed decision. In practice, a balance must be determined between the need for the specific technical expertise of providers and their potential dominant role in the decision process.

It is apparent that certificate of need considerations initially require some understanding of the technology. The biomedical engineering improvements must then be translated into clinical implications. By some methodology, the true costs of public resources must be weighed with regard not only to public benefit from a new technology such as digital radiography methods, but also in relation to other medical imaging alternatives. For example, improvements in ultrasound real-time pulsed Doppler technology, computed tomography, and single photon and PET nuclear medicine advances also offer patient advantages and the potential for improved health care delivery. One can thus appreciate that in many circumstances, only the petitioning and competing providers have sufficient expertise to supply the decision makers with the data required to render an informed determination. Given this environment, the detection of and subsequent evaluation of, bias and provider manipulation is exceedingly difficult. The fiduciary capacity of providers with regard to consumers, as well as to their representatives is inherent in the CON process regarding medical instrumentation such as digital equipment.

The state action doctrine (Parker vs. Brown) and immunity provided by Noerr-Pennington appear to protect involvement of providers in the CON process. However, antitrust application to develop the logic of co-conspirator exceptions will be necessary to offer appropriate public protection (41,42). The official organizations of the health care delivery system may have the prerequisite understanding of the technology and its most appropriate application to develop guidelines of distribution and usage. The alternative of regulation by groups outside the health care system must be weighed against the risks of providers formulating guidelines and providing information to serve self-interests. These alternatives will become increasingly difficult to evaluate as the technological advancements and consumer expectations are to be accommodated by distribution of finite resources for such costly methods as digital radiology. The principles of digital radiology outlined in the initial chapters of this text and elsewhere (43–45) emphasize the technical value of this method. Many clinical reports have appeared recently to emphasize its clinical importance (46–48). Thus, it becomes the responsibility of the users to employ both sound judgement and legal principles to appropriately employ this technology.

ACKNOWLEDGMENTS

We are appreciative of the encouragement from Dean John Chapman of the Vanderbilt School of Medicine and Dean Denton Bostick of the Vanderbilt School of Law, as well as to the Vanderbilt Institute for Public Policy, Erwin Hargrove, Director and Frank Sloan as acting Director. We recognize the advantage of the environment of Vanderbilt University created by Chancellor Alexander Heard and President Emmett Fields.

REFERENCES

1. Holder, A.R., "Medical Malpractice Law," Wiley & Sons, New York, (1975).
2. Curran, W.J., and Shapiro, E.D., "Law, Medicine, and Forensic Science," 2nd ed., Little, Brown and Co., Boston, (1970).
3. American Law Institute, "Restatement (2nd) of the Law of Agency," American Law Institute Publishers, (1959).
4. Seavey, W.A., "The Law of Agency," West Publishing Co., (1964).
5. James, A.E., Jr., Johnson, B.A., and Hall, D.J., Informed consent: Some newer aspects and their relation to the specialty of radiology, Radiology 123, 809-813 (1977).
6. Crane, J.A., and Bromberg, A.R., "Law of Partnership," West Publishing Co, (1968).
7. James, A.E., Jr., Hall, D.J., and Johnson, B.A., Some applications of the law of evidence to the specialty of radiology, Radiology 124, 845-848, (1977).
8. James, A.E., Jr., and Sherrard, T.J., The law of agency as applied to radiology, Radiology 128, 257-260 (1978).
9. James, A.E., "Legal Medicine: With Particular Reference to Diagnostic Imaging," Baltimore, Urban & Schwarzenberg, (1980).
10. Smith vs. Grant, 29 Chicago Legal News 145.
11. Bruce vs. Beall, 99 Tenn. 303, 41 S.W. 445 (1897).
12. Haynes, 56 Alb. L.J. 309, 15 Medico-Legal Journal 246 (1897).
13. Hickey vs. Chicago Transit Authority, 52 Ill. App. 2d 132, 201 N.E. 2d 742 (1964).
14. Rheingold, The basis of medical testimony, 15 Vanderbilt Law Review 473, 1962.
15. Howell vs. George, 210 Miss. 783, 30 So. 2d 603 (1947).
16. 3 Wigmore, Evidence, 795.

17. Chadbourn Rev., 1970.
18. Kimball vs. the Northern Electric Company, 159 Cal. 225, 113 Pac. 156 (1911).
19. Wosoba vs. Kenyon, 215 Iowa 226, 243 N.W. 569 (1932).
20. Vale vs. Campbell, 123 Ore. 632, 263 Pac. 400 (1928).
21. Rawleigh vs. Donoho, 238 Ky. 480, 38 S.W. 2d 227 (1931).
22. Whipple vs. Grandchamp, 261 Mass. 40, 158 N.E. 270 (1927).
23. Call vs. City of Burley, 57 Idaho 58, 62 Pac. 2d 101 (1936).
24. Baker vs. Norris, 248 S.W. 2d 870, Mo. App. (1952).
25. Eckels vs. Boylan, 136 Ill. App. 258 (1907).
26. Reeder vs. Thompson, 120 Kan. 722, 245 Pac. 127 (1926).
27. Fed. Rules Evid. Rule 1003, 28 U.S.C.A.
28. Chicago City Railway Co. vs. Smith, 226 Ill. 178, 80 N.E. 716 (1907).
29. Baltimore & O.R. Co. vs. Zapf, 192 Md. 403, 64 A 2d 139 (1949).
30. Eastern Railroad Presidents Conference vs. Noerr Motor Freight, Inc., 365 U.S. 127 (1961).
31. United Mine Workers vs. Pennington, 381 U.S. 657 (1965).
32. Parker vs. Brown, 417 U.S. 341, 350–351.
33. Posner, R., The proper relationship between state regulation and antitrust laws, 49 NYU L. Rev. 693, 697–698 (1974).
34. Miller, F.H., Antitrust and certificate of need, The Georgetown Law Journal 68, 873–917 (1980).
35. The antitrust laws and professional discipline in medicine, Duke L. Rev. 443, (1978).
36. Holzer, An analysis for reconciling the antitrust laws with the right to petitions: Noerr–Pennington in light of Cantor vs. Detroit Edison, 27 Emory L. J. 673, (1978).
37. Application of antitrust law to the health care delivery system, Cum. L. Rev. 9, 685 (1979).
38. Parker vs. Brown: A presumption analysis, 84 Yale L.J. 1164, 1164–65 (1975).
39. Office of Technology Assessment, Congress of the United States, Policy implications of the computed tomographic (CT) scanner, 63–64 (1978).
40. Huron Valley Hospital, Inc. vs. City of Pontiac, 466 F. Supp 1301, E.D. Mich. (1979).
41. Symposium: CON Laws in Health Planning, Utah L. Rev. 1 (1978).
42. Bovbjerg, Problems and prospects for health planning: The importance of incentives standards and procedures in certificate of need, Utah L. Rev. 83 (1978).

43. Mistretta, C.A., Crummy, A.B., and Strouther, C.M., Digital angiography: A prospective, Radiology 139, 273-276 (1981).
44. Baily, N.E., Video techniques for x-ray imaging and data extraction from roentgenographic and fluoroscopic presentations, Med. Phys. 7, 472-91 (1980).
45. Roehrig, H., Nudelman, S., Fisher, H.D., Frost, M.M., and Capp, M.P., Photoelectronic imaging for radiology, IEEE Trans. Nucl. Sci. NS-28(1) (1981).
46. Ovitt, T.W., Christensen, P.C., Fisher, H.D., et al., Intravenous angiography using a digital video subtraction x-ray imaging system, AJNR 1, 287-390 (1980).
47. Chilcote, W.A., Modic, M.T., Pavlicek, W.A., et al., Digital subtraction angiography of the carotid arteries, Radiology 139, 287-295 (1981).
48. Coulam, C., Erickson, J.J., Rollo, F.D., and James, A.E., Jr., "The Physical Basis of Medical Imaging," Appleton-Century-Crofts, New York, (1981).

9

INJECTION TECHNIQUE AND CONTRAST MEDIA FOR DSA

Joseph F. Sackett
Frederick A. Mann
Patrick A. Turski
Charles M. Strother

Department of Radiology
University of Wisconsin Medical School
Madison, Wisconsin

I. INTRODUCTION

Intravenous digital subtraction angiography, as in the case with any subtraction technique, suffers from image artifacts resulting from misregistration between the mask and the post-injection image. Even with instruments which allow remasking, frequently no suitable mask can be found. Patient motion probably accounts for the majority of technically unsatisfactory studies using intravenous DSA. The intravenous injection of some contrast media can often induce a swallowing reflex as well as a sensation of heat. Both of these can result in patient motion. The characteristic of the contrast media being used and the mode of administration will therefore have significant effects on patient motion and ultimately on the technical adequacy of the examination.

II. INJECTION TECHNIQUES

For digital subtraction angiography using the intravenous technique, the following factors must be considered in selecting an injection technique. The contrast medium bolus must remain intact. There should be adequate pressure connectors and apparatus to withstand the high pressures that occur with power injections of high viscosity contrast media.

There should be minimum risk of venous injury. Patient discomfort must be reduced to minimize subtraction artifact.

A peripheral needle injection is fast and inexpensive. If a 16 gauge needle is selected, the injection rate and contrast medium bolus will be adequate. Because of the needle size, local anesthetic at the injection site is recommended. If venous access will not allow placement using a 16 gauge needle and a 19 gauge needle is selected instead, we have found it necessary to inject both arms in order to obtain adequate arterial opacification. This, of course, results in a very cumbersome system. A short catheter (5-6 cm) can also be used provided that it has a large enough size to permit a rapid injection. Placing side holes in such a short catheter reduces the pressure at the catheter tip and may reduce the risk of venous injury from extravasation.

Hand-injection techniques do not produce adequate arterial opacification for DSA. If the contrast medium bolus is to remain intact to give a high iodine concentration, an injection of 10-15 cc per second is necessary. If the peripheral vein is small, there is a significant risk of extravasation. A physician is thus required to monitor the injection site during pressure injection and terminate the injection if he detects extravasation. Due to a high iodine concentration (370-400 mg iodine/ml), the contrast agents have a high toxicity which may cause endothelial injury and may result in delayed venous thrombosis.

If a peripheral venous injection is used in an antecubital vein, it is necessary to follow this immediately with a saline bolus to force the contrast medium centrally. We found in using this flushing technique that a good portion of the contrast medium remained in peripheral veins even distal to the injection site. Using this saline bolus flush technique, one is required to reload the injector after each injection. The decision to use peripheral injection techniques has financial (see chapters by Evens and Freedman) and legal (see chapter by James) implications. If the catheter tip is passed more centrally into the subclavian vein or superior vena cava, then it is not necessary to follow the contrast agent bolus with a saline bolus. With a central injection, the contrast medium bolus remains intact, which improves the arterial visualization. There is less risk of venous extravasation or venous thrombosis from contrast medium injury. A disadvantage of this longer catheter technique is that it requires guide wire manipulation which increases the expense and time for the procedure.

With a central catheter injection technique, increased time is required for catheter placement. It is necessary to check the catheter tip placement to be certain that it is in the subclavian vein or superior vena cava. The tip of the catheter must be in the central lumen—not directed into the wall of the central vein. With the injection rate of 12-14 cc per second, there remains some risk of extravasation, even in a central vein. More elderly subjects with more fragile veins are the ones (2 cases in our experience) in whom we have had central extravasation. The extravasation caused immediate pain—a signal to terminate the injection. No other difficulty resulted in these two instances.

Patient throughput can be improved if the venous catheter can be placed before the subject is brought into the dedicated room for DSA. If a central catheter is used, it can usually be passed from the basilic vein directly, without the assistance of image intensification fluoroscopy. The tip position can then be checked just prior to DSA with the fluoroscopic system. The subjects can then be prepared in a room without fluoroscopy prior to DSA. If the cephalic vein must be used, which is often necessary in subjects who have had prior coronary arteriography by brachial artery approach, guide wire manipulation is necessary. In this situation the catheter tip is placed in the cephalic vein and not passed centrally until the fluoroscopy is available.

The central venous placement has been found to have many advantages. Personnel do not have to remain in the room to monitor the injection site and be exposed to radiation. A greater range of injection rate is also available with a central catheter position. In selected subjects an injection rate of 25 cc per second can be used if necessary. There is less risk of venous injury from either extravasation or endothelial injury with the central venous catheter technique.

If there is no venous access in either arm, a femoral venous approach can be used using the same catheter materials. At the University of Wisconsin, the femoral venous approach has been performed on an outpatient basis. Patients remain in the department for one hour for observation following the procedure.

III. CONTRAST MEDIUM FOR DIGITAL INTRAVENOUS ARTERIOGRAPHY

Contrast medium must be of high iodine concentration. Of equal importance to the high iodine concentration is a low toxicity to minimize cardiac changes and systemic discomfort that results in motion and registration artifacts. The viscosity of the medium must be low enough to allow its use with a standard pressure injector connector and catheter material. With imaging of the extracranial carotid arteries, there are three motion registration difficulties encountered. The first is generalized motion because of heat and pain experienced when the contrast medium enters the systemic capillary circulation. The second phenomenon, which occurs at the same time, is a reflex swallowing. If the larynx is superimposed over the carotid artery bifurcation, the image is degraded severely. A third registration artifact results from vessel pulsation if the vessel wall has calcification in it or a metallic clip in a post endarterectomy patient (Fig. 1).

The non-ionic contrast media have a low systemic toxicity and, for this reason, may result in better image quality. The University of Wisconsin performed a controlled study comparing two ionic media—Renografin 76 and Conray 400—to a non-ionic medium, Amipaque. Renografin 76 is diatrizoate-meglumine 66% and sodium 10%, with 370 milligrams iodine per milliliter. Conray 400 is sodium iothalamate-66.8% and has 400 milligrams of iodine per milliliter. The Amipaque is reconstituted to 370 milligrams iodine per milliliter. The patients were all studied in a similar technique, using a catheter passed from the antecubital vein into the superior vena cava. Injection rates and volumes are 10 to 12 cc per second for a total of 30–40 cc per injection. Electrocardiogram, pulse rate, and blood pressure are compared to control of vital signs up to 15 minutes following each injection.

The results show that all three contrast media are tolerated without major difficulty. The patients' spontaneous response after questioning indicated that Conray 400 created the greatest pain sensation, with Renografin 76 somewhat better and Amipaque caused the least pain and discomfort. An analysis of EKG data shows that there are fewer EKG changes with Amipaque and the greatest EKG changes with Conray 400 (Table 1). Comparison of image quality shows that there is less motion and swallowing with Amipaque (Fig. 2).

DSA, because of its ability to detect small iodine concentration, has resulted in a modification of intra-arterial techniques; also an aortic root injection with a small catheter (15 cc) often obviates the need for selection catheterization in elderly subjects at risk of embolization from selective catheter placement. Vertebral artery circulation in elderly subjects can be studied with low dose (5 cc) subclavian artery injection.

Using intra-arterial DSA does allow selection of smaller catheters, use of smaller injection rates and volumes, and reduces the need for selective catheter placement. These result in improved patient comfort and, probably, in reduced risk compared to conventional angiographic procedures.

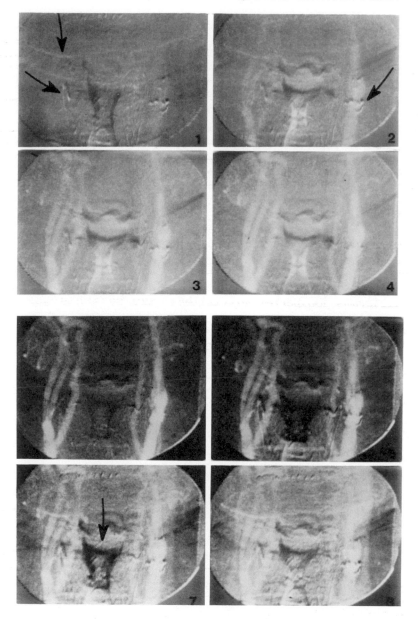

FIGURE 1. *Serial frontal neck images in a standard DSA study illustrate several registration artifacts. Calcified plaques (arrow in Image 2) illustrate motion artifacts from vessels pulsation. Swallowing artifact is clearly illustrated in Image 7 (note arrow). General patient motion artifacts can be seen in image as incomplete subtraction of the vertebral bodies and facial bones (Image 1).*

TABLE I. EKG Response to Contrast Media

	Amipaque	Renografin	Conray
HR (△10%)	2/6	5/5	5/6
Ectopy - APC	0/6	3/5	4/6
VPC		1/5	1/6
ST (△> 1 mm)	3/6	2/5	5/6
persistent at			
end trace	0/3	0/2	1/5
T-waves △'s	2/6	0/5	3/6
QT (> 40 mSec)	1/6	2/5	4/6
Rhythm	0/6	1/5 (SVT)	0/6

Image quality is often improved over film techniques because of less patient motion with reduced contrast medium injection.

Central venous pressure is increased by 2–4 cm of water in most subjects, following 2 or 3 intravenous injections. If a

VISUALIZATION

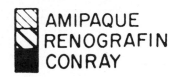

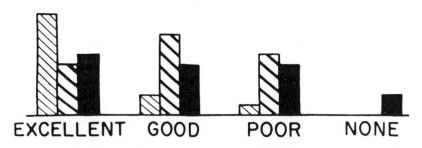

FIGURE 2. Comparison of Image Quality using 3 contrast media--50 subjects.

patient has marginal left ventricular function, the usual study may create enough osmotic and fluid load to cause congestive heart failure. The need for DSA in such a patient must be balanced against such a risk.

Renal toxicity had not been detected in the inpatients in whom the Wisconsin studies have compared pre- and post-DSA serum creatinine. Patients with known renal disease or diabetics would be at risk of renal injury from standard DSA contrast agent volumes.

Arrhythmias occur from peripheral or central contrast medium injection. This is probably the greatest risk from DSA in the elderly population selected for study. It is best to perform DSA procedures in a hospital so the skills of an entire resuscitation team are available to manage a severe adverse reaction.

The present state of digital subtraction angiography is in its infancy. Contrast media will be improved as the technology developments occur, as may injection and image recording techniques.

REFERENCES

1. Mistretta, C.A., The use of a general description of the radiological transmission image for categorizing image enhancement procedures, Opt. Eng. 13, 134–137 (1974).
2. Kruger, R.A., Mistretta, C.A., Lancaster, J., et al., A digital video image processor for real-time x-ray subtraction imaging, Opt. Eng. 17, 652–657 (1978).
3. Strother, C.M., Sackett, J.R., Crummy, A.B., et al., Clinical applications of computerized fluoroscopy. The extracranial carotid artery, Radiology 136, 781–783 (1980).
4. Crummy, A.B., Strother, C.M., Sackett, J.F., et al., Computerized fluoroscopy: Digital subtraction for intravenous angiocardiography and arteriography, AJR 135, 1131–1140 (1980).
5. Robb, G.P., and Steinberg, I., Visualization of the chambers of the heart, the pulmonary circulation and the great blood vesels in man, AJR 41, 1–17 (1939).
6. Berg, G.R., Hutter, A.M., and Pfister, R.C., Electrocardiographic abnormalities associated with intravenous urography, N. Engl. J. Med. 289, 87–88 (1974).
7. Lindgren, P., Hemodynamic responses to contrast media, Invest. Radiol. 5, 424–445 (1970).

8. Wildenthal, K., Mierzwiak, D.S., and Mitchell, J.H., Acute effects of increased serum osmolality on left ventricular performance, <u>Am. J. Physiol.</u> 216, 898–904 (1969).
9. Stadalnik, R.C., Vera, Z., DaSilva, O., et al., Electrocardiographic response to intravenous urography: prospective evaluation in 275 patients, <u>AJR</u> 129, 825–830 (1977).
10. Newell, J.D., Higgins, C.B., Keley, M.J., et al., The influence of hyperosmolality on left ventricular contractile state: Diagnostic effect of nonionic and ionic solutions. <u>Invest. Radiol.</u> 15, 363–370 (1980).
11. Fischer, H.W., and Thompson, K.R., Contrast media in coronary arteriography: A review, <u>Invest. Radiol.</u> 13, 450–459 (1978).
12. Popio, K.A., Ross, A.M., Oravec, J.M., and Ingram, J.T., Identification and description of separate mechanisms for two components of Renografin cardiotoxicity, <u>Circulation</u> 58, 520–528 (1978).
13. Almen, T., and Aspelin, P., Cardiovascular effects of ionic monomeric, ionic dimeric and nonionic contrast media, <u>Invest. Radiol.</u> 10, 557 (1975).
14. Tragardh, B., Lynch, P.R., and Tragardh, M., Coronary angiography with diatrizoate and metrizamide: Comparison of ionic and nonionic contrast medium effect on coronary blood flow in dogs, <u>Acta Radiol.</u> (Diagn.) 17, 69 (1976).

10

DIGITAL SUBTRACTION ANGIOGRAPHY (DSA) OF THE HEAD AND NECK

Michael T. Modic
Meredith A. Weinstein

Department of Diagnostic Radiology
Cleveland Clinic Foundation
Cleveland, Ohio

I. INTRODUCTION

Digital subtraction angiography has been shown to be safe, accurate, and reproducible when compared with conventional arteriography. In the evaluation of the extracranial carotid arteries, the accuracy rate was 97% in technically satisfactory studies. In the evaluation of intracranial vasculature, intravenous digital subtraction angiography was as accurate as conventional arteriography in 65% of cases. In 22%, intravenous digital subtraction angiography provided important diagnostic information, but because of vessel overlap, spatial resolution, or patient motion, there was a significant chance for error. In situations where high spatial resolution or selectivity is required, intra-arterial injections can be made which will increase the contrast media concentration in the region of interest and will also increase the overall accuracy.

Recent progress in the development of computers, television systems, x-ray intensifiers, and digital electronic storage devices has permitted a reassessment of intravenous angiography in the evaluation of vascular structures. The images obtained with DSA are comparable to those of conventional arteriography and its accuracy and safety has been documented in comparative studies of the extracranial carotids, intracranial, renal arteries, abdominal aorta, and cardiac systems (1-5).

155

II. TECHNIQUE

Patients who are reported in this chapter were examined on a commercially available production unit with a 512 matrix. The x-ray tube has a nominal focal spot selection of .6/1.2 mm and a heat unit capacity of 400,000 heat units. A 1,000 mA generator is used and x-rays are detected using a trimodal 9, 6, 4.5" cesium iodine image intensifying tube. A 12:1 grid with 40 lines per cm is employed. The output phosphor of the image tube is scanned with a video camera with a lead oxide tube. The video signal from the camera is logarithmically amplified and digitized for storage in the imager, which has two 512 X 512 X 12 bit memories. A digital PDP 11/34 computer is used for image processing.

An 8", 16-gauge angiocatheter is inserted in an arm vein by a nurse in a holding area to expedite patient throughput. The catheter is attached to a 50 cc bag of D5W with constant infusion to maintain patency. The catheter position and vein are examined fluoroscopically with a small test injection. If the cannulated vein is tortuous or very small, the catheter is repositioned. If a central injection is warranted, a 5-French, 65 cm straight catheter is introduced into the inferior vena cava via the femoral vein or the superior vena cava from an arm vein.

With the injector syringe in the inverted position, 25 cc of D5W is layered over the contrast material. The injection rate is 12-20 cc per second. A layered D5W solution acts to flush the contrast material and decrease the time and concentration of contrast material within the vein. With careful loading of D5W and contrast in the inverted position, there is no significant mixing of the two solutions. Forty to fifty cc of Renografin-76 is the usual bolus dose and 3 cc per kilogram or five injections is the usual limit, depending on the patient's weight, age, and renal function.

Radiographic exposures start 5-8 seconds after the beginning of an injection and 10-15 images are collected in the digital mode with acquisition rates depending on the area and type of abnormality suspected. A 128 X 128 matrix can acquire frames at 16 per second. There is a 6 second maximum at 256 X 256 and 1 per second maximum of 512 X 512. The average time for an examination is 30-40 minutes with 15-18 patients examined per day.

III. CAROTID ARTERIES

Confidence in the accuracy of intravenous digital subtraction angiograms (IV-DSA) of the carotid bifurcations was gained from a comparative study with conventional arteriography in 100 patients. When the quality of the IV-DSA examination was good or excellent, there was excellent correlation (accuracy 97%) (Fig. 1). In situations in which the carotid bifurcation was not well visualized, there was a substantial chance for error (accuracy 64%). The most common causes for a technically poor study were swallowing artifacts, patient motion, and superimposition of adjacent vascular structures over the proximal internal carotid artery (Fig. 2). Currently over 85% of these studies are considered good or excellent.

The 4" image intensifier is used for the evaluation of the carotid bifurcation. Smaller intensifier field sizes produce better images because of reduced light scatter. Seventy-degree LAO and RAO projections are obtained. If the separate origins of the internal and external carotids are not identified on either oblique, an AP projection is obtained. The frontal projection, however, is the least useful because of frequent overlap of the proximal internal carotid artery by either the ipsilateral external carotid or vertebral artery. In the RAO position and LAO positions, the contralateral carotid is often obscured by swallowing artifacts (Fig. 3).

The indications for an IV-DSA study of the carotid bifurcations have been: transient ischemic attacks, episodes of amaurosis fugax, nonspecific symptoms of cerebral ischemia, or asymptomatic carotid bruits. Less common indications are the evaluation of fibromuscular disease, nonspecific neck masses, suspected chemodectomas of the carotid body or other vascular lesions of the neck, such as traumatic aneurysms, or arteriovenous malformation.

IV. INTRACRANIAL VESSELS

A comparative study with conventional arteriography was performed in 55 patients. Entities studied include tumors, aneurysms, arteriovenous malformations, carotid cavernous sinus fistulas, occlusive vascular disease and extracranial-to-intercranial bypass grafts. In 65%, the diagnosis was achieved with an IV-DSA study. In 22%, the DSA examination provided important diagnostic information, but there was a significant chance of misinterpreting the results

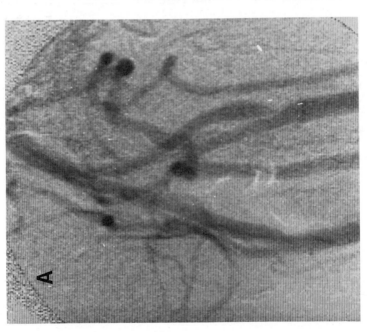

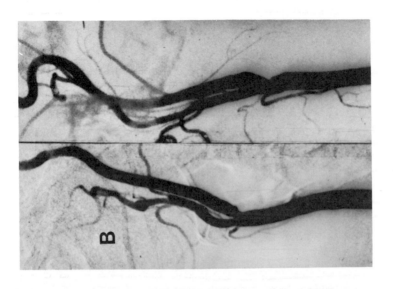

FIGURE 1. A 60-year-old female with a left carotid bruit. (A) IV-DSA study. (B) Composite of a film subtraction of a conventional arteriogram demonstrating moderate stenosis of the proximal portion of the left internal carotid artery.

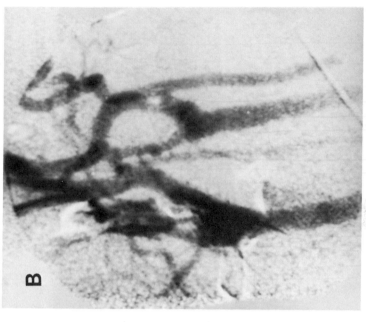

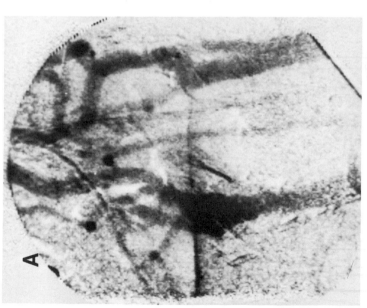

FIGURE 2. A 57-year-old male with a left carotid bifurcations. The left vertebral overlaps the proximal portion of the left internal carotid artery. Because of this, (B) 70° LPO view was obtained. This projected the ipsilateral vertebral off the proximal portion of the internal carotid artery demonstrating a moderate to severe stenosis.

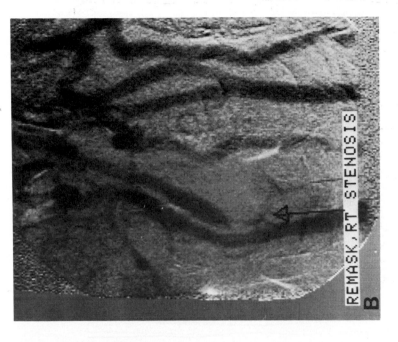

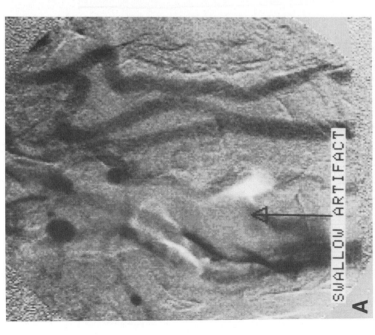

FIGURE 3. (A) A 60° LPO view with a swallowing artifact obscuring the right carotid bifurcation. (B) A resubtraction utilizing a later frame for the mask demonstrates a moderate to severe stenosis of the proximal portion of the right internal carotid artery.

of the study. This was usually a result of patient motion or overlap of opacified structures.

Positioning for intracranial studies is tailored to the type and area of suspected abnormality. For sella and parasellar lesions, AP, lateral, and 25° obliques appear to be the most useful views. A submentrovertical view is sometimes helpful, but swallowing artifacts and patient motion are increased by the awkward position. Oblique views in the AP projection may be necessary in cases of suspected aneurysms. Caldwell, Towne's, and lateral views are used for the evaluation of the posterior fossa vessels, particularly the basilar artery. A 25° oblique view is used for evaluation of the carotid siphon (Fig. 4). An AP and 25° oblique view centered over the jugular bulbs are useful in evaluating venous outflow abnormalities. A 4" image intensifier field is used whenever possible, but when larger regions such as the dural venous sinuses are examined, a 6 or 9" image intensifier field is necessary.

Intravenous digital subtraction angiography (IV-DSA) has become the exclusive examination of the juxtasellar carotids in patients prior to transphenoidal surgery (Fig. 5). It is

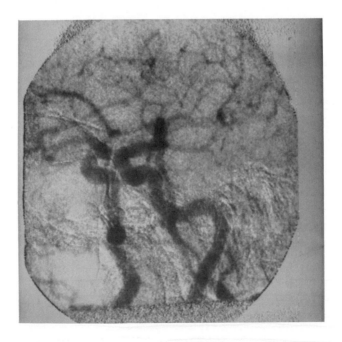

FIGURE 4. A 25° off lateral oblique view of the carotid siphons.

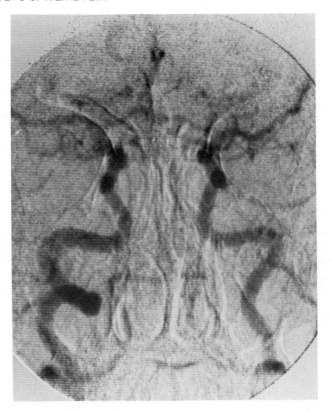

FIGURE 5. A 28-year-old female with a large enhancing
sellar lesion on CT. The IV-DSA in the AP projection shows
lateral displacement of the internal carotid arteries in their
juxtasellar portion and no evidence of an aneurysm or ectatic
carotid.

used for the evaluation of the patency of extracranial-
to-intracranial anastomoses. In combination with computed
tomography, it is adequate for determining the extent and
vascularity of most intracranial tumors preoperatively
(Fig. 6). Intravenous angiography is capable of
distinguishing between tumors and aneurysms and is accurate in
the initial diagnosis of aneurysms or arteriovenous
malformations, but it cannot replace conventional
arteriography preoperatively, where selectivity and greater
spatial resolution is necessary. It can replace conventional
arteriography in the postoperative evaluation (Fig. 7). The
intravenous injection is ideal for the evaluation of the
intracranial dural venous sinuses. Filling defects from

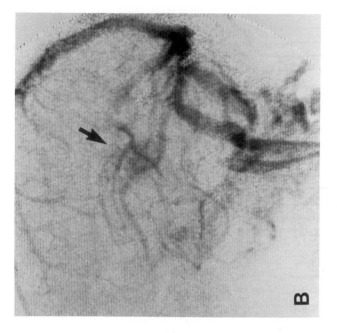

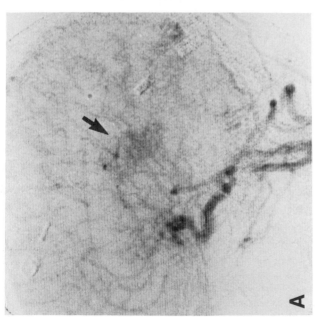

FIGURE 6. A 20-year-old white male with a large enhancing mass in the region of the posterior third ventricle. (A) Arterial and (B) venous phase DSA's in the lateral projection demonstrating a tumor blush in the region of the posterior third ventricle. Unlike the CT, these images completely differentiate between a tumor mass and an aneurysm. In addition, one can appreciate the extraventricular location by the relationship of the blush to the arterial and deep venous structures.

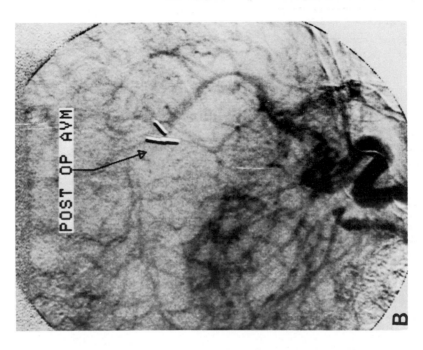

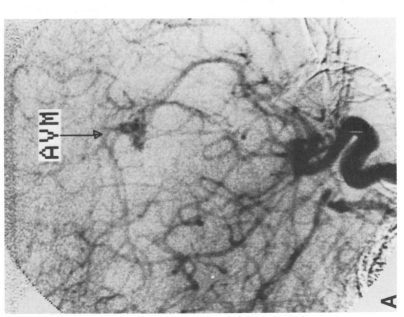

FIGURE 7. A 28-year-old female with a history of subarachnoid hemorrhage. (A) Lateral IV-DSA demonstrates a small arteriovenous malformation fed by branches of the pericallosal artery. (B) Postoperative IV-DSA demonstrates complete surgical obliteration of the lesion.

incomplete mixing, seen with conventional selective arteriography, are eliminated because of the simultaneous bilateral opacification. It is particularly useful in the evaluation of the size and position of the jugular bulb and venous drainage of the brain.

V. DISCUSSION

The basic principles of digital subtraction angiography have been reported (6-14). Vessels can be visualized with DSA following intravenous injections of contrast material because the low contrast detectability of the DSA equipment is superior to that of conventional film/screens. This improved low contrast detectability is a result of a number of factors, such as high quality image TV camera systems and improved image tubes with relatively noiseless electronic amplification. These produce a more faithful detection of small differences in radiation exposure.

The subtraction process is the most important factor in making possible diagnostic examinations from an intravenous injection. Subtraction offers a marked increase in contrast and conspicuity (the degree to which an area of interest stands out from its surroundings) (See chapter by Mistretta). Without the use of subtraction, 8-10 times the concentration of contrast material would be required to provide images of equally diagnostic value. Subtraction with a digital apparatus is more accurate than conventional film subtraction. This is because constant signal levels for iodine, even over areas of widely varying densities such as air and bone, are achieved because the log amplification of the video signal is valid over the entire range of radiation intensity absorbed in the input phosphor of the cesium iodide tube. This results in a more accurate contrast transfer in the toe and shoulder regions of the H and D curve and greater sensitivity to small exposure differences.

The digital memory and computer interface produce real-time subtracted images and the capability to remask instantly, obviating the time consuming and expensive manual registration and re-registration required for film subtraction.

A significant cost saving is achieved by utilizing the digital apparatus. An IV-DSA study can be stored on tape and hard copies with a cost of approximately $10 per examination. Conventional angiography requires $60-100 in film costs alone (see chapters by Evens and by Freedman).

The major limitations of digital subtraction angiography are related to the overlap of opacified structures, spatial resolution, contrast concentration in the region of interest, image intensifier field size and motion artifacts. However, experience has shown that certain maneuvers can minimize these problems.

Monitoring of the examination and tailored oblique views can usually offset the effect of overlap of opacified structures. The theoretical spatial resolution of the system is 2.2 line pairs per millimeter at a 512 X 512 matrix. Factors affecting the spatial resolution are the television line system, matrix size, image intensifier blur and the concentration of iodine in the region of interest from an intravenous injection. When high spatial resolution is required, a selective intra-arterial injection can be made which will increase the contrast concentration in the region of interest and also allow selectivity. In this fashion, high quality examinations can be generated utilizing only one-half the amount of contrast material typically used for a conventional arteriogram.

The field of study is limited by the image intensifier size. Recently, a 14" image intensifier has become available for clinical use which can utilize a larger image intensifier field size without degradation of the image.

Patient motion remains the most common cause of technically unsatisfactory examinations. Intravenous contrast material induces a swallowing reflex in many patients and a sensation of heat which is uncomfortable and often produces patient motion (see chapter by Sackett). Swallowing moves the hyoid bone and larynx in the area of the carotid bifurcation and creates artifacts because of misregistration between the mask and contrast frames. Remasking can offset the effect of motion, but there are often changes in motion between all frames of the study (Fig. 3). Software programs are being evaluated that can change the alignment of the mask and contrast frames electronically. Recently, preliminary reports on a non-ionic contrast material (metrizamide) seem to indicate that it is associated with marked reduction in the number of swallowing artifacts and patient motion (15). Restraining devices may also prove to be useful.

Because of its ease, safety, and accuracy, IV-DSA has gained widespread clinical acceptance as a valuable angiographic procedure. The examination can be performed on an outpatient basis, requiring less material and personnel than conventional arteriography. No serious complications have resulted in over 2,500 examinations. Patients with asymptomatic carotid bruits and high risk patients who have not been studied with conventional arteriography are being studied with DSA. As surgeons gain more confidence in the accuracy of DSA, they are operating on patients without confirming DSA findings with conventional arteriography. Thus, it appears that we are in the preliminary clinical applications of a most exciting and promising clinical technique.

REFERENCES

1. Buonocore, E., Meaney, T.F., Borkowski, G.P., Pavlicek W.A., and Gallagher, J., Digital subtraction angiography of the abdominal aorta and renal arteries, Radiology 139, 281–286 (1981).
2. Buonocore, E., Borkowski, G.P., Meaney, T.F., Tarazi, R.C., Shirey, E.K., and Fuod, F.M., Computerized angiography of the human heart, Presented at the Fifty-third Scientific Session of the American Heart Association, Nov. 17–20, 1980, Miami, Florida.
3. Chilcote, W.A., Modic, M.T., Pavlicek, W.A., Little, J.R., Furlan, J.A., Duchesneau, P.M., and Weinstein, M.A., Digital subtraction angiography of the carotid arteries: A comparative study in 100 patients, Radiology 139, 287–295 (1981).
4. Modic, M.T, Weinstein, M.A., Chilcote, W.A., Pavlicek, W.A., Duchesneau, P.M, Furlan, J.A., and Little, J.R., Digital subtraction angiography of the intracranial vascular system—A comparative study in 55 patients, AJNR 2, 527–534, (1981).
5. Modic, M.T., Weinstein, M.A., Buonocore, E., Pavlicek, W.A., and Meaney, T.F, Intravenous digital angiography of the head and neck: A clinical update, SPIE 314, 244–449, (1981).
6. Christensen, P.C., Ovitt, T.W., Fisher, H.D., Frost, M.M., Nudelman, S., and Roehrigh, H., and Seeley, G., Intravenous angiography using a digital video subtraction: Intravenous cervicocerebrovascular angiography, AJNR 1:379–387 (1981).
7. Ergun, D.L., Mistretta, C.A., Kruger, R.A., Riederer, S.J., Shaw, C.G., and Carbone, D.P., A hybrid computerized fluoroscopy technique for noninvasive cardiovascular imaging. Radiology 132, 739–742 (1979).

8. Kruger, R.A., Mistretta, C.A., Houk, T.K., Riederer, S.J., Shaw, C.G., Goodsitt, M.M., Crummy, A.B., Swiebel, W., Lancaster, J.C., Rowe, G.G., and Flemming, D., Computerized fluoroscopy in real time for noninvasive visualization of the cardiovascular imaging, Radiology 130, 49–57 (1979).

9. Meaney, T.F., Weinstein, M.A., Buonocore, E., Pavlicek, W., Borkowski, G.P., Gallagher, J.R., Sufka, B., and MacIntyre, W.E., Digital subtraction angiography of the human cardiovascular system, SPIE 233, 272–278 (1980).

10. Meaney, T.F., Weinstein, M.A., Buonocore, E., Pavlicek, W., Borkowski, G.P., Gallagher, J.H., Sufka, B., and MacIntyre, W.J., Digital subtraction angiography of the human cardiovascular system, AJR 139, 1153–1160 (1980).

11. Mistretta, C.A., Digital videoangiography, Diagnostic Imaging 14–25 (1981).

12. Mistretta, C.A., Crummy, A.B., and Strother, C.M., Digital angiography: A perspective. Radiology 139, 273–276 (1981).

13. Ovitt, T.W., Christensen, P.C., Fisher, H.D., Frost, M., Nudelman, S., Roehrig, H., and Seeley, G., Intravenous angiography using a digital video subtraction x-ray imaging system, AJNR 1, 287–390 (1980).

14. Strother, C.M., Sackett, J.R., Crummy, A.B., Lillaes, F.G., Swiebel, W.J., Turnipseed, W.D., Javid, M., Mistretta, C.A., Kruger, R.A., Ergun, D.L., and Shaw, C.B., Clinical applications of computerized fluoroscopy, Radiology 136, 781–783 (1980).

15. Sackett, J.R., and Strothers, C.M., Contrast media for computerized fluoroscopy, Presented at the 66th Scientific Assembly and Annual Meeting of the Radiological Society of North America, Nov. 16–21, 1980, Dallas, Texas.

11

CARDIAC DIGITAL RADIOGRAPHY

Clyde W. Smith
Marvin W. Kronenberg

Department of Radiology and Radiological Sciences
Vanderbilt University School of Medicine
Nashville, Tennessee

I. INTRODUCTION

Visualization of cardiac chambers and the great vessels by intravenous contrast administration was originally described by Castellanos in 1937 and Robb and Steinberg in 1939 (1,2). A large volume of contrast material was necessary for a successful study. Image improvement by film subtraction was possible but not convenient. The ability to generate subtracted video images rapidly with high contrast sensitivity has made it possible to apply the digital subtraction technique to cardiac images utilizing smaller amounts of contrast material.

II. ANATOMY-PHYSIOLOGY

In our experience, the assessment of normal and pathologic cardiac physiology and anatomy is feasible with the digital technique. It should be pointed out, however, that the imaging requirements may differ between anatomic and physiologic studies. An anatomic study may require only a few frames (5-10 per sec); however, relatively high spatial resolution is essential. On the other hand, a higher frame rate (15-30 per sec) is required for physiologic examinations, but spatial resolution need not be as great. Anatomy studies require as high resolution images as are available; but for physiologic studies, an image matrix of 128 x 128 picture elements may be adequate. Consequently, the computer memory requirement per frame in physiologic studies may be less than required for anatomic studies, thus permitting the storage of a larger number of frames (Fig. 1).

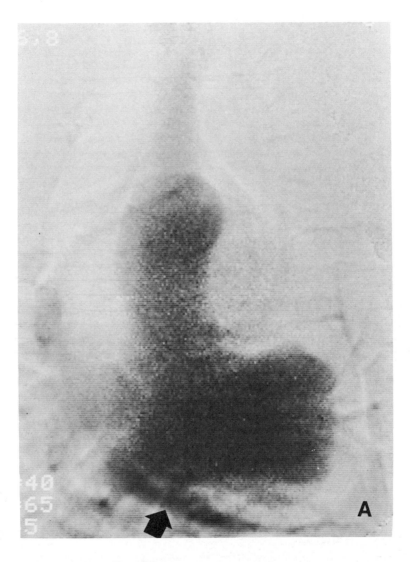

FIGURE 1. A canine left ventricle and aorta are demonstrated with an image matrix of 256 X 256 picture elements (A) and 128 X 128 picture elements (B). The image quality in B is adequate for physiological studies. Note the subtraction artifact in A due to misregistration (arrow).

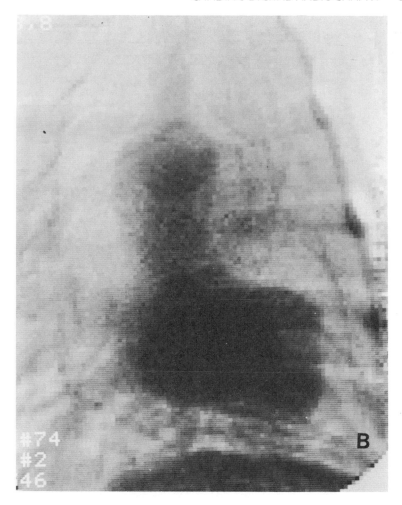

FIGURE 1 (continued).

III. <u>MASK SELECTION</u>

Because of the continuous cardiac motion, the proper selection of the mask for subtracting cardiac images is problematic. Several types of mask image selection are possible. A single frame may be chosen at random or triggered by the electrocardiogram. Several consecutive frames may be summed to form an average mask. This averaged mask has been called the "mask mode" by Kruger, et al. (3). Multiple frames exposed at the same point in the cardiac cycle may be summed and subtracted from contrast filled frames exposed at the same point in the cardiac cycle. The mask may be continually updated with subtraction of sequential or nearly sequential frames. This method has been called "time interval difference" subtraction by Kruger, et al. (3).

In spite of the many different potential mask images, the periphery of the cardiac silhouette is frequently not subtracted properly due to the misregistration caused by cardiac motion (Fig. 1). To overcome this problem, it has been proposed that multiple mask images from several cardiac cycles be obtained and stored for subtraction from contrast filled frames. While theoretically possible, this methodology is cumbersome and is not likely to be practical.

IV. TECHNIQUES

In adult patients, 30 to 40 cc of contrast material are injected at 15 to 20 cc per sec through a "pig tail" catheter in the superior vena cava or right atrium. This volume and flow rate provides adequate visualization of right and left heart chambers with the digital technique. One half to one cc of contrast material per kilogram is adequate for children. Since children have faster heart rates and faster flow than adults, the contrast bolus should be injected within 1 to 1.5 sec. Prolonged circulation time due to cardiac failure or incompetent cardiac valves may preclude adequate visualization of cardiac chambers.

V. CLINICAL EXPERIENCE

Digital intravenous cardiac angiography has multiple uses for the evaluation of patients with ischemic heart disease. The initial experience at Vanderbilt and several other institutions indicates a significant positive correlation between digital intravenous studies and cineangiographic studies for the evaluation of left ventricular volumes and ejection fractions (4,5). Utilization of an end-diastolic frame as the mask with subtraction of subsequent frames produces a visual representation of the ejection fraction (Fig. 2). Wall motion abnormalities secondary to myocardial infarction are identified readily by digital intravenous studies (Fig. 3). Evaluation of myocardial perfusion using iodinated contrast material and the digital technique is currently being evaluated and is discussed in more detail in the chapter by Monahan.

In addition to intravenous injections of contrast material, intraventricular injections of small volumes of contrast media to evaluate left ventricular function have been successful (Fig. 4) (4). Multiple small injections before and after exercise or drug administration can provide useful information about the functional reserve of the left ventricle with minimal perturbation of hemodynamics. Small volumes of contrast are particularly desirable in patients with significant impairment of cardiac function or poor renal function.

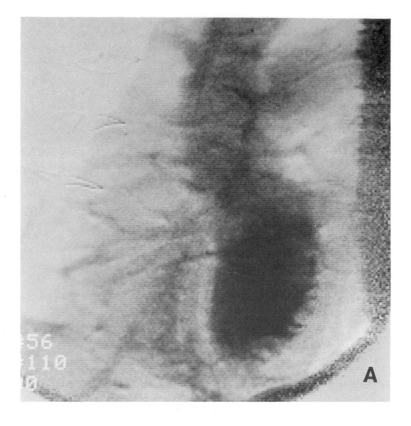

FIGURE 2. The left ventricle is depicted in the left anterior oblique projection in diastole (A), in mid-systole (B), and in end-systole (C). In B and C, the systolic images are subtracted from the end-diastolic image. Thus, the darkened areas at the periphery represent the ejection fraction (arrows).

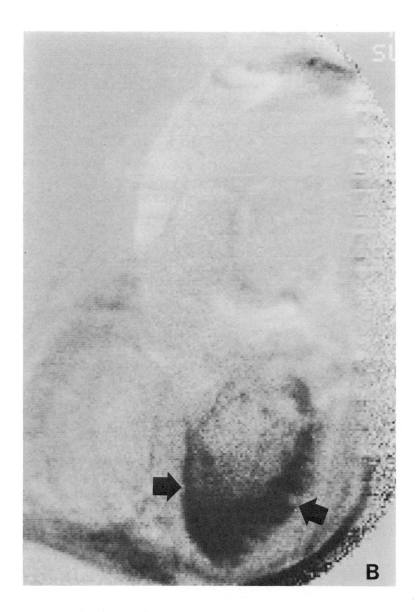

FIGURE 2 (continued).

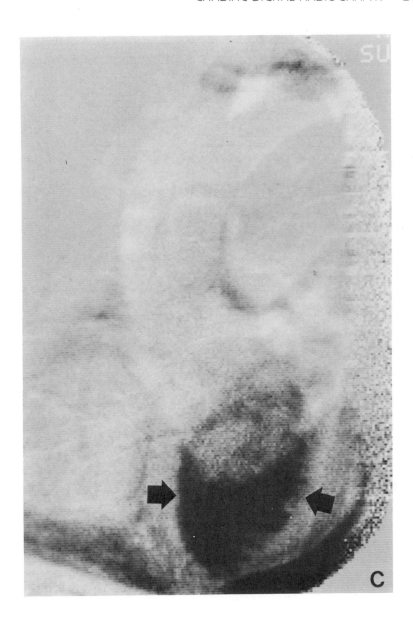

FIGURE 2 (continued).

Cardiac digital studies provide functional information about the ventricle similar to gated isotopic (MUGA) cardiac studies. Digital studies have the advantage of greater spatial resolution than isotopic studies. However, pre- and post-exercise studies are more conveniently performed with the isotopic technique since only a single isotopic injection is required. Digital studies present a problem in that they would require separate injections of contrast agents before and after exercise. Isotopic and digital examinations are likely to be competitive for the evaluation of cardiac function.

Digital intravenous subtraction images of the coronary arteries have been disappointing. However, intra-aortic and

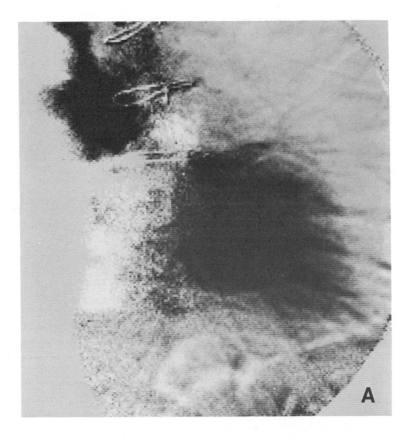

FIGURE 3. *Right anterior oblique views showing the left ventricle in diastole (A) and systole (B) in a patient with a segmental akinetic segment secondary to infarction (arrows).*

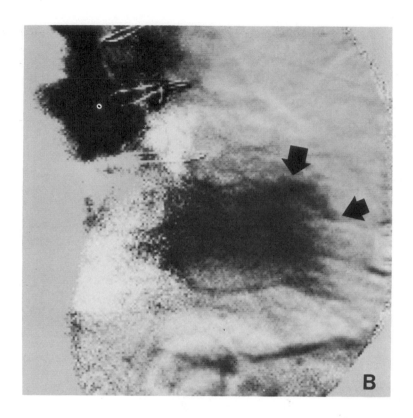

FIGURE 3 (continued).

intracoronary injections with the digital technique have been promising (Fig. 5). Small volumes of contrast media (2-3 cc) have produced spectacular images of the coronary arteries.

Patency of coronary artery bypass grafts has been demonstrated by intravenous digital angiography. Myerowitz, et al. correctly identified eleven of fifteen patent grafts and eleven of eleven occluded grafts (6). As opposed to computed tomography which demonstrates bypass grafts in cross section, digital studies demonstrate bypass grafts longitudinally (Fig. 6). Visualization of grafts as they course over the myocardium and distal graft anastomoses have not been successful because of the large volume of contrast agents in the myocardium which obscures the grafts.

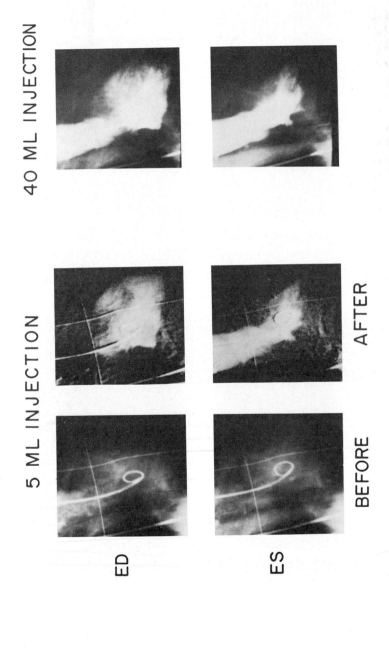

FIGURE 4. *End-diastolic and end-systolic frames of a 5 cc injection of a contrast media in the left ventricle are shown before and after subtraction. The chamber is not identified prior to subtraction but is easily seen following subtraction. A 40 cc injection in the same ventricle is demonstrated for comparison.*

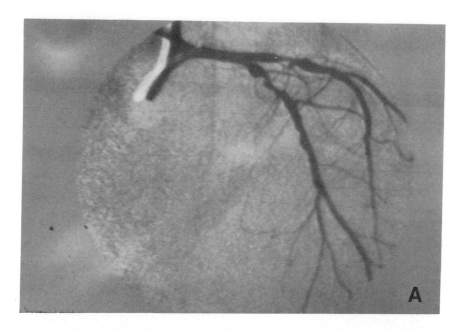

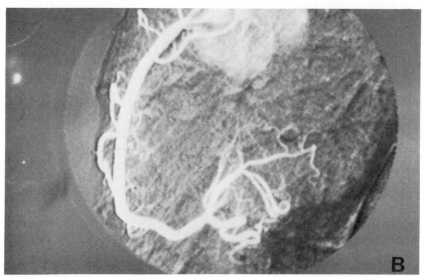

FIGURE 5. Digital subtraction images of intracoronary injections of contrast material are shown in the left coronary artery (A) and the right coronary artery (B). Images courtesy of Philip's Medical Systems.

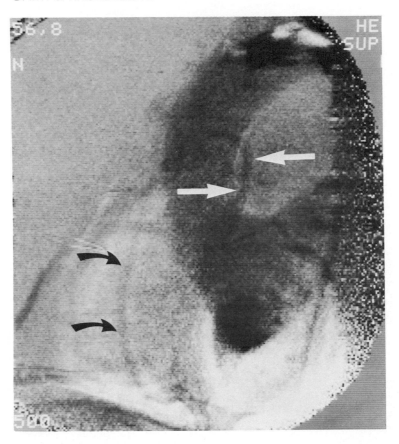

FIGURE 6. Coronary artery bypass grafts to the right coronary artery (curved arrows) and the left anterior descending coronary artery (straight arrows) are demonstrated.

VI. <u>SUMMARY</u>

Several quantitative assessments of cardiac function and anatomy may be possible with the digital technique. Cardiac chamber volumes and ventricular wall mass can be derived from digitized cardiac images. The severity of shunt lesions and valvular insufficiencies can be assessed by the quantification of chamber volumes. The interventricular septum in patients with idiopathic hypertrophic subaortic stenosis (IHSS) can be outlined and measured with the digital technique.

Considerable potential for the evaluation of congenital anomalies of the heart and great vessels exits. The size and shape of cardiac chambers and their anatomic relationships with each other and the great vessels can be demonstrated by the digital technique. Systemic and pulmonary veins may be demonstrated. Coarctation of the aorta and supracardiac total anomalous pulmonary venous return are readily diagnosed.

Bogren, et al. have shown that atrial and ventricular septal defects can be demonstrated with the intravenous digital technique (7). There is hope that cardiac shunts can be quantitated by the digital technique if corrections for scattered radiation and veiling glare within the image intensifier can be found.

Digital intravenous cardiac angiography, although in its infancy, has already demonstrated considerable potential for the evaluation of cardiac anatomy and physiology. It can be expected to be of major importance in the future for the evaluation of cardiac disorders.

REFERENCES

1. Castellanos, A., Pereiras, R., and Garcia, A., La angiocardiografia radioopaca, Arch Soc Estud Clin (Habana) 31, 523 (1937).
2. Robb, G.P., and Steinberg, I., Visualization of the chambers of the heart, the pulmonary circulation and the great blood vessels in man, AJR 41, 1–17 (1939).
3. Kruger, R.A., Mistretta, C.A., Houk, T.L., et al., Computerized fluoroscopy in real time for noninvasive visualization of the cardiovascular system, Preliminary studies, Radiology 130, 49–57 (1979).
4. Kronenberg, M.W., Price, R.R., Smith, C.W., et al., Evaluation of left ventricular performance using digital subtraction angiography, Am J Cardiol (in press).
5. Martin, E.C., Nichols, A.B., Stugenkey, K., et al., Low dose ventriculography with digital subtraction fluoroscopy, Presented at Radiology Society of North America Meeting, November 17, 1981.
6. Myerowitz, P.D., Turnipseed, W.D., Shaw, C.G., et al., Computerized fluoroscopy: New technique for the noninvasive evaluation of the aorta, coronary artery bypass grafts, and left ventricular function, J Thorac Cardiovasc Surg 83, 65–73 (1982).
7. Bogren, H.G., Bursch, J.H., Brennecke, R., and Heintzen, P.H., Intravenous angiocardiography using digital image processing: Experience with axial projections in normal pigs, Circulation 64 (IV), 220 (1981) (abstr).

12

DIGITAL SUBTRACTION ANGIOGRAPHY OF THE CHEST

Edward Buonocore
Michael T. Modic

Division of Radiology
Cleveland Clinic Foundation
Cleveland, Ohio

I. INTRODUCTION

The noninvasive nature and proven accuracy of intravenous digital subtraction angiography (1-3) is ideal for the evaluation of vascular chest abnormalities, particularly since the usual chest radiographic densities are combinations of vascular structures and air. DSA readily determines if unexpected radiographic findings are vascular, their relation to adjacent vital structures, and whether they are clinically significant.

Classification of chest abnormalities suited for examination by digital subtraction include cardiac, thoracic aorta, pulmonary vascular and hilar structure abnormalities, and disturbances of pulmonary ventilation and perfusion.

The purpose of this chapter is to illustrate the applications of digital radiography in the evaluation of chest disorders. Discussion will include the current practical applications, the near future expectations, and the future aspirations.

II. METHOD

The examinations are performed on a production DSA unit (DR 960 Technicare Corporation) with a 512 X 512 matrix. The x-ray tube (2-292 EIMAC, Salt Lake City, Utah) has a nominal focal spot selection of .6/1.2 mm and a heat capacity of

L I

400,000 heat units. A 1,000 mA generator (Septar, CRG Medical Corporation, Baltimore, Maryland) is used. X-rays are detected by using a 9 or 6, or 4.5 inch (22.5, 15, 11.25 cm) cesium iodide image-intensifying tube (Thompson-CSF Boulogna-Billancourt, France) and a 16:1 grid with 40 lines per centimeter is utilized. The output phosphor of the image tube is scanned with a lead oxide video camera tube. The video signal from the camera is logarithmically amplified and digitized for storage in each of two imagers with 512 X 512 X 12 bit memories. A PDP-11/34 computer (Digital Equipment Corporation, Maynard, Mass.) is used for image processing.

To expedite the procedures, a nurse inserts an 8", 16 guage angiocatheter in the arm vein while the patient waits in a holding area. The catheter is attached to a 50 cc bag of D5W with constant infusion to maintain patency. The catheter position and vein are examined fluoroscopically with a small test injection so that if the cannulated vein is tortuous or very small, the catheter can be repositioned.

With the injector syringe in the inverted position, 25 cc of D5W is layered over the contrast material. The injection rate is 12-20 cc per second. The layered D5W solution acts to flush the contrast material and decreases the time and concentration of contrast material within the vein. With careful loading of the D5W and contrast media while the syringe is in the inverted position, there is no significant mixing of the two solutions. Forty cc of Renografin-76 is the usual bolus dose and 3 cc per kilogram or five separate injections are the limit, depending on the patient's weight, age, and renal function. In children, doses are accordingly reduced to 10-20 cc per bolus at rates of 2-10 cc per second, according to the patient's size and available vein.

The T.V. signals can be digitized with different matrix formats depending on the acquisition rates. A 128 X 128 matrix can be acquired at 24 frames per second, 256 X 256 at 6 per second, and 512 X 512 at 1.2 frames per second. The mask frame is stored in the first memory and the subtracted images are viewed in real time from the second memory. The digital memory and computer interface produce real-time subtracted images and the capability to easily select and subtract other masks. Hard copies are made on a multiformat camera for record keeping. The average skin dose per study has been from 1 to 5 rads depending on the framing sequence.

III. APPLICATIONS

A. Cardiac

As an anatomic imaging modality, DSA is able to document accurately the transit of contrast material through the chambers of the heart and clearly outline their contribution to the configuration of the mediastinum (Fig. 1). Enlarged cardiac chambers, which may mimic mediastinal masses, are differentiated from masses adjacent and contiguous to the heart. Imaging of the course of media through the cardiac, arterial and venous structures eliminates the confusion

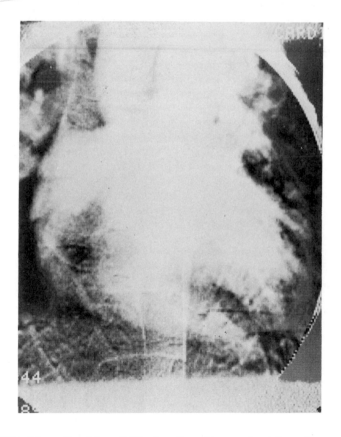

FIGURE 1A. Cardiac DSA in the AP projection demonstrating filling of the right and left ventricles through an interventricular septal defect. Note that the ventricular chambers are well identified in their contribution to the mediastinum.

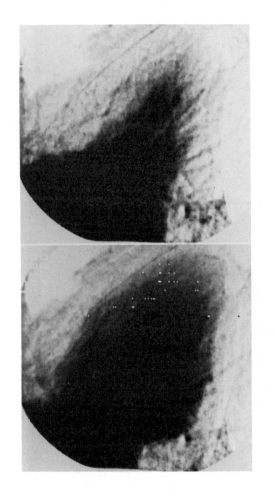

FIGURE 1B. Diastolic and systolic left ventricular digital subtraction angiograms in the RAP projection. Anatomic and physiologic data are retrieved from this study, total wall motion as well as contour of the left ventricular cavity.

produced by benign anomalous vascular structures, misinterpreted as abnormalities. Frequent examples include presence of dilated pulmonary veins (pulmonary varix) and arteries which mimic mediastinal tumors.

Masses discovered in the juxta-cardiac area often are difficult to separate from cardiac chambers (Fig. 2). Conversely, dilated selected chambers may distort the mediastinal outline and produce confusion with mediastinal neoplasms. These findings are clarified by angiography which is made available to outpatient care by the intravenous technique of digital subtraction studies.

Visualization of coronary artery bypass grafts is possible, but the distal run-off has not been demonstrated. Identification of the native coronary arteries has been observed, but it is usually the right and never with any consistency. However, intra-aortic supravalvular injections

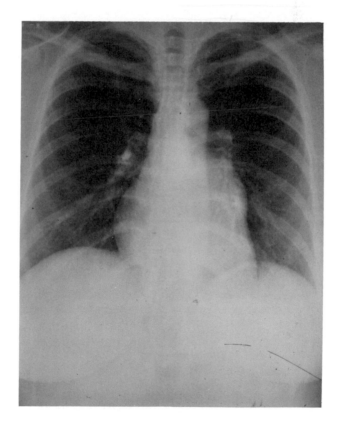

FIGURE 2A. PA examination of the chest showing unusual convexity of the left heart border.

of small doses of contrast material with and without EKG
gating has produced clinically satisfactory images of the
entire coronary circulation and this has been accomplished
with significantly lower doses of media and without the
hazards of selective arterial opacification.   Most notably,
anomalous coronary arteries originating from the pulmonary
circulation have been readily diagnosed by both arterial and
intravenous DSA studies (Fig. 3).

The acquisition of digital data has also been used to
provide quantitative information concerning cardiac dynamics.
Recirculation of contrast media in patients with congenital
heart defects is visualized directly and further documented by
timed appearance of contrast media curves.   Accurate
determination of intracranial shunts has been documented and
has compared favorably with those of nuclear medicine.
Quantification of the digitized data is useful in studying
dynamics of the left ventricle, including wall motion,
ejection fraction and stroke volume.   Congenital heart defects
such as single left ventricle, double chambered hearts,
anomalous pulmonary venous drainage, ASD's and VSD's have been
diagnosed by intravenous DSA, and the images have compared

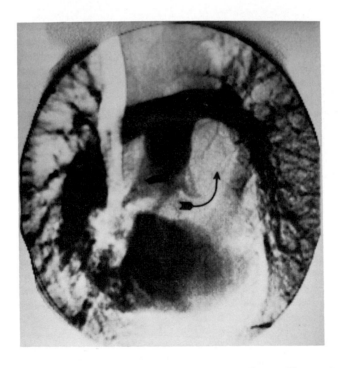

FIGURE 2B. *Right ventricular phase of cardiac DSA.*

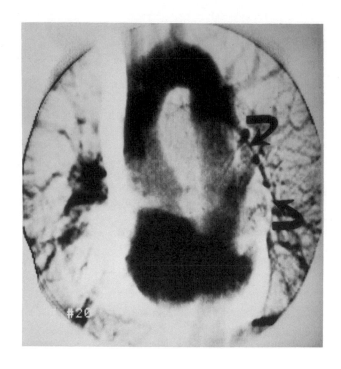

FIGURE 2C. Left ventricular phase. Note a large avascular mass is bordering the left heart border, paracardial cyst was found at surgery. DSA study clearly showed the mass was adjacent to but not a portion of the left ventricular cavity.

favorably with conventional catheterization studies on the same patients.

B. Thoracic Aorta

Tortuosity of the thoracic aorta, coarctation, and aneurysms, including traumatic and dissecting, can provide a variety of configurations that may be confused with mediastinal neoplasms. DSA consistently differentiates these entities (Fig. 4). This is particularly useful if a needle biopsy is contemplated. Occlusive atherosclerotic disease involving the origin of the great vessels from the aortra can be identified and frequent examples of great vessel occlusion,

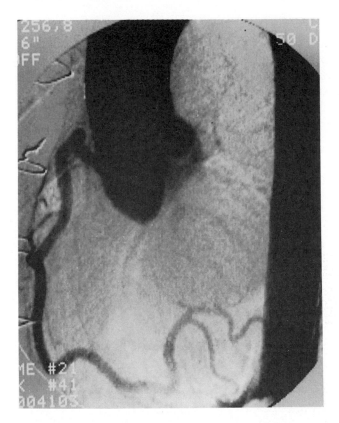

FIGURE 3. Digital subtraction angiogram after intra-aortic injection of 20 cc of contrast media; a solitary right pulmonary artery with retrograde filling into the anterior descending branch of the left coronary artery is identified.

including subclavian steal syndromes, have been recorded (Fig. 5). Normal anatomic variations of the great vessels and aberrant origins are readily identified.

C. Pulmonary Vessels

Unusual configurations of the main pulmonary arteries and veins which mimic hilar adenopathy are clarified by IV-DSA. In the evaluation of pulmonary embolic disease, DSA has identified the right ventricular chamber, outflow tract, main pulmonary artery, and the central pulmonary branches (Fig. 6). More peripheral vascular defects have been identified in isolated cases, but most have remained elusive to diagnosis by DSA. The inability of the patient to suspend respiration and involuntary motion and the overlap of numerous vessels have made evaluation of distal pulmonary branches unproductive.

Pulmonary nodules are readily separated into vascular and avascular densities on the basis of intravenous digital subtraction angiography examinations. One pulmonary lesion was identified that was initially thought to be a sequestration because of its abundant arterial supply from subdiaphragmatic vessels. The pulmonary mass was subsequently found to be an inflammatory process. Hence, the vascularity of pulmonary masses from either the pulmonary arterial system or bronchial arteries is discernable with the use of digital subtraction angiography.

D. Pulmonary Ventilation and Perfusion

Future hopes and expectations of digital radiography will be to identify regional air exchange and pulmonary perfusion without injection of contrast media and using the same system

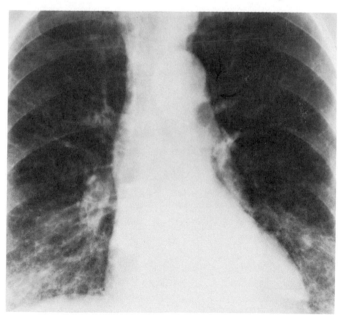

FIGURE 4A.   Chest x-ray in PA projection.   Small arrows delineate a suspicious density adjacent to the aortic arch, initially thought to be a metastatic nodule.

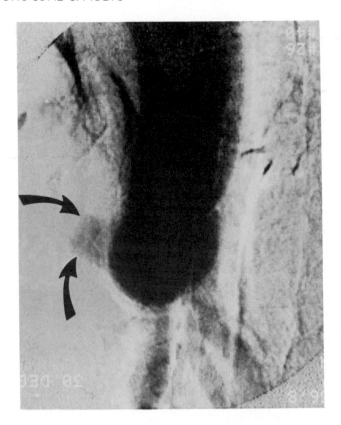

FIGURE 4B. *DSA of the aortic arch in AP projection*
demonstrates this to be an unusual aortic aneurysm.

that yields the studies of digital subtraction angiography.
The basis of this premise is that normal pulmonary densities
depend solely on vascular structures for identification. Air
spaces and normal interstitial structures do not attenuate the
x-ray beam. Radiographic pulmonary density depends on the
concentration of pulmonary vessels within a region. With
inspiration, the ingress of air will spread pulmonary
arteries, and with expiration, the depletion of air will
concentrate the pulmonary vascularity within the region of
observation.
    Pixel values reflect the linear attenuation coefficient
and correlate with the concentration of blood (vessels) in the
region of interest. Separate values for inspiration and
expiration represent the regional ventilation of the observed
area, if overlying attenuation by the chest wall can be
eliminated. Since the 1950's, pulmonary physicians have

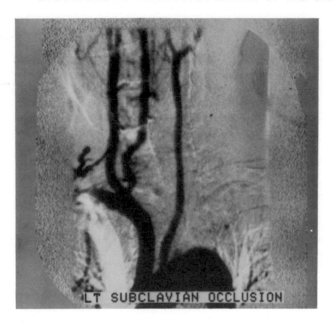

FIGURE 5A. DSA of the aortic arch after intravenous injection. Note complete occlusion of left subclavian artery.

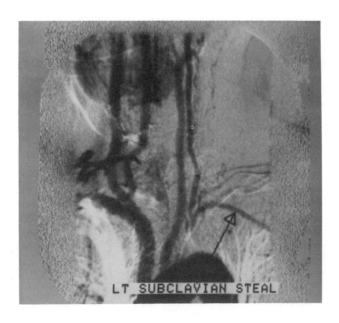

FIGURE 5B. Retrograde filling of the distal left subclavian is achieved through the left vertebral artery.

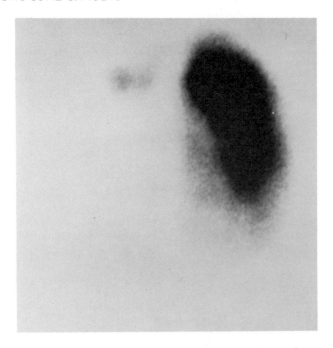

FIGURE 6A. Perfusion scan of the lungs showing almost total absence of isotope in the right lung except for a small accumulation in the right pulmonary apex.

using video densitometry through small intercostal windows achieved similar results (4).

Computer analysis of x-ray transmission through the chest has identified the contribution to pulmonary density by the pulmonary structures with selective elimination of the chest wall. Attempts have been made to correlate inspiraton/expiration ratios with the results of standard pulmonary ventilation tests in patients with a host of pulmonary diseases. Unfortunately, strict comparisons are impossible since conventional pulmonary function tests are global studies, which test mixing affect of both lungs and cannot take advantage of the regional examination possible with DSA.

Neoplasms may be identified by unexpectedly high pixel values during the expiratory phase of breathing resulting from localized air trapping. The sensitivity of electron imaging also will identify the contribution of pulmonary blood flow when a selected area is examined. A cyclic variation in pixel values overlying a portion of lung in suspended respiration has been identified and is attributed to the systolic and diastolic pulmonary flow.

Various entities including emphysema, restrictive lung disease and chronic obstructive pulmonary disorders have been studied with digital radiography and have produced consistent results. A further refinement of technique is required to make this a clinically useful entity.

IV. DISCUSSION

The exquisite sensitivity of improved electronic equipment including image intensifiers, T.V. systems, and computer

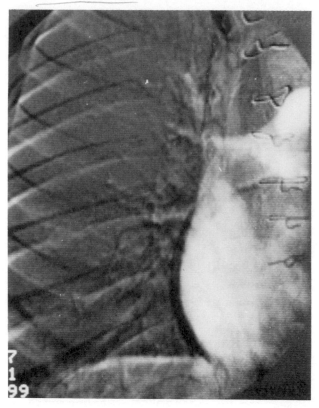

FIGURE 6B. Pulmonary DSA in 9 inch mode, showing occlusion of the main right pulmonary artery and nonperfusion of the major portion of the right lung. Note the close correlation with the isotope perfusion scan.

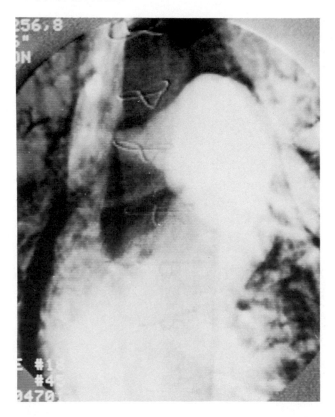

FIGURE 6C. Pulmonary DSA in 6 inch mode.

recording has simplified angiography in general, and has been
shown to be particularly applicable to the evaluation of the
chest. Rapidity, safety, accuracy and reproducibility after
intravenous injections have qualified digital subtraction
angiography as an outpatient technique. The current practical
application is the ready identification of all the vascular
structures of the chest, including intracardiac chambers.
    The expectations for the near future will be the ready
utilization of the digital data to produce quantitative
physiologic information. In progress is a study to correlate
the pixel flow curves of the cardiac chambers and great
vessels with the standard techniques of angiography and
nuclear medicine. Preliminary experience has indicated that
the flow data curves have compared favorably with the
information retrieved from nuclear medicine and angiographic
studies. A distinct advantage over nuclear medicine studies
is the consistently higher spatial resolution achieved with

digital subtraction angiography. Further experience with a larger number of patients is required before more definitive statements may be made.

Aspirations for the future include the conversion of the radiographic signal to digital data so that conventional radiographic examinations of the chest may be converted to physiologic evaluations. The differential evaluation of ventilation and perfusion in selected regions of interest should become readily available. This would convert the currently used subjective analysis of common chest radiographs to a more precise science. Descriptive picturesque terms of the past will be replaced by definitive quantitative values.

REFERENCES

1. MacIntyre, W.J., Pavlicek, W., Gallagher, J.H., Meaney, T.F., Buonocore, E., and Weinstein, M.A., Imaging capability of an experimental digital subtraction angiography unit, Radiology 139, 307-313 (1981).
2. Buonocore, E., Meaney, T.F., Borkowski, G.P., Pavlicek, W., and Gallagher, J.H., Digital subtraction angiography of the abdominal aorta and renal arteries: Comparison with conventional aortography, Radiology 139, 281-286 (1981).
3. Meaney, T.F., Weinstein, M.A., Buonocore, E., Pavlicek, W., Borkowski, G.P., Gallagher, J.H., Sufka, B., and MacIntyre, W.J., Digital subtraction angiography of the human cardiovascular system, AJR 135, 1153-1160 (1980).
4. Kourilsky, R., Marchal, M., Marchal, M.T., A new method of functional x-ray exploration of the lungs: Photo- electric stati-densigraphy, Diseases of the Chest 42(4), 345-358 (1962).

13

PULMONARY APPLICATIONS OF DIGITAL RADIOGRAPHY

Howard Jolles[1]
Rosalyn Reilley
Ronald R. Price[1]
Peter L. Lams[1,2]
Clyde W. Smith
A. Everette James, Jr.

Department of Radiology and Radiological Sciences
Vanderbilt University Hospital
Nashville, Tennessee

I. INTRODUCTION

The ability to convert x-ray attenuation data from analog to digital form offers a great deal of promise for diagnostic evaluation; the pulmonary area is no exception.

A common lung ailment affecting hospitalized patients is pulmonary embolic disease, a disorder that is often misdiagnosed. Presently, contrast pulmonary angiography is the most definitive technique for investigation of suspected pulmonary thromboembolic disease. This procedure has approximately a 4% risk of morbidity and mortality. Pulmonary angiography is contraindicated if the right ventricular end diastolic pressure exceeds 20 mm Hg at catheterization. Obviously, one would wish to have a noninvasive or less invasive procedure to provide this information. To some extent, radionuclide perfusion and inhalation studies fulfill this need. However, the radionuclide lung scan pattern may not provide a conclusive diagnosis but rather suggest the

[1]Supported by: Biomedical Research Support Grant RR-05424
[2]Present address: Brompton Hospital, London, England

probability of this or some other disease. False positive radionuclide lung scans may be recorded in lung zones poorly perfused because of impaired ventilation, even if no vascular obstructive lesions are present but resistance to blood flow is increased. Thus, in patients with COPD, congestive heart failure, or asthma, one may have to perform pulmonary arteriography to establish the diagnosis of embolism with certainty.

Digital techniques applied to radiographic imaging offer the potential of replacing catheter arteriography with a relatively noninvasive procedure requiring only intravenous injection of contrast media. In addition, arteriographic procedures can be performed with smaller amounts of contrast media. These advantages have been noted throughout this text and we are equally enthusiastic about its promise in evaluating the pulmonary vasculature. At most of the institutions using digital subtraction angiography (DSA), much of the work to date has been applied to studying peripheral arteries, especially the carotid and renal circulation. These techniques, when successfully applied to the pulmonary arteries, will make it possible to obtain high resolution images with an intravenous injection of reasonable amounts of contrast material. Actual clinical experience has been limited; most studies have been performed on animals. We have been fortunate to have access to three different types of digital systems, including one with bi-plane capability.

II. EXPERIMENTAL INVESTIGATION

We are currently investigating the diagnostic utility of digital subtraction angiography in the evaluation of pulmonary embolus using an animal model. Magnification (2x) pulmonary arteriography and pulmonary DSA are performed prior to and following gelfoam embolization of a selected pulmonary artery in the dog. With the catheter tip positioned in the iliac vein, the pulmonary DSA images were obtained in the six inch image intensifier mode and 512 X 512 matrix. This technique has produced the greatest detail with the least compromise in the size of the area of interest.

Figs. 1-3 illustrate the pulmonary images that are possible with current DSA equipment and how they compare with conventional angiography. Figs. 1A and 1B are conventional magnification pulmonary arteriograms (2x) of the right lower lobe vessels in a dog. Fig. 1A is the pre-embolization study and 1B is the study performed after the gelfoam embolization.

The occluded vessel is clearly seen and measures approximately 2.5 mm in diameter.

The DSA images corresponding to the selective pulmonary angiogram in Fig. 1 are shown in Figs. 2A and 2B. The study was performed with the image intensifier operating in the six inch image intensifier mode, with the injection of 15 cc of

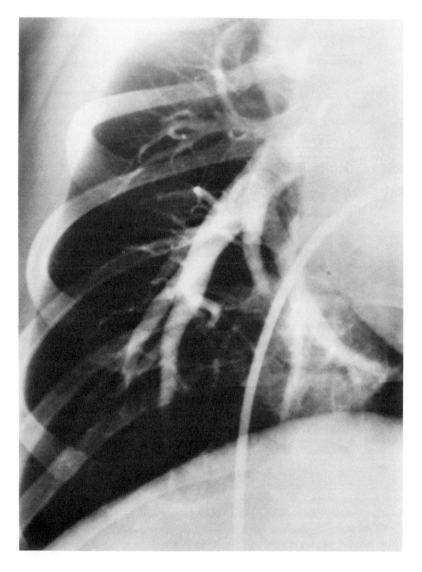

FIGURE 1A. Pre-embolization magnification (2x) arteriogram of right lower lobe vessels in a dog.

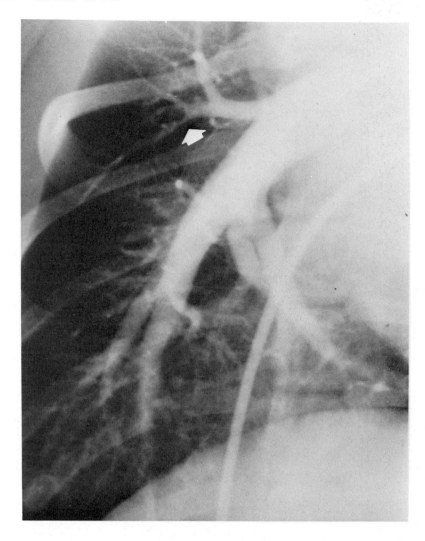

FIGURE 1B. Post-gelfoam-embolization magnification (2x) arteriogram of right lower lobe in dog.

contrast media into the right iliac vein of a 20 Kg dog. The images were acquired in a 512 X 512 matrix size at 1.2 images per second with suspended respiration. The comparison of the post-embolization DSA image clearly demonstrates the same embolus shown by the conventional arteriogram. Fig. 3 is a magnified view of Fig. 2B.

Although the digital intravenous pulmonary arteriogram is a very appealing procedure, it suffers from a number of shortcomings. These include motion artifacts, a limited field-of-view, and resolution somewhat inferior to film systems with arterial contrast media injections. Motion artifacts result both from respirations which might occur during the imaging portion of the study and from pulsations of the heart and aorta. The field-of-view, as has been noted, is dictated by the size of the image intensifier. In our laboratory, the maximum field-of-view is small, only 9 inches; however, the DSA images have been very promising provided the

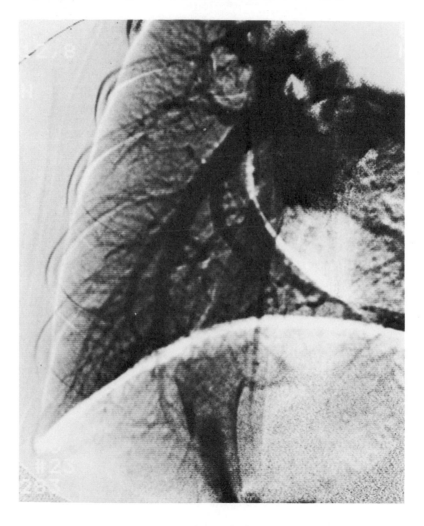

FIGURE 2A. Pre-embolization digital pulmonary angiogram 6-inch mode 512 X 512 matrix with catheter in right iliac vein.

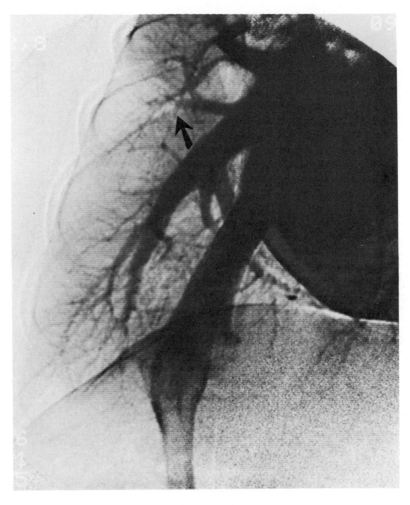

FIGURE 2B. Post-gelfoam-embolization pulmonary DSA 6-inch mode 512 X 512 matrix with catheter tip in right iliac vein.

suspect region has been defined prior to the DSA study. A preliminary perfusion radionuclide lung scan would be most helpful in this regard. Even though there are larger image intensifiers available, the field-of-view is closely coupled to the third shortcoming, resolution, so that as the field-of-view is increased, the resolution (for a fixed matrix size) is decreased. Larger field-of-view image intensifiers with an associated increased matrix size should obviate this problem. It is possible to visualize the pulmonary vessels with smaller amounts of contrast material than needed with

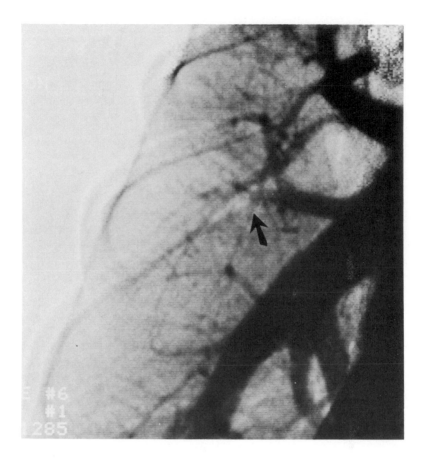

FIGURE 3. Post-gelfoam-embolization pulmonary DSA magnified view of Figure 2B.

carotid or extremity studies. This is because the arrival time of the contrast media in the pulmonary arteries is much shorter than in the peripheral arteries and the contrast bolus remains relatively intact.

As discussed earlier in the chapters by Price and Mistretta, framing rates at image matrix sizes greater than 512 X 512 are limited in data acquisition time to about 1 image per second. At this relatively slow imaging rate, one may find that without EKG gating of the image acquisition, images at peak concentration of the contrast media may not be recorded. This mistiming becomes more of a problem as the heart rate increases. We have, in our experience, however, been able to obtain excellent quality images in most cases without the aid of EKG gating. From comments made elsewhere in this text this seems to have been the experience of other groups.

In the chapter by Price, a number of applications of the different modes of data acquisition are discussed and how these might be advantageously utilized. Bi-plane imaging in the digital fluoroscopic mode has the potential to improve our assessment of the contrast filled pulmonary vessels (1).

Our bi-plane video-fluoroscopic and digital image-processing system is shown diagrammatically in Fig. 4. The system is capable of digitizing a video frame into an image matrix of 512 X 256 picture elements. By combining the independent video images from the anterior and lateral imaging systems into a single video image, we are able to digitize images simultaneously from both intensifying chains of a standard bi-plane system. Images generated in this manner are illustrated in Fig. 5.

The manner in which the combination image is digitized and subtraction protocols are employed is the same as that used for systems with a single video input. The video combiner module is inserted into the video chain to receive as input the signals from both image intensifying video camera systems and to generate a single standard video frame that contains selected portions of each input image.

The three-dimensional information provided by the real-time bi-plane imaging techniques described here should improve the accuracy of a number of DSA procedures. It should also minimize the number of contrast injections needed for an adequate clinical study.

III. DIGITAL ANALYSIS OF CHEST FILMS

In our laboratory, digital analysis of the mediastinum has demonstrated practical applications in chest radiography (Fig. 6) (2). For this assessment, the film is placed on an illuminator. A vidicon camera positioned over the illuminated film carries the image through a log amplifier and then to a video digitizer. The video signal is processed in a PDP-11/55 computer and displayed on a matrix of 512 X 256. Twenty-five normal PA radiographs have been digitized. Regions of interest for this study were drawn over the mediastinum, and density measurements obtained. The same process was carried out in selected radiographs of patients with known mediastinal disease (i.e., adenopathy, other masses, and carcinoma of the esophagus). By defining the normal density patterns of the mediastinum, we found it possible to predict mediastinal

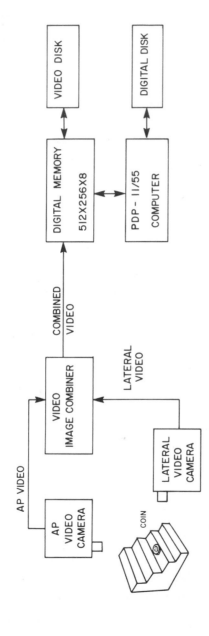

FIGURE 4. A schematic diagram of the digital video-fluoroscopic bi-plane system. Video images from both AP and lateral imaging chains are merged into a single video image before digitization. Digital images are stored on digital disk for further processing.

pathology on the basis of increased density alone, even when a contour abnormality could not be seen on the plain films. This capability could be extended to investigation of other intrathoracic areas.

IV. SCAN PROJECTION RADIOGRAPHY OF THE LUNG

With its scout film capability, computer tomography (CT) units, as noted elsewhere in this text, produce a digital scan projection radiograph. By keeping the x-ray tube and detector system in a fixed position (i.e., frontal, lateral, oblique), the patient is moved through the gantry while the x-ray beam is pulsed. In this manner, conventional format radiographs of the chest are obtained.

This system was compared with conventional radiography of the chest by Foley, et al. (3). The advantages of digital CT system were: 1) superior contrast resolution, due to better scatter rejection; 2) the intrinsic sensitivity, linearity, and dynamic range of the ionization detectors; and 3) the ability to manipulate the digital data by the computer, i.e., windowing and edge enhancement. The major disadvantage of the digital CT system was inferior spatial resolution of 0.5 line pairs/millimeter, compared to the 3-8 line pairs per millimeter capability of conventional radiography. Foley and

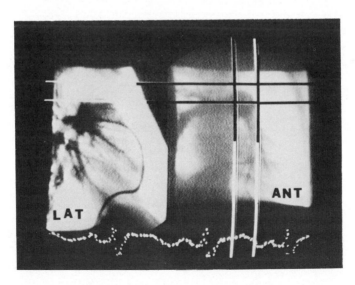

FIGURE 5. An example of a digitized bi-plane image following a ventricular injection of contrast media.

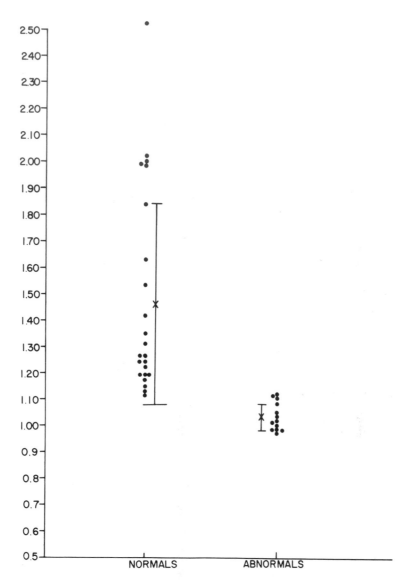

FIGURE 6. The numbers on the left represent the ratio of the density of the lower portion of the mediastinum, below the carina, to the upper portion where the trachea overlies the thoracic spine. Normally, this ratio is greater than one. In the abnormal group, this ratio is approximately one, the upper mediastinum being just as dense as the lower mediastinum.

his associates concluded that small, low contrast details in
the chest which were both linear and nodular were resolved
best by conventional radiography. When nodules could be
resolved utilizing the CT digital system, however, perception
was improved over plain radiography, due to superior contrast
discrimination and edge enhancement.

In addition to studies of contrast and spatial resolution
of computed tomography, lung density has also been measured by
Wegener, et al. (4). In this method, the CT numbers on one
slice are averaged together over the area of the lungs. A
histogram of lung density is then developed. This method
provides a quantitative measurement of the density of lung
parenchyma and has been proposed as a means to study diffuse
interstitial diseases. For example, the average CT number of
lung density has been found to be higher in renal failure
patients prior to dialysis and then became more negative
following dialysis. This difference could not be discerned on
the conventional chest radiographs. Wegener's data suggests
greater potential sensitivity of digitally obtained CT
measurements of lung density than chest radiographs, in this
instance, demonstrating the presence of increased
extravascular pulmonary water. Certainly this measurement is
of great clinical importance; special x-ray techniques, dual
indicator radionuclide dilution techniques, video densitometry
and microwave imaging have also been employed to make this
assessment (5).

V. OTHER DIGITAL SYSTEMS

In addition to the scan projection radiographic units
which are used as an adjunct to transverse section computed
tomography, a number of stand-alone units are now appearing in
the marketplace. One unit being developed (Picker
Corporation, Miner Road, Cleveland, Ohio) and now under
clinical evaluation is designed specifically for the chest.
The system uses a vertical array of detectors which are
opposed by an x-ray fan beam source which is mechanically
scanned across the patient's chest. Being a mechanically
scanned system, the imaging rate is relatively slow (a few
seconds), thus precluding the general use of the system for
DSA. The spatial resolution of the system is of the order of
1 mm.

Another unit for chest procedures (Fuji Corporation,
Tokyo, Japan) utilizes an "imaging plate" with heavy metal
halide salts as a detector. The most innovative aspect of
this system is that the plate is "developed" by a scanning

laser beam. The output of the laser scan is digitized, and the resulting information stored as a digital image. An advantage of this approach is that extremely high spatial resolution can be achieved because of the great scan precision provided by the laser beam. Unfortunately, the time required for the digitizing and transfer process is sufficiently long that DSA is not currently possible. Further discussion of the scan projection process can be found in the chapter by Heller.

Dual-energy subtraction techniques popularized by Brody and co-workers also promise to have several applications in chest radiography (6-9). For a given change in x-ray photon energy, the x-ray attenuation coefficient of various body tissues will differ. This basic principle has been applied by the Stanford group to produce images from which either bone or soft tissue have been subtracted. The patient is moved linearly through a modified CT scanner in which the x-ray source rapidly alternates between 85 and 135 KVp. This produces a combined image created by two different x-ray energies. Computer processing of this interlaced image results in cancellation of either soft tissue or bone density.

It is expected that this technique will enhance the detection of pulmonary parenchymal abnormalities by subtracting out the overlying bony thorax. Conversely, bone lesions may become more obvious on soft tissue cancellation images. Because the dual-energy estimates the mean atomic number of materials constituting the radiographic images, tissue characterization may be possible by appropriate analysis based on the dual-energy images. Characterization of such lesions as lung nodules may be achieved on the basis of their mean atomic numbers. One might also use this technique to evaluate extravascular pulmonary water. Applications of this technique to DSA are presently limited as only a narrow area of interest can be scanned at relatively slow frame rates.

The principles of dual-energy imaging have been expanded to triple-energy radiography. With the former, either soft tissue or bone can be subtracted, but not both. The triple-energy process allows both to be cancelled. If this could be adapted to current DSA systems, it would be possible to image only the iodinated contrast filled vessels, eliminating the overlying bone and soft tissues of the chest wall (10,11).

VI. CONCLUSION

Preliminary results of pulmonary DSA are very encouraging. It is believed that this relatively noninvasive technique has the potential to fill a great diagnostic need. At this time, it is possible to visualize small embolic vessel occlusions of about 2.5 mm. Future improvements needed are a larger field of view with an increased matrix size and a faster framing rate.

Bi-plane imaging has the potential to yield more diagnostic information with decreased radiation and contrast burden to the patient. Dual and triple-energy subtraction techniques are expected to provide better detection of parenchymal abnormalities and enhance visualization of contrast filled pulmonary vessels.

The major limiting factor of digital images of the lung parenchyma appears to be inferior spatial resolution when compared with conventional radiography. It is expected that future technical refinements will diminish this problem. Advantages of digital images of the chest include superior contrast resolution and the potential for computer manipulation of the image. A quantitative measurement of lung density is also possible, which may reflect diffuse abnormalities not apparent on the conventional chest radiograph. Digital evaluation of the mediastinum has broadened our understanding of the normal radiographic anatomy and made it possible to detect abnormalities entirely on the basis of density (rather than contour) aberrations.

REFERENCES

1. Price, R.R., Radiology 143, 255-257 (1982).
2. Lams, P.M., Unpublished data.
3. Foley, D.W., et al., Digital radiography of the chest using a computed tomography instrument, Radiology 133, 231-234, (1979).
4. Wegener, O.H., Koeppe, P., and Oeser, H., Measurement of lung density by computed tomography, J. Comput. Assist. Tomogr. 2, 263-273 (1978).
5. Nudleman, S., Capp, M.P., Fisher, H.D., Frost, M.M., and Roehrig, H., Photoelectronic imaging for Radiology, IEEE Trans. on Nuclear Science NS-28(1), 190-204 (1981).
6. Sommer, F.G., Brody, W.R., Macovski, A., and Alvarez, R.E., Dual-energy scanned projection radiography, Applied Radiology (March/April 1982).

7. Brody, W.R., Cassel, D., Sommer, F.G., et al., Dual-energy project radiography: Initial clinical experience, AJR 1347, 201-205 (1981).
8. Brody, W.R., Butt, G., Hall, A., et al., A method for selective so tissue and bone visualization using scanned projection radiography, Med. Phys. 8, 353-357 (1981).
9. Lehmann, L.A., Alvarez, R.A., Macovski, A., et al., Generalized image combinations in dual kVp digital radiography, Med. Phys. 8, 659-667 (1981).
10. Brody, W.R., Hybrid subtraction for improved intravenous arteriography, Radiology 141, 828-831 (1981).
11. Macovski, A., Alvarez, R.E., Lehmann, L.A., et al., Iodine imaging using three energy spectra, SPIE Proc. 314, 140-142 (1981).

14

DIGITAL VIDEO SUBTRACTION ANGIOGRAPHY
OF THE RENAL CIRCULATION

Bruce J. Hillman

Department of Radiology
University of Arizona College of Medicine
and Health Sciences Center
Tucson, Arizona

I. INTRODUCTION

Since 1974, University of Arizona researchers have pursued
the development of a digital radiographic system suitable for
performing intravenous angiography. The result—digital video
subtraction angiography (DVSA)—is based on a sequence of
highly sensitive electronic components which make possible the
visualization of vascular structures containing less than 2%
radiographic contrast material concentration. Initial efforts
were oriented toward imaging the cervical circulation, because
of its superficiality and relative freedom from superimposed
structures. In the past eighteen months, however, attention
has been redirected to include the challenges presented in
imaging the renal circulation. In so doing, DVSA has been
applied to the diagnosis of a variety of renal vascular
abnormalities. These have included: investigation of
possible renovascular etiology of hypertension (1-3),
characterization of renal masses, evaluation of unexplained
hematuria, depiction of the arterial circulation of renal
transplant donors and recipients (1,4), and evaluation
following surgical or transluminal renal angioplasty (5).
University of Arizona's reports to date, and those of
other authors (6-8), have largely related anecdotal
experiences or small series. Now, however, University of
Arizona investigators have compiled the results of 100 digital
intravenous angiographic examinations of the renal
circulation. These results indicate that DVSA is a safe,

215

quickly performed, inexpensive method for angiographic examination of outpatients, and is suitable for screening and diagnosis of renal vascular abnormalities.

II. DVSA SYSTEM AND INJECTION TECHNIQUE

Renal intravenous angiography is performed by first inserting a 16 G angiocatheter into an antecubital vein, then, by Seldinger technique, advancing a 7 French pigtail catheter with sideholes into the distal superior vena cava. There follows the mechanical injection of 76% meglumine-sodium diatrizoate, 45 cc's (30 cc's per second for 1.5 seconds). The central injection site and the rapidity of the injection serve the purpose of presenting a concentrated bolus of contrast to the region of interest, improving visualization of small vascular structures and abnormalities. This is particularly important in patients with poor cardiac function, in whom a successful diagnostic examination may be impossible using a more prolonged injection method. This injection method varies from those reported by other institutions; however, this method has been developed with the intent to optimize image quality while minimizing risk. The group at the University of Wisconsin also is now advancing a catheter into a central vein prior to injection (see chapter by Sackett). This catheter, however, is smaller (5 French), and they administer a more prolonged injection, delivering a similiar contrast load (9). Buonocore et al., at the Cleveland Clinic, have focused their efforts on keeping the examination as "non-invasive" as possible. They continue to inject contrast at a rate of 10-12 cc/second via an antecubitally-placed 8 inch angiocatheter. Contrast is layered onto a volume of 5% dextrose to assist its transit centrally (8) (see chapter by Buonocore). The advantage of this technique is that the procedure may be performed by nurses or technologists, requiring only that the images be monitored by the radiologist prior to the conclusion of the study. Despite this, University of Arizona scientists believe that studies of diagnostic quality may be more consistently achieved by taking the additional effort to place a central catheter. In addition, their work indicates that intravascular contrast levels and arterial demonstration may be improved by administering contrast as a compact bolus, rather than by more prolonged injection.

Exposing images begins immediately upon injection, directly onto an image intensifier, at a rate of one per second for 15-20 seconds. Images are transmitted by a frogshead plumbicon camera to an A/D converter, are digitized, and sent to our computer-memory complex (Fig. 1). At the behest of a radiologist-operated interactive keyboard, images obtained prior to the appearance of contast in the renal arteries are subtracted from those containing contrast material; resulting images are variably enhanced to depict anatomical detail, then undergo post-processing to optimize diagnostic content (Fig. 2). Software programs designed to improve diganostic reliability include, among others: smoothing and edge enhancing filtration, magnification, noise reducing image averaging, reference frame shift to improve pre- and post-conttrast image registration. The use of such programs has proven invaluable in extracting initially obscured diagnostic information and in salvaging examinations which might otherwise have been nondiagnostic (Fig. 3).

III. CLINICAL EXPERIENCE

The Arizona group has previously reported several series dealing with renal vascular abnormalities. One early publication discussed the reliability of intravenous angiography in investigating a variety of renal circulatory lesions (1). In this work, 36 of 39 examinations (92%) were of diagnostic quality. Twenty of 21 examinations (95%), for which correlation with subsequent clinical, radiographic, or pathologic diagnoses were available, were proven accurate.

Another series dealt with the efficacy and cost-effectiveness of digital intravenous angiography in case-finding for renovascular hypertension (3). The examinations of 38 patients were prospectively evaluated, at the time of their performance, and assigned to one of three groups: a) definitely showing one or more stenoses--15 cases (41%) (Fig. 4); b) definitely normal--17 cases (46%); or c) possibly abnormal, requiring catheter angiography--5 cases (13%). Thirteen of the 15 positive cases subsequently underwent radiologic or surgical procedures which verified the intravenous angiographic diagnosis. However, only one of the 17 negative cases--negative on catheter angiography--has born similar scrutiny.

Applying this experience to the broader question of the efficacy of case-finding for renovascular hypertension has yielded interesting results. The projected costs incurred in examining one hundred newly discovered moderately or severely hypertensive patients by DVSA, and treating those whose hypertension is related to renal artery stenoses by percutaneous transluminal angioplasty (PTA), are comparable to

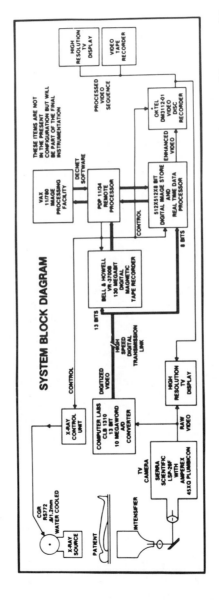

FIGURE 1. System block diagram for University of Arizona digital video subtraction angiography.

those costs expected for a lifetime of medical therapy. In addition, the lowered morbidity associated with PTA should compare favorably with medical therapy in view of the severity of potential drug side effects and published rates of non-compliance.

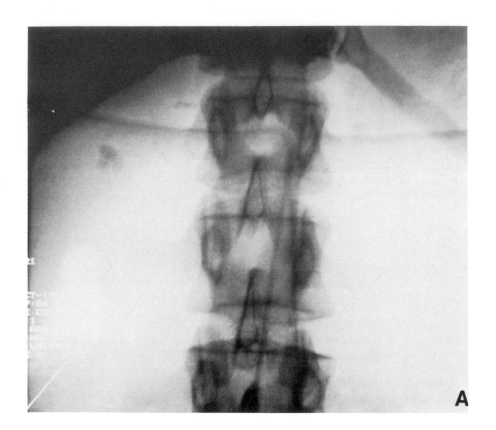

FIGURE 2. Digital intravenous angiogram of a potential renal donor. (A) Pre-contrast raw data image--contrast was mechanically injected one second previously but has not yet reached the abdominal arterial circulation. (B) Post-contrast raw data image--seven seconds following administration, contrast material is faintly seen in the abdomen. (C) Subtraction image. (D) Electronically enhanced subtraction image improves visualization of the renal arteries (arrows). (E) Diagnostic image--the pre-contrast raw data image has been shifted into better registration ("reference shift"), removing artifact produced by patient motion of the spine. A weighted, nine-point smoothing filter also improves image sharpness.

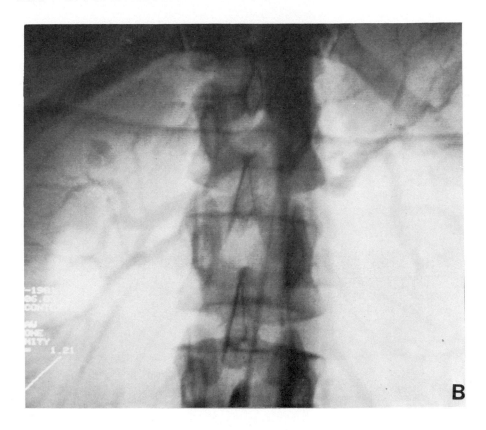

FIGURE 2 (continued).

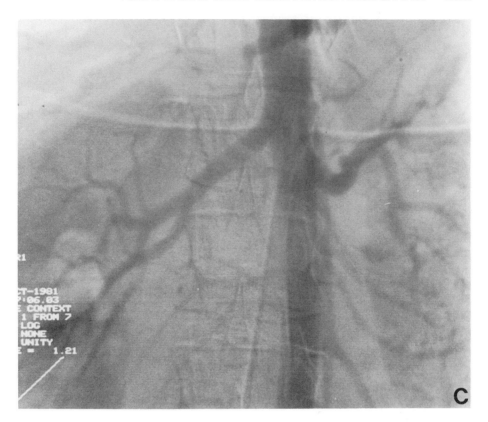

FIGURE 2 (continued).

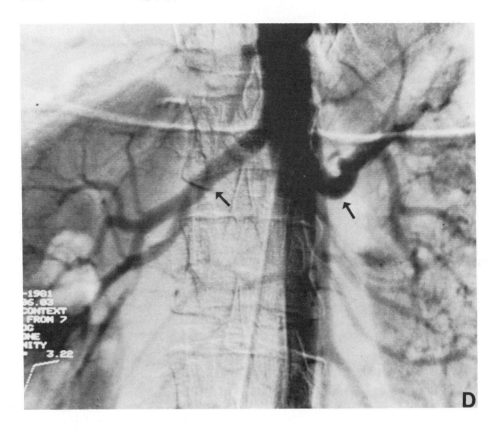

FIGURE 2 (continued).

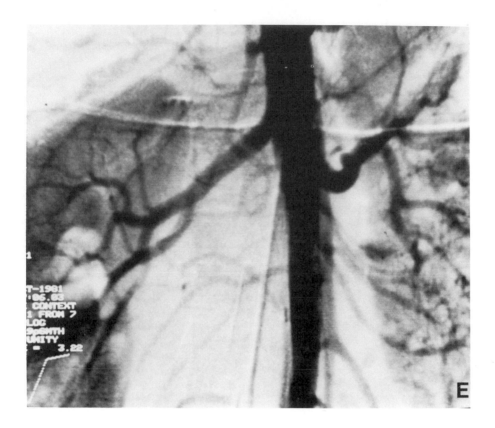

FIGURE 2 (continued).

Recently, the series of 30 examinations relating to the clinical area of renal transplantation has been evaluated (4). For indications relating to potential donor evaluation and investigation of transplant recipients, digital intravenous angiography has become the preferred examination at the University of Arizona's Health Sciences Center. In the case of preoperative evaluation of renal donors, intravenous angiography has accurately depicted the number, position, and lengths of the renal arteries and has excluded the presence of significant atherosclerotic or fibromuscular disease. In so doing, it saves the potential donor the discomfort and morbidity of arterial catheterization and the expense of

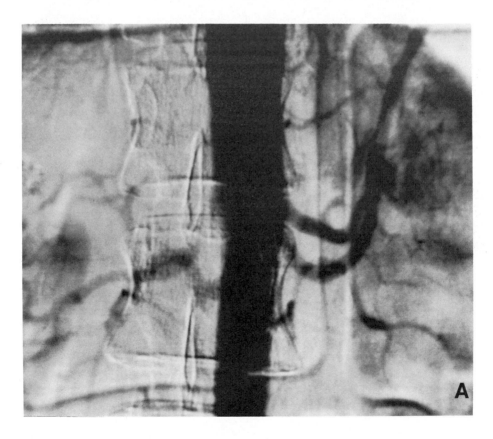

FIGURE 3. An elderly woman presented with accelerating hypertension. (A) The patient moved considerably between pre- and post-contrast exposures, resulting in spinal artifact overlying the region of interest. (B) Following "reference shift", a severe right renal artery stenosis (arrow) is clearly visualized.

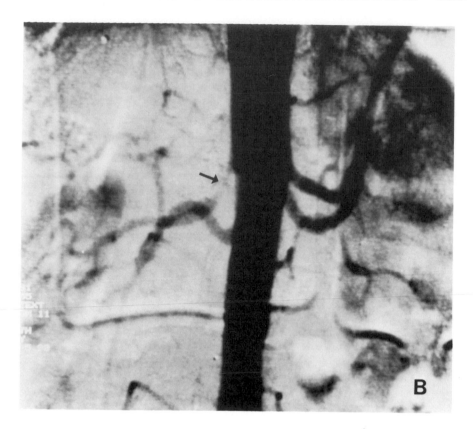

FIGURE 3 (continued).

associated hospitalization. Digital intravenous angiography
has been particularly valuable for investigating the problems
of renal allograft recipients. This population group is
particularly subjected to repeated and prolonged
hospitalizations and discomforting procedures. Digital
intravenous angiography has been successfully applied to the
indications of hypertension (Fig. 5), evaluation following
transplant artery angioplasty, masses, and unexplained
worsening of allograft function in the clinical setting of
renal transplantation (4).

In all, 100 DVSA examinations of the renal circulation
(Table I) have been performed. Of these 50 have been
interpreted, at the time of the examination, as demonstrating
some abnormality. Forty-four examinations were believed
normal, while in 6 others, no diagnosis was possible.
Seventy-six attempted examinations which resulted in
anatomical information comparable to that achievable by

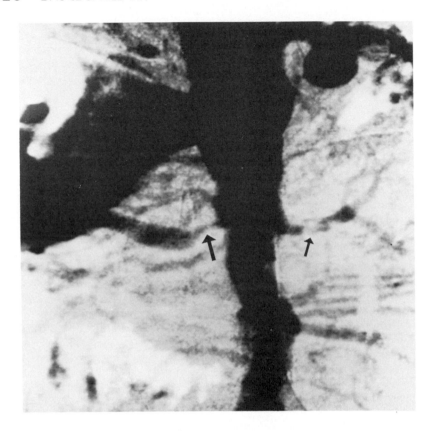

FIGURE 4. A hypertensive middle-aged man had a positive intravenous urogram performed at an outside hospital. His digital intravenous angiogram demonstrates a long right renal artery (large arrow) stenosis (the normal kidney on urography), and a mid-left renal artery stenosis (small arrow).

conventional angiography. In 18, images were considered to be of suboptimal quality; however, sufficient information was obtained to either make a diagnosis or suggest an ensuing step in the patient's evaluation. Problems resulting in this assessment largely related to uncontrollable patient or bowel gas motion, patient obesity, or poor cardiac output. No diagnostic information was produced in 6 examinations. In 3 of these, cardiac function was so poor as to preclude visualization of the renal circulation sufficient for diagnosis. Two patients had non-displaceable bowel gas. One early patient, examined via a direct antecubital injection, suffered a rupture at the injection site. However, neither in

TABLE I.   Referrals for Performance of Renal DVSA

	100 Cases[a]
Hypertension	*53*
Renal allografts	*21*
Characterization of mass	*12*
Potential renal donors	*10*
Unexplained hematuria	*7*
Postoperative evaluation	*6*
Post-embolization evaluation	*3*
Preoperative vascular anatomy	*1*

[a]*Some patients had more than one indication
for referral.*

this case, nor in any other renal DVSA examination, has a patient suffered any lasting morbidity. Among the 40 cases which have gone on to a definite radiologic, surgical or pathologic procedure, the DVSA etiologic diagnosis has been corroborated in 36 (90%).

IV. PROBLEMS AND SOLUTIONS

Although the central concept of digital video subtraction angiography remains the same for the abdomen as with the neck, abdominal, and particularly renal, intravenous arteriography presents a new set of challenges not encountered in these other areas (Table II). Specifically, these include a wider variation in radiographic techniques, superimposition of vasculature, and respiratory and peristalsing bowel gas motion. We have overcome difficulties with variations in patient size and vascular superimposition by careful attention to radiographic technique and the performance of multiple injection–exposure sequences in varying obliquities. However, as noted by Buonocore et al., positioning the patient in such a way that the renal artery origins are seen in tangent is a procedure of trial and error, and may prove difficult in actual practice (8). Since we prefer to make no more than three injection–exposure sequences during an examination, patients with more than three renal arteries may require arterial catheterization to avoid missing concealed

TABLE II. Problems with Digital Intravenous Angiography and their Potential Solutions

Problem	? Solution
Small intensifiers	Research and development
Motion artifact	Multiple reference-subtraction pairs; reference shift
Overlying vessels	Multiple projections
Low cardiac output	Central catheter bolus injection
Bones/s.t./gas differences	Logarithmic subtraction
Noise	Filtration, averaging
Bowel gas motion	Compression, glucagon

atherosclerotic lesions near renal artery origins. The possibility of bi-plane as noted by Price et al. (see chapter by Jolles) may assist with this problem.

One potential problem with abdominal intravenous angiography, which is frequently cited, is the need for patient cooperation. This is because a cessation of patient motion—respiratory and corporeal—is necessary for proper registration of mask and post-contrast images, so that satisfactory digital subtraction may be performed. In clinical practice, this has proven less of a problem than

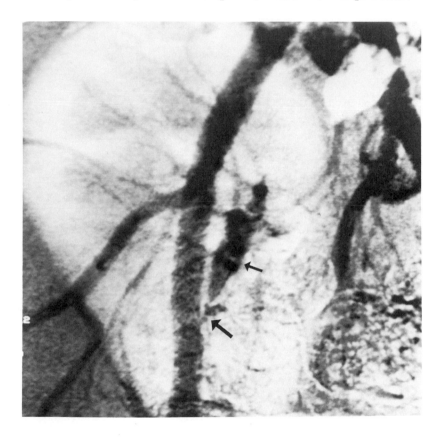

FIGURE 5. This patient developed hypertension one year following renal transplantation in which the transplant renal artery was anastomosed directly to the external iliac artery. There is a long severe stenosis of the allograft artery (large arrow) with post-stenotic dilation (small arrow). The nephrogram is shown simultaneously by using as a reference frame an image exposed following the passage of contrast through the arterial circulation.

originally supposed, permitting intravenous angiographic evaluation of severely ill patients, who might benefit most from the relative benignity of this procedure.

We have described successful performance of digital renal intravenous angiography on patients with severe respiratory compromise (1). The effects of motion are ameliorated by careful selection of mask-contrast image pairs and the use of a software program which permits the radiologist-operator to shift the position of the mask image into better registration. The former is facilitated by beginning exposures immediately, resulting in the exposure of 5-10 potential mask images prior to contrast reaching the renal circulation. Storage of all raw data images in digital form permits rapid and faithful retrieval of each image for registration with post-contrast raw data images. The latter technique of "reference shift" has salvaged numerous examinations in which the ability of the patient to cooperate was compromised and it has been most useful in correcting misregistration artifacts due to corporeal or respiratory motion (Fig. 3).

Finally, bowel gas peristalsing over the region of interest will produce artifacts which obscure vascular detail. Again, the problem is one of misregistration due to motion between the exposure of mask and post-contrast images. However, since the motion is local, rather than generalized, shifting the position of the reference image is unlikely to improve image quality. In our own experience, a urographic compression device, inflated over the area of interest prior to injection, has been nearly universally successful in displacing bowel gas and permitting visualization of the renal circulation (1) (Fig. 6). We have also administered 1 mg of glucagon, IV, in an effort to halt peristalsis of non-displaceable bowel. This has been successful occasionally, but not in all cases.

V. POTENTIAL FOR PHYSIOLOGIC QUANTIFICATION

Perhaps the most exciting area of current research is the application of photoelectronic imaging modalities to the quantification of physiologic processes. As Crummy et al. have noted, this is feasible because "the iodine contrast...is proportional to the products of iodine concentration and the vascular thickness along a path normal to the image plane" (7). Thus, temporal alterations in the density of an anatomic structure through which contrast is passing should reflect characteristics of its flow. Using this concept, they have been able to plot changes in ventricular volume during the course of the cardiac cycle, and hence, calculate cardiac ejection fraction. Drs. Heintzen and Brennecke of Keil, Germany, have been working in this area for a number of years. Their preliminary work has been in analyzing video tapes, obtained simultaneously with cine angiocardiograms, and in performing cardiac output measurements, shunt calculations and vascular flow studies (10). They have designed, and are now in the process of building, a digital video subtraction system for imaging and physiologic quantification of the heart.

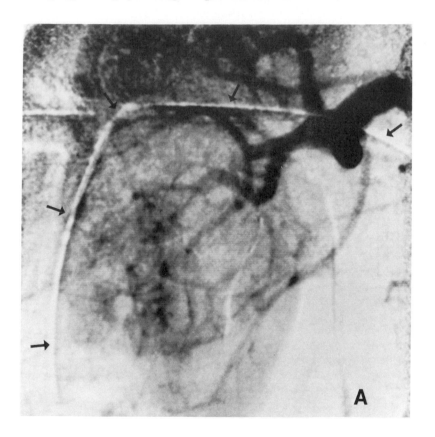

FIGURE 6. (A) An excretory urogram showed this middle-aged man to have a right renal mass. A urographic compression balloon (arrows) displaced bowel gas from the area of interest on digital intravenous angiography. The arterial phase of the digital intravenous angiogram demonstrates distorted renal arterial arborization and neovascularity, indicative of hypernephroma. (B) The venous phase demonstrates a patent main renal vein (large arrow).

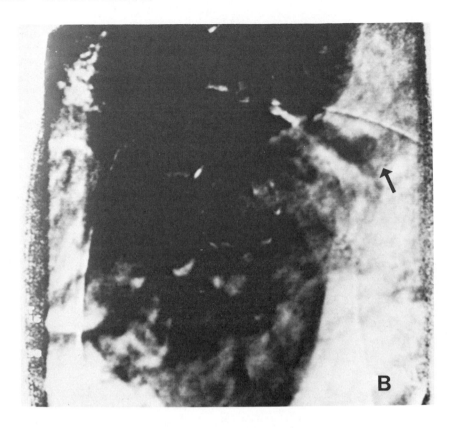

FIGURE 6 (continued).

Meaney et al. have reported experiments investigating the relationship among videodensitometric measurements of renal artery, cortex and medulla in transplant patients (6). This technique bears considerable promise for the estimation of contrast transit times through vascular and tissue compartments, which will aid in the diagnosis of arterial and parenchymal disease. Similarly, University of Arizona researchers are currently investigating methods for the non-invasive quantification of total renal and renal cortical blood flow, using experimental contrast agents and digital fluorography. These efforts have met with some success; however, as indicated by Mistretta et al., one must yet contend with sources of error peculiar to digital radiography before such methods of measurement become feasible. These authors cite particularly the problems of veiling glare and x-ray scattering related to the use of image intensifiers in imaging opaque structures. One must also contend with signal variation as well as image amplifier output drift (9). In addition, the more mundane consideration of consistency of the tissues the beam must traverse at one locus, relative to another, needs also to be taken into account. Baily has written an excellent review of the early work done in this area, which critically evaluates the problems associated with adapting digital fluorography to physiologic quantitation (11).

VI. SUMMARY

Experience with renal digital intravenous angiography remains at best preliminary, but is likely to burgeon in the near future with the incipient dissemination of commercial systems. To date, these results with the DVSA system indicate that digital intravenous angiography is a safe, quickly performed, accurate method for screening and diagnosing a variety of renal vascular abnormalities in outpatients. In addition, the relatively low cost of examination and its potential for physiologic quantification should make it an attractive alternative to conventional arteriography in appropriate clinical situations. Other experiences detailed in this text will support this concept.

REFERENCES

1. Hillman, B.J., Ovitt, T.W., Nudelman, S., et al., Digital video subtraction angiography of renal vascular abnormalities, Radiology 139, 277-280 (1981).
2. Hillman, B.J., Ovitt, T.W., Chirstenson, P.C., et al., Diagnosis of vascular disease by photoelectronic intravenous angiography, JAMA (in press).
3. Hillman, B.J., Ovitt, T.W., Capp, M.P., et al., The potential impact of digital video subtraction angiography (DVSA) on screening for renovascular hypertension, Radiology (in press).
4. Hillman, B.J., Zukoski, C.F., Ovitt, T.W., et al., Digital video subtraction angiography in the evaluation of potential renal donors and renal allograft recipients. Manuscript submitted for publication.
5. Osborne, R.W., Jr., Goldstone, J., Hillman, B.J., et al., Digital video subtraction angiography: Screening technique for renovascular hypertension, Surgery (in press).

6. Meaney, T.F., Weinstein, M.A., Buonocore, E., et al.,
    Digital subtraction angiography of the human
    cardiovascular system, AJR 135, 1155–1160 (1980).
7. Crummy, A.B., Strother, C.M., Sackett, J.F., et al.,
    Computerized fluoroscopy: Digital subtraction for
    intravenous angiocardiography and arteriography, AJR
    135, 1131–1140 (1980).
8. Buonocore, E., Meaney, T.F., Borkowski, G.P., et al.,
    Digital subtraction angiography of the abdominal aorta
    and renal arteries, Radiology 139, 281–286 (1981).
9. Mistretta, C.A., Crummy, A.B., Strother, C.M., Digital
    angiography: A perspective, Radiology 139, 273–276
    (1981).
10. Brennecke, R., Hahne, H.J., Moldenhauer, K., et al.,
    Improved digital real-time processing and storage
    techniques with applications to intravenous contrast
    angiography, Comput. Cardiol., pp. 191–194 (1978).
11. Bailey, N.E., Video techniques for x-ray imaging and
    data extraction from roentgenographic and fluoroscopic
    presentations, Med. Phys. 7, 472–491 (1980).

15

USE OF DIGITAL SUBTRACTION ANGIOGRAPHY TO ASSESS FUNCTION

Thomas F. Meaney
Joe H. Gallagher

Cleveland Clinic Foundation
Cleveland, Ohio

I. INTRODUCTION

The digitization of serial video images from the television camera during the digital subtraction angiography process provides a sequence of images containing numerical information. Numerical data for each pixel within the sequence can be used to provide functional information either from a defined region of interest within the image or from the entire image itself.

The acquisition of accurate quantitative information derived from the x-ray attenuation of x-rays by iodinated contrast media, e.g., ejection fraction determination, is limited primarily by Compton scatter and veiling glare within the image intensifier tube. These factors, without correction, may make the measurements invalid for clinical purposes when the quantitative information is required. However, parameters based upon relative measurements such as time of contrast arrival, transit through a vessel or organ, distribution of contrast within an organ as a function of time, recirculation times of contrast material within the heart in congenital heart disease, and frequency and amplitude of myocardial wall motion are all parameters which can be assessed from the digital subtraction angiography images without absolute calibration.

The measurement of absolute blood flow within the various vessels, particularly those which are narrowed due to disease, has been a long sought for goal for noninvasive techniques. Unfortunately, factors such as very high velocity of blood flow in vessels such as the carotid and renal arteries would require exceedingly high framing rates, beyond the capability of current digital subtraction angiography equipment. Despite such limitations, clinically useful assessments can be made taking advantage of the usual paired nature of most of the arteries in the body which are of clinical interest. These are the internal carotid arteries, the renal arteries, and arteries to the extremities. Placement of region–of–interest cursors over such paired vessels gives one the opportunity to assess the arrival time, peak concentration, and "wash–out" of contrast in one artery relative to its paired vessel, and also to assess the slope of the inflow and outflow of contrast material through the region of interest. These measurements can be made using cursors to indicate the region of interest where the average attenuation of iodine per pixel or the total attenuation is to be determined.

In the assessment of congenital heart disease, both pre- and postoperative, the presence of right–to–left or left–to–right intracardiac shunts may be evaluated using time–density curves generated from regions–of–interest over the right or left side of the heart. Such information is usually difficult, if not impossible, to determine from simple inspection of serial images.

The dynamics of ventricular wall motion may be assessed in several ways, using the digital information derived from intravenous digital subtraction techniques. Gated systolic and diastolic images provide a gross representation of myocardial wall motion. In addition, standard nuclear cardiology techniques can be used to detect alterations in frequency and amplitude of left ventricular wall motion.

Parametric images may also be obtained using the digital subtraction data. The time at which the maximum attenuation of the contrast media occurs in each pixel during the series of images can be determined and a single parametric image may be displayed using either the numerical data or color coding of each pixel to indicate the time at which the maximum attenuation occurred. This type of parametric image is particularly useful in studying organs such as the kidney, where inhomogeneities within the organ's blood flow might result in a spurious assessment of the transit of contrast material should only a small region of interest be selected. One of the advantages of the parametric image is that it prevents incorrect sampling of a portion of the organ which may not be representative of the organ as a whole.

Even though the digital pixel values are not calibrated to the absolute concentration of contrast material, the maxima and minima of the time-concentration curves will occur at exactly the same times as the true concentration curves.

Such parametric images have been applied to the assessment of renal transplants. We have found that the time-to-maximum parametric image clearly differentiates normal from abnormal renal function and, with the addition of time-to-half-maximum images, provides a useful aid in differentiation between acute tubular necrosis and rejection.

II. PARAMETERS FOR RENAL TRANSPLANT EVALUATION

In the past decade, there has been continued improvement in the success rates following renal allotransplantation. This has been due, in part, to improved management of patients who experience early and late transplant complications. In the post-transplant period, differentiation between acute tubular necrosis, acute rejection, and surgical complications is essential to assure proper therapy. Acute tubular necrosis (ATN) may occur because of damage sustained during the interval between removal of the kidney from the donor and reimplantation into the recipient. During this interval, the kidney may not receive sufficient oxygen and nutrients, and some of the renal tubular cells die. No direct therapy is administered for ATN, but the patient is supported until the kidney recovers from the trauma and begins functioning again. In acute rejection, the body's immune system recognizes the presence of a foreign organ and begins attacking the transplanted kidney. This condition is characterized by fever, pain, swelling of the graft, and acute deterioration in the level of kidney function. Rejection is treated with immunosuppressive drugs which impair the body's ability to mount an attack against the transplanted organ. Surgical complications are rare but may occur if either the kidney's artery, vein, or ureter is not properly reconnected or if these structures become obstructed or blocked. Many renal transplant patients will experience some degree of ATN and almost every patient, except those who receive their own kidney (autotransplant), will experience some form of rejection.

The flow of blood through the kidney and the kidney's ability to remove waste products (such as iodinated radiographic contrast material) from the blood is one physiological measure of how well a transplanted kidney is functioning. Normally, when a bolus of contrast material enters the kidney, most of the contrast material is removed from the blood and is rather rapidly transported to the renal collecting system, through the ureter, to the bladder. The characteristic "wash-in" and "wash-out" of normal kidney function is illustrated in Fig. 1. In ATN, the flow of blood to the kidney is usually only mildly or moderately impaired. The blood carries the contrast material to the kidney; but, because of the damage to the tubules, the kidney is unable to excrete the contrast material as rapidly as it arrives. Typical moderate ATN has a slow rise in contrast material, as illustrated in Fig. 1. In rejection, there are local patchy areas which have markedly decreased blood flow. The swelling and the attack of the white blood cells cause the vessels to become stenosed. The very slight accumulation of contrast material characteristic of rejection is also shown in Fig. 1.

A graph of the concentration of radiographic contrast material as a function of time is a useful measure of the function of the kidney, but such a graph represents the average function of the region of the kidney which has been selected for analysis. What is needed is a measure of how each part of the kidney is performing.

A parametric image is a pictorial representation of some parameter of the time-concentration curve at each pixel. From a time sequence of images, the concentration as a function of location and time, $C(x,y,t)$, is used to derive a parametric image as a function of location, $P(x,y)$. The derived parameter may be a slope, a rate constant, an extremal value, a time of occurrence, etc.

Patients who had undergone renal transplantation or autotransplantation were evaluated by digital subtraction angiography. An intravenous injection of 40 ml of contrast material, Conray 400 or Renografin-76 was introduced into an antecubital vein at the rate of 12 to 15 cc per second by a pressure injection technique previously described (1,2). Digital images of 256 x 256 by 8 bits were acquired by a pre-prototype digital subtraction angiography (DSA) x-ray unit (3) or by a Technicare DR-960 digital subtraction unit. The start of the study sequence was delayed for several seconds after the injection but was begun before the contrast material arrived in the area of the pelvis. Examinations ranged from 11 to 37 seconds in duration, with the typical examination being 20 seconds. All image frames were acquired in the logarithmically amplified mode at frame rates of 1 to 6 frames per second.

Images acquired by the pre-prototype unit were converted to the DR-960 storage format, in which images are stored as frames rather than difference frames. In this form, the pixel values (DSA numbers) are proportional to the logarithm of the signal intensity at that point. Mathematically, the DSA value at a pixel point x,y is

$$DSA(x,y) = C_1 \left[I_0(x,y)\exp(-\smallint u \ dz) + CS + VG \right] + C_2$$

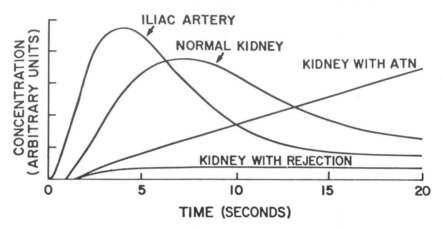

FIGURE 1.   Characteristic "wash-in" and "wash-out" curves of iodinated contrast media for normal kidneys, kidneys with ATN and kidneys with rejection.

where C_1 and C_2 are the gain and bias of the logarithmic amplifier, I_O is the incident x-ray intensity, u and z are the linear attenuation coefficient of and the path length through the imaged object, CS is the term due to Compton scattering and VG is the contribution from veiling glare in the imaging system. The dependence on the x-ray energy, which is quite important and mathematically complex, has been suppressed for simplicity. Changes in the concentration of iodinated radiographic contrast material are reflected as changes in the linear attenuation coefficient and changes in the DSA numbers. As long as variation in the Compton scattering and veiling glare terms are small compared to variation in the directly attenuated intensity term, the critical points (maxima and minima) of the curve of DSA values as a function of time occur at the same time as the critical points (minima and maxima) of the concentration as a function of time. Such a result can be shown by the differentiation of the equation. Thus, a peak in the concentration of radiographic contrast material occurs at a minimum in the DSA values. It is for this reason that a parametric image of when the minima in DSA values have occurred exactly describes when the maxima in concentration have occurred.

For each study sequence, three parametric images were computed, using a primitive image processing language. This

process is illustrated in Fig. 2. For each frame in the study
and for each pixel in the image, the minimum DSA value for
that pixel is found. When this image of minima (the "MINMIN"
image) is subtracted from the first image of the sequence, a
parametric image is produced which represents the maximum
concentration that has occurred at each pixel, irrespective of
when that maximum occurred. Such an image is called in this
paper the "MAXMAX" image. To compute the second parametric
image, each pixel of each frame of the sequence is compared
with "MINMIN" image. If the pixel value of a frame is less
than or equal to the pixel value in the "MINMIN" image, the
frame number plus a large positive number replaces the pixel
value in the "MINMIN" image. The large positive number may be
any number which is greater than the largest possible number
which could occur in the "MINMIN" image, which in this case is
255. After the "MINMIN" image is compared with each image of
the sequence and appropriate replacements made, the large
positive number is subtracted, leaving the parametric image
which is the frame number at which each pixel reached its
minimum in DSA value or maximum in concentration. This image
would be called "FRAME-TO-MAX". When the "FRAME-TO-MAX" image
is scaled by the number of frames per second in the study, the
resultant parametric image is the time at which the maximum
occurs and has been called "TIME-TO-MAX" or "T-TO-MAX". Such
a parametric image has been described previously for digital
radiographic images (4,5) and has been used in nuclear
medicine for studies of the kidneys (6), head (7), and central
cardiovascular system (8). The third parametric image is
computed by first deriving an image which is one-half of the

FUNCTIONAL IMAGES

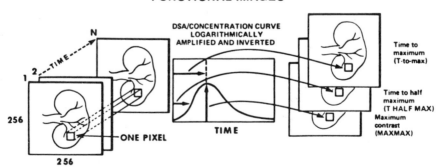

FIGURE 2. Diagram illustrating how functional images of
time-to-maximum concentration, time-to-half-maximum and
maximum contrast images are created using the time-density
curve.

minimum. This is calculated by subtracting one-half of the "MAXMAX" image from the first image of the sequence. Each image of the sequence is then compared with this half-minimum to derive, in a similar way as for "T-TO-MAX", an image which is the time at which the concentration has reached one-half of its maximum. This parametric image is called "TIME-TO-HALF-MAX" or "T HALF-MAX". When comparing the functional images "T-TO-MAX" and "T HALF-MAX", it is convenient to use the same color or gray scale to display them. The image two times "T HALF-MAX", which is called "2* T HALF MAX", has the same time scale as "T-TO-MAX", and it is, therefore, more appropriate to compare with the "T-TO-MAX" image.

When the three parametric images from each study were separated by diagnostic class into normal, ATN, rejection, and complete renal nonfunction (called here shutdown), some rather striking patterns emerged. The kidney is well visualized in the "MAXMAX" image for normal and ATN, slightly less well for rejection, and poorly to not at all for renal shutdown. The "MAXMAX" image contains almost no significant diagnostic information for differentiating normal, ATN, and rejection. Only the lack of visualization of the kidney in the "MAXMAX" image identified renal shutdown. However, considering the "T-TO-MAX" and "2* T HALF MAX" as a pair, the four diagnostic states are surprisingly well differentiated by the visualization of the kidney in the images. These four situations are described in Table 1.

In the "MAXMAX" images, the images are produced so that white represents more contrast material. In the "T-TO-MAX" and "2* T HALF MAX" images, white is early and black is late.

An organ such as the kidney is visualized in the parametric images "T-TO-MAX" and "2* T HALF MAX" because the

TABLE 1. Visualization of Kidney in Parametric Images

	T-TO-MAX	*2* T HALF-MAX*
Normal	*well visualized*	*well visualized*
ATN	*not visualized*	*well visualized*
Rejection	*poorly visualized*	*poorly visualized*
Shutdown	*not visualized*	*not visualized*

max and half-max arrival times are sufficiently different for the corresponding times in the tissues surrounding the kidney. When the kidney is functioning normally, there is a high blood flow rate to the kidney, and the kidney is able to excrete the contrast material rapidly. The maximum concentration is reached within a few seconds of the bolus arrival; but in the tissue surrounding the kidney, the maximum occurs many seconds after the end of the 20- to 30-second study. In ATN, in which it is difficult for the kidney to excrete the contrast material as fast as it arrives, the maximum concentration measured within the study sequence is the last frame, since both the kidney and surrounding tissue experience their true maxima many seconds after the end of the study. Thus, the kidney with ATN is not distinguished from the surrounding tissue in the "T-TO-MAX" image. However, the kidney is still more vascular than the surrounding tissue, and the rate of accumulation of the contrast is initially greater in the kidney than in the surrounding tissue. Thus, the kidney with ATN is visualized in the "2* T HALF MAX" image. In rejection and shutdown, the blood flow to the kidney is markedly impaired, and the measured time-concentration curves for the kidney are almost flat or rise very slowly. In either case, the kidney and the surrounding tissue are nearly indistinguishable.

Both ATN and rejection are not simple, single-disease states. Both can be described as chronic or acute and may be mild, moderate, or severe. Thus, ATN and rejection encompass a whole range of states from completely normal to complete irreversible failure. Thus, a parametric image pair in which the kidney was moderately well visualized on the "T-TO-MAX" and well visualized on the "2* T HALF MAX" image would correspond to mild ATN. Moderate visualization on both the "T-TO-MAX" and "2* T HALF MAX" corresponds to mild to moderate rejection. Nonvisualization of the kidney on both parametric images is renal dysfunction, but the cause cannot be determined. Only a repeated set of studies in which there is some renal function can distinguish very severe ATN, complete rejection, and complete obstruction.

In the past, there has been concern expressed about the potential nephrotoxic effects of radiographic contrast materials on the transplanted kidney. In these case series, no patient experienced an increase in the creatinine levels after the intravenous DSA study. In a recent study of angiograms in renal transplant patients (9), administration of contrast for performance of these studies did not increase the likelihood of rejection.

REFERENCES

1. Meaney, T.F., Weinstein, M.A., Buonocore, E., et al., Digital subtraction angiography of the human cardiovascular system, AJR 135, 1153-1160 (1980).
2. Buonocore, E., Meaney, T.F., Borkowski, G.P., et al., Digital subtraction angiography of the abdominal aorta and renal arteries: Comparison with conventional aortography, Radiology 139, 281-286 (1981).
3. MacIntyre, W.J., Pavlicek, W., Gallagher, J.H., et al., Imaging capability of an experimental digital subtraction angiography unit, Radiology 139, 307-313 (1981).
4. Brennecke, R., Hane, J.H., Moldenhauer, K., et al., A special purpose processor for digital angiocardiography: Design and application, Computers in Cardiology 343-346, IEEE(CH1452-1) (1979).
5. Hoehne, K.H., Boehm, M., Nicolae, G.C., The processing of x-ray image sequences, in Advances in Digital Image Processing, Stucki P, editor. Plenum Pub Corp, 1980, pp. 147-163.
6. Agress, H., Green, M.V., Redwood, D.R., et al., Computer-generated functional mapping - Utility of multiple approaches to imaging of dyamic data, Proceedings of the Sixth Symposium on Sharing of Computer Programs and Technology in Nuclear Medicine, Society of Nuclear Medicine, January 25-26, 1976, Atlanta, Georgia, pp. 430-449.
7. Toyama, H., Ito, M., Iisaka, J., et al., Color functional images of the cerebral blood flow, J Nucl Med 17, 953-958, 1976.
8. Gallagher, J.H., Fouad, F.M., Cook, S.A., MacIntyre, W.J., Automatic ROI selection for first transit nuclear cardiology, IEEE Trans Nucl Sci NS-27, 513-518 (1980).
9. Ahlmen, J., Blohme, I., Brynger, H., and Nilsson, A.E., Acute rejection and angiography in renal transplantation, Transplantation 31, 452-453 (1981).

16

CLINICAL EXPERIENCE AT THE UNIVERSITY OF WISCONSIN

Charles A. Mistretta

Departments of Medical Physics and Radiology
The University of Wisconsin
Madison, Wisconsin

The use of digital subtraction angiography will, for the purpose of this discussion, be divided into intravenous applications and nonselective arterial injection applications.

I. INTRAVENOUS ANGIOGRAPHY

A. Injection Technique

A large number of injection techniques have been attempted by various groups. The University of Wisconsin's initial attempts at intravenous angiography involved the use of hand injections, first in a single antecubital vein and eventually using antecubital veins in two arms. Although some successful results were obtained, the uniformity of the results was not acceptable. The next technique we tried involved power injection through a single 2 inch angiocath inserted preferably in the basilic vein. The first three hundred patients were done in this manner. Using injection rates up to 18 cc per second, 3 extravasations of contrast were experienced. The injection rate was later reduced to between 12 and 14 cc, after which there were no further extravasations. Subsequently the catheter was placed in the superior vena cava. It was felt that this procedure would be safer and it was hoped that it would improve image quality. The investigator's subjective impression is that the best images obtained using the SVC placement are quite similar to those obtained using the short 2 inch angiocath when similar

injection volumes are kept the same. However, the SVC
technique probably reduces the number of inadequate
examinations by eliminating those deteriorated by poor venous
flow between the injection site and the superior vena cava, or
by Valsalva maneuvers. The SVC technique also reduces the
amount of reflux into other venous structures. Such reflux
can be objectionable in aortic arch examinations. At this
institution injection rates are typically kept at 12 to 14 cc
per second. However, with the catheter placed in the SVC it
is possible to use higher injection rates if desired.
Injection rates up to 30 cc per second have been reported by
some groups. Another technique which seems to be quite
effective is the use of a somewhat longer catheter, on the
order of 8 inches, which is inserted in the antecubital
region. This has the advantage that the catheter can be
placed by a technician. The radiologist may then check the
venous flow fluoroscopically before making the injection. This
technique has been developed at the Cleveland Clinic. It
should be emphasized that none of these injection techniques
should be identified with any particular digital subtraction
angiography apparatus. The choice of injection technique can
be made independent of the particular subtraction apparatus
available to each investigator.

B. Extracranial Carotid Arteries

For intravenous studies of the extracranial carotid
arteries, the University of Wisconsin scientists (1,2) usually
use the serial mode, in which images are taken at a rate of
about 1 per second (Fig. 1). The radiologists prefer using
the 6 inch mode for studying the carotid bifurcations. An
injection of 40 cc of Renografin 76 at a rate of 12 to 14 per
second is ordinarily used. Typically, an AP and one or two
oblique projections will be made in order to ensure proper
profiling of the bifurcations. Motion artifacts due to
swallowing are a well known problem in this examination.
Preliminary studies at this institution suggest that the use
of non-ionic contrast materials, when they become economically
feasible, will greatly reduce motion in the extracranial
carotids (see chapter by Sackett). The carotid studies are
generally done at 60 to 70 kVp, using 200 to 400 mA of x-ray
tube current. Generally between 32 and 250 msec of exposure
are integrated in the digital memory. The University of
Wisconsin is presently conducting a study which compares
intravenous angiographic results with conventional angiography
and surgical specimens. Regarding the timing of the injection
for this examination, it is usually best to take the mask

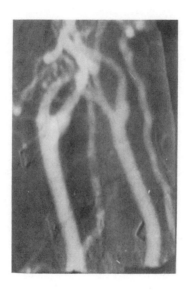

FIGURE 1. Intravenous angiogram of the extracranial carotid arteries obtained using a 40 cc injection of Renografin 76 at a rate of approximately 14 cc per second. Eight frames of video integration were obtained with a 512 X 256 matrix.

immediately thereafter so that a number of pre-opacification images are available as alternate masks to be used in the event that motion occurs.

C. Intracranial Vessels

The technique used for intracranial vessels is similar to that used for the extracranial carotid arteries except that higher kVp's and mA's are used. A typical examination might use 500 mA at 75 to 80 kVp (Fig. 2 & 3). Somewhat higher tube current capabilities might be beneficial in this instance in order to avoid having to raise the x-ray tube voltage to a level which might compromise iodine contrast.

Three projections are most commonly used. An AP projection, a base projection and a 25° off-lateral projection. The AP projection has been useful for determining the position of the carotid arteries in patients to be operated on for pituitary tumors. However, in this projection it is difficult to evaluate the carotid siphon because of the orientation of the vessels. This is better accomplished in the 25° off-lateral in which where the carotid arteries are more favorably profiled. The basilar artery can often be seen clearly in this projection and in the base projection.

D. The Aortic Arch

When imaging the aortic arch using intravenous injection, it is preferable to take the mask image before injection of contrast so as to avoid venous structures persisting in the subtraction display (Fig. 4). Another consideration worth keeping in mind is that a large amount of contrast is present in the aortic arch. If one is using a system employing analog storage of the digitally processed information, it is desirable to use a moderate degree of contrast enhancement so that the information is not clipped to a maximum black or white level. When such clipping occurs, redigitization and reprocessing of the image is not effective in the areas where saturation has occurred. In practice, this does not present a serious problem. One simply knows that for arch injections the contrast enhancement factor should be reduced by a factor

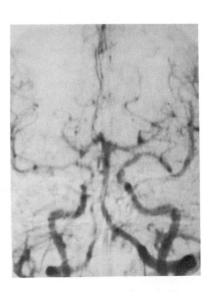

FIGURE 2. Intracranial vasculature obtained using an intravenous injection of 50 cc of Renografin 76. An eight frame video integration was used. X-ray factors were approximately 300 mA and 80 kVp.

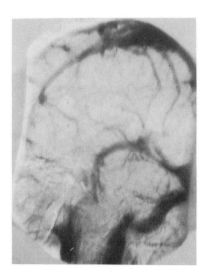

FIGURE 3. *Venous return following typical intracranial intravenous examination.*

of 2 relative to that used for carotid examinations.   Another consideration in the area of the aortic arch is that image bright spots should be eliminated as much as possible through collimation or the use of bolus material, such as saline bags. Bright spots can deteriorate the image by producing scatter, but perhaps more importantly by supressing the signal-to-noise ratio in the darker portions of the image.   This occurs because most systems detect the brightest portion of the image in order to determine what x-ray exposure to use.   If one portion of the image is extremely bright the x-ray exposure will be reduced, leaving insufficient exposure in the darker portions of the image.

There is presently some question about the utility of EKG gating in studies involving the aortic arch.   Using exposure times as long as 64 msec, extremely sharp images of the aortic arch have been obtained.   However, it is possible that some blurring may occur during a portion of the cardiac cycle. Certainly EKG gating is a reasonable way to prevent this from occurring.

E. Lungs

Because the contrast arrives at the lungs very early, the concentration is still quite high and adequate images can be

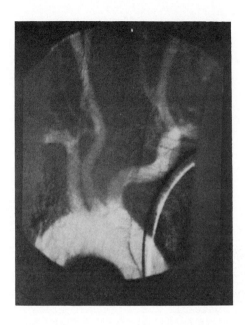

FIGURE 4. Aortic arch obtained using 40 cc of Renografin 76 at 14 cc per second. This image was obtained with a 512 X 512 matrix and a single frame video read-out. The intravenous catheter in the superior vena cava is seen to have moved between the time of the mask and the post-opacification image.

obtained using considerably less iodine than may be required for more peripheral vessels. Good images of the lungs can be obtained using 10 to 20 cc of Renografin 76. The comments made with respect to EKG gating for the arch also apply to the lungs. However, excellent images of the lungs have been obtained without using EKG gating. Motion is a particular problem in the lungs. Any respiration which occurs during the examination will have disastrous effects on the image quality. It is in the lungs that the largest variation in image quality has probably been experienced. These variations are directly related to the extent to which the patient is able to cooperate during the examination. Studies of the lungs, using a 9 inch intensifier have been limited to imaging one lung per injection. For this application the use of a larger format image intensifier would be particularly useful (see chapter by Jolles).

F. Left Ventricle

For studies of left ventricular wall motion, the mask should be taken before injection of contrast so as to eliminate right heart and venous structures (Fig. 5). Because of the low resolution required, a modest x-ray current, typically a few mA, is probably adequate for this examination. The continuous mask mode or the TID mode can be used for these studies. Generally the real-time data is taken in the continuous mode and the information stored either on disk or tape. The TID display is then done, avoiding further patient exposure by reprocessing the stored data. Preliminary quantitative studies to determine cardiac ejection fraction have been done using data from the continuous mode. Drs. Ludwig and Engels at St. Anthony's Hospital in Utrecht, Holland have done a comparison of ejection fractions, using the area length method from TID and have found that these correlate well with similar calculations based on conventional cine angiography (see also references 3 and 4). The TID signals are easily interpretable in all areas except the border between the left atrium and left ventricle. Here confusing signals can arise because of the uncertain amount of ventricle and atrium contributing to the signals in that region.

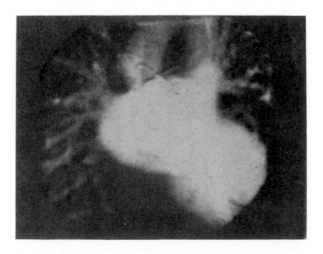

FIGURE 5. Image of the heart following a 40 cc intravenous injection. Note the residual opacification in the pulmonary structures. Such backgrounds interfere with the determination of coronary graft patency.

G. Coronary Bypass Grafts

EKG gating has been tried for the evaluation of coronary bypass grafts in order to obtain static images at end-diastole using the continuous mode. Because of simultaneous opacification of the ventricle and residual opacification of pulmonary structures, it has been felt that the continuous mode provides better information than the static images, which sometimes are difficult to interpret because of the overlying pulmonary structures. In order to obtain acceptable images, more x-ray exposure is needed than in the case of observing left ventricular wall motion. However, to keep the patient exposure to a minimum, the continuous mode is done using two separate doses: a low dose during the right heart phase, and then a higher dose during the left heart phase. During this high exposure, typically 100 to 300 mA, 30 images per second, at 512 X 512, are stored on videotape or on video disk. Then, in order to provide a display which gives sufficient time for orientation, the disk is operated in forward and reverse directions, between an upper and lower track number so that an indefinitely long repetitive dynamic display is available. In this display the correlation of the motion of the vessels with that of the left ventricle helps to separate the bypass grafts from the overlying backgrounds. There has been moderate success with this technique in the determination of graft patency. However, this particular exam is one of the more difficult tasks performed by the digital subtraction angiography apparatus. The visualization of native coronary vessels is rarely of high quality, especially in the distal portions of these vessels. It is in this area that better algorithms and improved equipment may be most beneficial.

H. Abdominal Vessels

For imaging abdominal vessels, the mask can be taken sometime after the injection of contrast. The post-mask pictures are taken beginning rather early, in order to give greater flexibility in terms of choosing alternate masks (5). The largest problem in abdominal imaging comes from bowel gas which moves during the examination. In order to decrease the effects of this, an abdominal band is used to displace bowel gas as much as possible. In addition, 1 cc of intravenous glucagon is also given to supress bowel peristalsis. The results in this area have been mixed, ranging from excellent examinations of the renal vessels to examinations in which bowel motion has been a serious problem (Fig. 6). Usually,

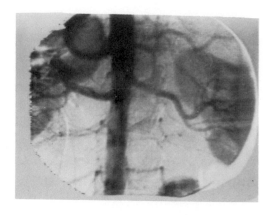

FIGURE 6. Intravenous study of the renal arteries following a 40 cc injection of Renografin 76 at 14 cc per second.

successful examinations can be made by repeating injections in different projections.

I. The Extremities

For imaging vessels in the pelvic area or the arms and legs, the mask is again taken after the injection of contrast material and, depending on the type of flow expected, the imaging rate might be reduced below 1 per second.   In addition, depending on the flow expected, the amount of contrast is sometimes increased to 60 cc per injection. Motion is a lesser problem in these examinations and adequate studies are almost always obtained. A large number of the studies have been postoperative examinations of the results of graft surgery (Fig. 7). The largest limitation for this application lies in the small format of most image intensifiers. Larger image intensifiers are useful in these applications in that they may be used to reduce the number of injections required for examination of the entire area of interest.

II. NON-SELECTIVE ARTERIAL INJECTION SUBTRACTION TECHNIQUES

A. Carotid Arteries

Excellent images of extracranial and intracranial vessels have been obtained using 10 to 15 cc of contrast injected at

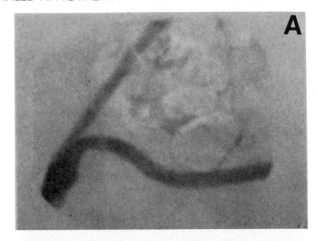

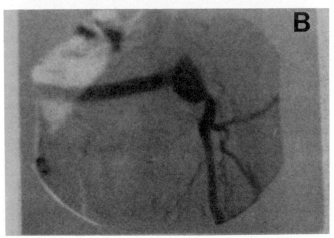

FIGURE 7. *Image of a femoral to femoral bypass graft obtained using two separate injections.*

12 to 14 cc per second into the aortic arch. Because of the short injection times, it is beneficial to use the continuous mode rather than the serial mode. Images are stored on videotape at a rate of 30 per second and are also recorded on a video disk at a rate of 6 images per second. The disk images are used for making hard copies. Because of the small time between the pre-injection and post-injection information, reprocessing using the intra-arterial injections is seldom necessary. Because of the small amount of contrast used, several projections may be made to minimize the superposition problems associated with nonselective injection. Because of

the high contrast achieved using arterial injection in conjunction with digital subtraction, the optimal spatial resolution for the digital system should be somewhat greater for this application than is necessary for intravenous applications, in which the lower contrast concentration reduces the requirements for the system spatial resolution. Matrix sizes of 512 X 512 covering a 6 inch field seem to be somewhat better than smaller sized matrix arrays. It is not clear yet whether even higher matrix densities will be beneficial (see chapter by Price).

B. Coronary Vessels

Preliminary studies using aortic root injection have been done in order to visualize the coronary circulation in animals. The results have been quite encouraging and indicate that, with some system improvements, considerable information might be obtained in humans using aortic root injections. It is not yet clear whether this will find application as a screening technique--to indicate which patients should go on to selective coronary angiography and which patients may eventually be diagnosed through this method.

C. Distal Runoff Studies

There are several clinical examples in which standard arteriography was unable to demonstrate viable vessels in the distal portions of the leg. Repeating these studies using digital subtraction angiography with a similar arterial injection has often yielded excellent images of vessels suitable for grafting. These comparisons should be made with film subtraction. However, this is not routinely done at the University of Wisconsin. In the one instance in which the digital subtraction results were compared with film subtraction, the image quality of the digital subtraction result was quite superior to the film subtraction result. The limitation of the film subtraction technique is that once the iodine has been isolated, there is no convenient way to increase the contrast to easily perceptible levels.

REFERENCES

1. Kruger, R.A., Mistretta, C.A., Riederer, S.J., Ergun, D., Shaw, C.G., Row, G.G., Computerized fluoroscopy techniques for noninvasive study of cardiac dynamics, Invest Radiol 14, 279-287 (1979).
2. Ergun, D.L, Mistretta, C.A., Kruger, R.A., Riederer, S.J., Shaw, G.G., Carbone, D., A hybrid computerized fluoroscopy technique for noninvasive cardiovascular imaging. Radiology 132, 739-742 (1979).
3. Meaney, T.F., Weinstein, M.A., Buonocore, E., Pavlicek, W., et al., Digital subtraction angiography of the human cardiovascular system, SPIE 233, 272-278 (1980).
4. Meaney, T.F., Weinstein, M.A., Buonocore, E., et al., Digital subtraction angiography of the human cardiovascular system, AJR 139, 1153-1160 (1980).
5. Ovitt, T.W., Christensen, P.C., Fisher, H.D., et al., Intravenous angiography using a digital video subtraction x-ray imaging system, AJNR 1, 287-290 (1980).

17

DIGITAL ANGIOGRAPHY IN THE DIAGNOSIS OF PEDIATRIC CARDIOVASCULAR DISORDERS

Barry D. Fletcher

Rainbow Babies and Childrens Hospital
University Hospitals of Cleveland
Cleveland, Ohio

Digital subtraction angiography promises to be an important, relatively noninvasive tool in the diagnosis of cardiovascular disorders of children. For children, however, a number of procedural and technical adjustments need to be made in order to accommodate smaller, less cooperative individuals in whom the diagnostic requirements of DSA are markedly different from those of the adult. In this chapter, I will discuss modifications, indications and problems we have encountered in applying digital angiographic techniques to the diagnosis of pediatric cardiovascular disorders.

I. EQUIPMENT

All pediatric digital subtraction angiography at Case Western Reserve University has been performed using the Technicare DR-960 system, which provides mask mode imaging at up to 6 frames per second on a 256 X 256 matrix. Four, six or nine-inch image intensifier field sizes are utilized depending on the size of the patient and specific anatomy which is to be studied. The x-ray tube and image intensifier are suspended on opposite ends of an L-C arm, allowing cardiac imaging in oblique and axial projections (1).

II. IMMOBILIZATION AND SEDATION

In order to obtain precise registration of mask and frame, very little motion can be tolerated. For pediatric DSA examinations, we have utilized methods of immobilization and sedation similar to those used for body CT scanning.

Infants approximately 2 years of age usually do not require sedation but can be immobilized on lucite boards or by means of elastic bandages and sandbags. It is helpful to quiet the infant by providing a nipple to suck. Most patients over age 5 are able to lie quietly on the table and even voluntarily suspend respirations for the duration of the exposure run. Between these ages, some form of sedation is usually needed and numerous regimens are available. Chloral hydrate 50-100 mg/kg is given orally or a combination of meperidine (Demerol) 2.0 mg/kg, chlorpromazine (Thorazine) 1.0 mg/kg and promethazine (Phenergan) 1.0 mg/kg is administered intramuscularly.

III. INJECTION TECHNIQUES

All the pediatric digital angiograms have been made following rapid intravenous injections of Renografin 76. The amount, method and site of injection vary with each patient. In general, peripheral venous injection sites have been satisfactory. Rapidity of injection rather than size of the bolus appears to be the more important factor in obtaining good images. Sheated 14 to 22 gauge needles are usually used depending on the size of the patient. An alternative method in patients with few superficial veins is venapuncture, carried out using a "butterfly" needle with the tubing removed. A short guide wire is inserted through the needle; the needle is removed and an introducer and sheath are subsequently threaded over the guide.

The contrast media is injected over a period of 2 seconds using a pressure injector and is followed by a small amount of 5 percent dextrose in water. Mechanical injection may, however, not be necessary for small infants. For example, a hand injection through a number 22 antecubital vein cannula resulted in an adequate bolus into the right atrium of a 2.5 kg newborn infant. For each injection, a dose of 0.5 to 1.0 ml per kg body weight is sufficient and can be safely repeated.

IV. INDICATIONS

The relative non-invasiveness of intravenous digital angiography makes it an attractive technique for diagnosis of many pediatric cardiovascular lesions, especially those in which diagnosis does not require collection of physiologic data during a formal heart catheterization procedure. Since a number of intracardiac lesions can be well visualized echocardiographically, the most frequent current use of DSA has been to diagnose aortic arch malformations such as vascular rings, coarctation of the aorta and to demonstrate patency of surgically constructed aortic-pulmonary arterial shunts (Fig. 1). In addition, the semilunar valves can be surprisingly well seen and abnormalities of the ascending

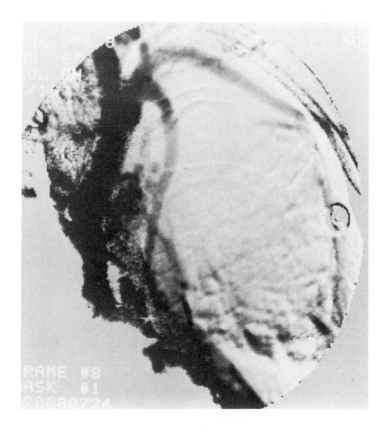

FIGURE 1. Patency of a surgically fashioned conduit between the origin of the left subclavian artery and the pulmonary artery as shown on a DSA frame.

aorta, which are often beyond the range of echocardiography, can be displayed (Fig. 2A).

Diagnosis and follow-up of certain intracardiac abnormalities is also possible. The ventricular septum can be well visualized on left anterior oblique projections (Fig. 2B). Interventricular and interatrial septal defects have been demonstrated on DSA studies of experimental animals (2). The right atrium, right ventricle and major pulmonary arteries are usually well demonstrated (Fig. 3). DSA would provide a relatively safe method to examine the pulmonary circulation, yet avoid direct pulmonary artery injection in patients with pulmonary hypertension.

In spite of some loss of spatial resolution, it has been found that the higher contrast resolution inherent in digital

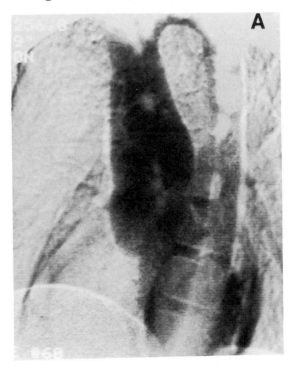

FIGURE 2. DSA of a 14-year old child with Marfan's syndrome shows dilation of the aortic valve ring, sinuses of valsalva and ascending aorta. The aortic valve also appears to be bifid. (A) Partial subtraction of left ventricular contrast aids visualization of the aortic valve. (B) The left anterior oblique projection displays pulmonary venous drainage from the left lung, the left atrium, the left ventricle and the ventricular septum.

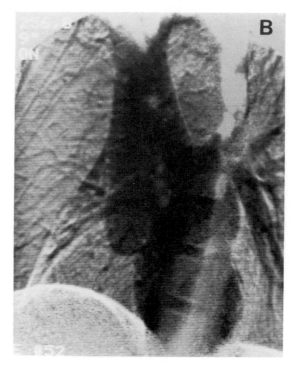

FIGURE 2 (continued).

angiography is useful in order to enhance images obtained during inferior or superior venacavography in small infants (Fig. 4). For this reason, DSA has also been used to demonstrate patency of Glenn shunts between the superior vena cava and right pulmonary artery.

Table I lists actual and potential applications for digital imaging of the cardiovascular system in children.

V. IMAGING PROBLEMS

As with any high technology equipment, digital imaging systems are subject to occasional technical failures. Aside from these, the results of an examination may be severely compromised by unforeseen pathophysiologic events. In spite of considerable preparation using experimental animals, investigators are still learning from experience and patients are counseled regarding the research nature of each examination. When studying the aorta, one should keep in mind

TABLE I. *Current and Potential Indications for DSA in*
          Diagnosis of Pediatric Cardiovascular Disorders

Aortic root abnormalities - Marfan's
Coarctation of aorta
Aortic arch anomalies
Acquired aortic disease - arteritis, aneurysms
Peripheral vascular anomalies
      A-V malformations
      Pulmonary sequestration
Systemic - pulmonary artery shunts
      Patent ductus arteriosus
      Patency of surgical shunts
Pulmonary circulation
      Pulmonic stenosis
      Peripheral pulmonic stenosis and banding
      Anomalous left pulmonary artery ("sling")
      Anomalous pulmonary venous drainage
Intracardiac lesions
      ASD
      VSD

---

that aortic contrast may be inadequate in patients who have large left-to-right shunts or reduced cardiac output. Moreover, it is at least theoretically possible, by subtracting an image obtained during earlier opacification of the chamber, to overlook reopacification to the right atrium or right ventricle due to a left-to-right shunt.

VI. RADIATION HAZARDS

In presenting DSA as a less invasive angiographic procedure, primarily because of the ease and safety of contrast injection, it is also necessary to compare radiation exposure to the patient with that produced by conventional cine imaging systems. Most modern pediatric cardiology installations consist of image intensifier tubes with video fluoroscopy and 35 mm cine recording at 60 to 90 frames per second.

The surface exposure dose rate calculated for our DSA system is approximately the same as that previously reported for similar equipment (3). Assuming cardiac angiography in a 10-year old patient at 80 KV and 82 cm from the x-ray source,

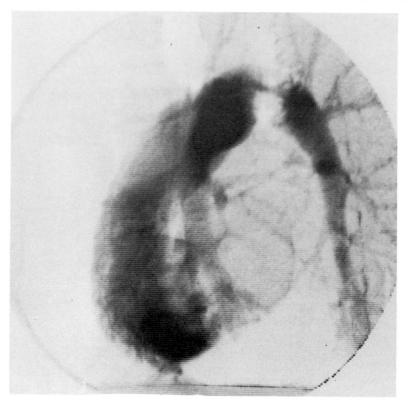

FIGURE 3. The right ventricle and pulmonary artery are well opacified following intravenous injection of contrast medium (LAO projection). Residual right atrial contrast has been subtracted. The apparent defect in the left pulmonary artery near its origin is an artifact due to excessive image brightness.

surface exposure was calculated to be 182 mR per image for DSA and 4.2 to 6.3 mR per image for single-plane cineangiocardiography. At 4 frames per second DSA imaging and 60 frames per second cine using 9 inch modes, the calculated exposure doses are 728 mR per second and 252 mR per second, respectively (4). This nearly 3-fold increase in exposure during digital angiography is ameliorated somewhat since the fluoroscopic time required for catheter placement for cineangiography is avoided with DSA. It is clear, however, that wide acceptance of DSA as a diagnostic tool in pediatric cardiology will require a reduction in patient exposure.

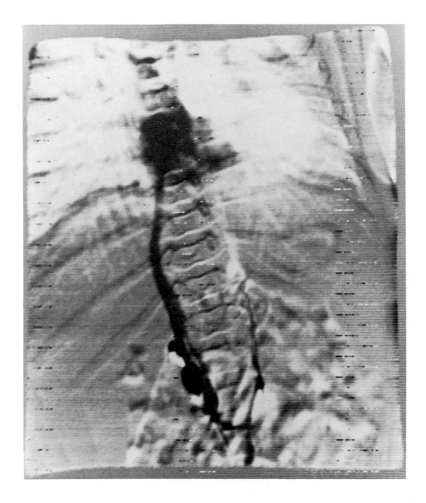

FIGURE 4. Partial inferior vena cava obstruction in a 4-month old infant. Injection was through a femoral vein catheter.

VII. CONCLUSIONS AND FUTURE CONSIDERATIONS

DSA is a currently useful imaging technique for diagnosis of a wide variety of pediatric cardiovascular disorders, especially those in which accurate angiographic depiction would eliminate the necessity of cardiac catheterization. Immobilization, sedation and rapid intravenous injection of contrast media can be accomplished in infants and small children. The quality and registration of the subtracted images are degraded by respiratory and cardiac motion and by the presence of significant cardiac diseases, which tend to dilute or delay the passage of contrast media. Moreover, radiation to the patient is higher than that produced during cineangiography.

It is expected that in the future, digital cardiovascular imaging will be improved by gating of exposures throughout the cardiac cycle. Ideally, frame rates approaching those used for conventional cineangiography will be able to be achieved at acceptable radiation exposure levels with adequate spatial resolution. When this is accomplished, it is expected that, due to its relative non-invasiveness, DSA will make a substantial contribution to pediatric cardiovascular diagnosis.

REFERENCES

1. Bargeron, L.M., Jr., Elliott, L.P., Soto, B., et al., Axial cineangiography in congenital heart disease. Section I. Concept, technical and anatomic considerations, Circulation 56, 1075-1083 (1977).
2. Bogren, H.G., Bursch, J.H., Brennecke, R., et al., Intravenous angiocardiography using digital image procesing: 2. Experimental studies in pigs with simple left-to-right shunts, Invest. Radiol. 16, 378 (1981).
3. Meaney, T.F., Weinstein, M.A., Buonocore, E., et al, Digital subtraction angiography of the human cardiovascular system, SPIE 233, 272-278 (1980).
4. Adams, R.B., Personal Communication, 1981.

18

PEDIATRIC NON-ANGIOGRAPHIC APPLICATIONS OF DIGITAL RADIOGRAPHY

Richard M. Heller
Jon J. Erickson
Ronald R. Price

Department of Radiology and Radiological Sciences
Vanderbilt University Medical Center
Nashville, Tennessee

I. INTRODUCTION

Digital radiography can be considered as being divided into two distinct categories: digital fluoroscopy and scanned projection radiography. Both techniques generate images in a digital format. In digital fluoroscopy, the image formation mechanism is a two dimensional position-sensitive detector such as an image intensifier video camera system. In the second category, the image is formed by either a one or two dimensional mechanical motion of an electronic detector and a specially collimated x-ray beam (1,2).

The advantages of digital fluoroscopy and scan projection radiography include the capability of long range image data transmission by telephone lines or satellite, flexible capability for image storage and retrieval, and image processing and manipulation to exploit the entire range of detected information.

The details of digital fluoroscopy are adequately covered in other chapters in this text and will not be repeated here. However, for the sake of completeness we will discuss the detection characteristics which are relevant to pediatric radiology. Table I provides a comparison of the various modes of digital radiography and the routine film/screen combinations. This table is by no means exhaustive but does provide the reader with an overview of typical system

TABLE I. Typical Performance Specifications for X-ray Imaging Systems

Device	F-O-V	Spatial resolution	Contrast detect.	SNR	Dose (R)	Frame rate
Film/Screen	11x19"	4-8 lp/mm	2%	100:1	0.2	6/sec.
Digital Video Fluoroscopy	4-10"	1-2	1%	300:1	0.1	1-30
Point Scanning (SPR)	20x20"	1-2	0.2%	500:1	0.004	0.2
Linear Scanning (SPR)	20x20"	1-2	0.2%	500:1	0.07	0.2
CT Scanner	20"	1	0.2%	2000:1	4	0.2

parameters that have an impact on the performance of clinical studies.

II. DIGITAL FLUOROSCOPY

In digital fluoroscopy the image from the image intensifier tube is viewed by a special low noise television camera. The output signal from this camera is digitized and stored in the computer memory for subsequent data processing. The details of the operation of the digital fluoroscopy systems are adequately summarized in other discussions in this book and they will not be repeated here except where required for comparisons with the other modes of imaging. The primary advantage of the digital fluoroscopy system is its ability to provide a high frame rate. Rates as high as 30 frames per second are possible with equipment available at the present time. One disadvantage of the digital fluoroscopy systems is that in order to obtain the higher spatial resolution indicated on the table, the field of view must be reduced to a relatively small value; this severely limits the value of digital fluoroscopy in studies other than the small or special procedure studies. As is shown in other chapters in this collection, the primary use of digital fluoroscopy is for high resolution, high speed subtraction angiograms which are performed for the determination of patency of blood vessels. The use of this type of study in the pediatric population is very limited.

III. SCANNED PROJECTION RADIOGRAPHY

As stated in the introduction, digital radiographs may be generated by the one or two dimensional mechanical motion of specially collimated detectors and x-ray generators. There are essentially two classes of scanned projection radiography: the so-called flying spot scanner and the scanned linear array. Both of these have been developed for clinical applications by commercial firms. Because of the difference in the techniques, they will be discussed separately. The characteristics pertinent to pediatric radiography are also shown in Table I.

IV. FLYING SPOT RADIOGRAPHY

The method currently receiving the most clinical interest is that which was developed by American Science and Engineering, Inc., in an attempt to significantly reduce the radiation dose delivered during routine radiographic procedures. Other techniques have been developed and reported in the literature (3-5) but have had limited clinical trials, and the reader is referred to the literature for more information. In the Micro-Dose® x-ray system developed by AS&E, the image is generated by a combination of mechanical motions and x-ray beam collimators (see Figs. 1 and 2). The output of a conventional x-ray source is collimated by a tungsten slit into a narrow fan beam. The fan beam is further collimated by a series of tungsten slits arranged radially on a chopper wheel. The wheel and large tungsten slit together attenuate all the x-rays except those passing through the small aperture formed by the overlap of the non-rotating slit in one other rotating slit. Thus, a thin pencil beam of x-rays emerges from the small aperture. Due to the rotation of the chopper wheel at a speed of 1800 rpm, the x-ray beam rapidly scans the patient in a direction transverse (i.e.,

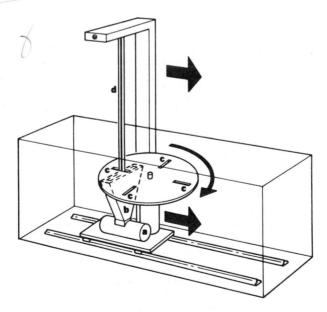

FIGURE 1. *Schematic representation of the Micro-Dose*® *unit. (A) X-ray tube. (B) Collimator. (C) Chopper wheel. (D) X-ray beam. (E) Detector.*

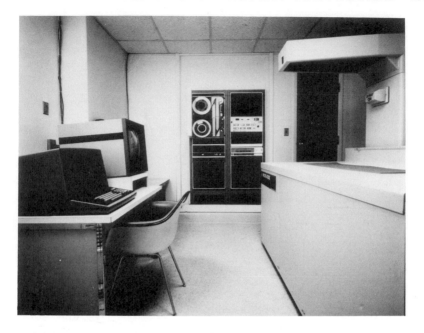

FIGURE 2. Installation of the Micro-Dose® unit at the Geisinger Clinic.

perpendicular) to the length of the table-bed and is detected by a linear detector system located over the patient couch. The entire assembly including the x-ray source, chopper wheel and detector, moves parallel to the long axis of the table-bed, resulting in a longitudinal scan of the patient. The patient remains stationary. The x-ray beam is partially attenuated by the patient and the remaining x-ray photons are detected with nearly 100% efficiency by the photon detector system. The detector is a sodium iodide scintillation crystal coupled to a photomultiplier tube. The single crystal intercepts all of the x-ray photons which penetrate the patient. At each instant of time, the electrical signal obtained at the output of the photomultiplier tube is proportional to the intensity of the attenuated x-ray beam. During one tranverse scan of the beam, the electrical signal from the detector corresponds to a radiographic "line image" of the patient. This line image is analogous to one scan line of a video system. The second dimension of the image is generated by virtue of the longitudinal movement of the source-collimator-detector with respect to the patient. A full radiographic scan of the patient initially requires 16 seconds and produces an image with a digital resolution of

512 X 480 pixels (see Figs. 3 and 4). All data processing occurs during this exposure. Thus, the complete radiographic display is available at the instant the scan is completed.

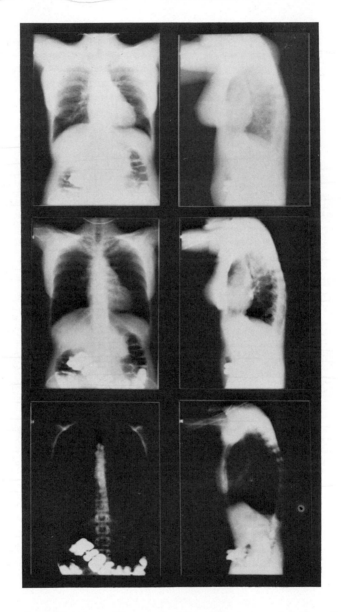

Figure 3. Chest radiograph of a 40 year old female. One image was obtained and displayed in various window settings so that the lungs, mediastinum and bones could be evaluated.

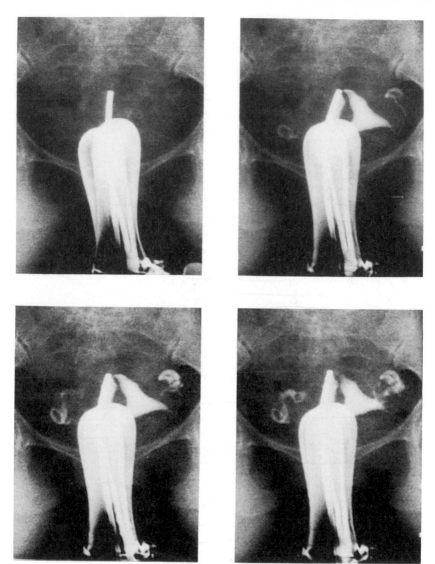

FIGURE 4. Hysterosalpingogram. Four images were obtained, each image requiring 0.7 mR for a total of 2.8 mR (scout image, initial filling, further filling, 2 minute delayed radiograph showing intraperitoneal spill).

Because the patient is exposed at any instant in time only to x-rays at the location from which the information is being read out of the dectector, the radiation dose is very low.

Doses of the order of 0.25 to 60 mR per scan are reported depending on the x-ray tube current, anode kilovoltage image field size and scan speed.

The concept of flying spot technology resulting in radiation dose reduction is most attractive in terms of pediatric medical imaging. Children have a life expectancy of many decades and are either capable of reproduction or soon will be. Reduction of exposure to ionizing radiation to the gonads and bone marrow without image degradation is a major advantage of this technology. Dosimetric studies have shown that diagnostic images can be routinely generated with SPR techniques which result in skin doses as low as 0.25 mR.

Due to the narrow x-ray detector aperture and extremely fine collimation of the x-ray beam, the adverse effects of scattered radiation are minimized. The advantages of this type of image generation include: the wide dynamic range of the electronic radiation detector system, low patient dose and the rejection of scattered radiation. The digital image format also provides the clinician with the ability to interact with the image after collection. The disadvantages of this mechanism include the relatively long image generation time which allows time for patient motion. Patient motion in this system is not evidenced as an overall blurring in motion as in conventional radiographs, but rather, appears as displacement of anatomical structures in adjacent scan lines. This means that structures with inherent motion such as the cardiac silhouette do not show continuous borders. New instrument designs have reduced the time required for image acquisitions to five seconds. This, in turn, reduces the problems of patient motion during the scan.

The wide dynamic range of the detection systems in these techniques provides the clinician with the ability to produce, in a single image, a detailed representation of both the low density soft tissue areas and the high density bony structures. This not only obviates the need for repeat exposures because of an error in the x-ray exposure techniques but also allows the use of a single exposure for screening procedures where both tissue types are to be examined.

V. LINEAR SCANNING ARRAYS

The second type of scanned projection radiography is that which was initially implemented to provide a method for localization of high resolution CT scanning procedures. This Scoutview or Scanogram technique makes use of a linear array of detectors. These detectors may be scintillation detectors, either sodium iodide or bismuth germinate coupled to photomultipliers, or, alternatively, they may be a single detector assembly constructed from a large segmented high pressure gas chamber. The latter detector assembly is the type used in several third generation CT scanners and represents a very high resolution, high reliability detector design with relatively good sensitivity. The x-ray source in both systems is a one-dimensional fan beam rather than the solid cone beam of conventional radiographic systems. In the present linear scanning arrays, the patient is moved through the space between the x-ray tube and the detector assembly. During the scan of the patient, the image is stored in the computer memory in a manner similar to the flying spot x-ray system. For this reason, it can be recalled immediately from display and manipulation.

The primary limitation of the scanned linear array is the spatial resolution which can be obtained with the basic design concept. The spatial resolution depends strongly on the ability of the manufacturer to pack a large number of detectors very tightly together so that each detector is collimated to view a very small anatomical region. A second problem with the scanned array is the difficulty in eliminating scatter from a particular detector from other parts of the fan-shaped x-ray beam. Mechanical collimation on both the source and the detector assemblies can serve to reduce this effect somewhat, but the requirement of high sensitivity limits the amount of collimation that can be placed in the system. The presence of the scatter component in the image will tend to reduce the image contrast in low contrast studies. It will not significantly effect high contrast studies such as skeletal imaging procedures. A third and very significant problem with the scanned linear array is that of the supporting electronics. Each individual detector in the system must have its own set of data processing electronics consisting of pre-amplifier, analog-to-digital converter and buffer register. For scanning systems with a large number of detectors, this electronic complement will represent a very expensive investment, comparable to that required for a conventional CT scanner. Innovative switching and mechanical construction techniques can perhaps reduce the cost, but at the expense of imaging speed.

The lateral resolution of this scanner depends on the packing density and collimation of the detector assembly. The longitudinal resolution depends on the mechanical scanning system and the pre- and post-patient collimation. Resolution of 1.5 X 1.5 mm is presently designed for prescanning patient alignment in CT scanners; this imaging modality should be considered for trauma screening applications as well as applications where multiple periodic examinations are required. In this use, the slightly less than optimal spatial resolution is offset by the ability to immediately view the images and by the reduced x-ray exposure, accomplished by the use of the high efficiency solid state or gas detectors.

The scanned linear array system represents a compromise between the digital fluoroscopy system and the total mechanical system represented by the flying spot imager. It suffers from a relatively high noise content unless the image time is extended to increase the proton count. The x-ray tube in SPR systems is one of the primary limitations of the techniques. Only a small fraction of the x-rays produced by the tube are actually allowed to pass through the patient and contribute to the image. The rest are stopped by the shielding and collimation. The tube loading, however, is a function of the total number of x-rays produced, so that the actual tube usage is significantly inefficient.

VI. PEDIATRIC APPLICATIONS OF FLYING SPOT RADIOGRAPHY

Exploration of the concept of radiation exposure reduction using SPR techniques in the pediatric population requires knowledge of the examinations which are repeated at frequent intervals and/or include the gonads in the radiated field, and/or include a large volume of bone marrow. These examinations include scoliosis radiographs, evaluation of the hips for the status of Legg-Perthes disease, excretory urography, and the long-term follow-up of children with congenital heart disease or chronic pulmonary disease. Another interesting application of scan projection radiography is computer alteration of the image in a child wtih malignant disease. With one exposure, the lungs can be evaluated. A change in the setting of the computer will permit the bones to be evaluated by generating an image that appears similar to an over-penetrated anteroposterior chest radiograph. Thus, radiation exposure reduction is achieved by manipulation of data captured at the time of a single exposure. Additional exposures at different x-ray factors are unnecessary!

REFERENCES

1. Katragadda, C.S., et al., Digital radiography using a computed tomographic instrument, Radiology 133, 83-87 (1972).
2. Foley, W.D., et al., Digital radiography of the chest using a computed tomography instrument, Radiology 133, 231-234 (1979).
3. Tateno, Y., and Tanaka, H., Low dosage x-ray imaging system employing flying spot x-ray microbeam (Dynamic Scanner), Radiology 121, 189-195 (1976).
4. Stein, J., and Swift, R., Flying spot x-ray imaging systems, Materials Evaluation 30, 137-148 (1972).
5. Stein, J., X-Ray imaging with a scanning beam, Radiology 177, 713-716 (1975).

19

NEURORADIOLOGIC APPLICATIONS OF DIGITAL SUBTRACTION
AUGMENTATION FOR INTRA-ARTERIAL ANGIOGRAPHY

Frank M. Eggers
Joseph H. Allen
Ann C. Price

Section of Neuroradiology
Department of Radiology & Radiological Sciences
Vanderbilt University
Nashville, Tennessee

I. INTRODUCTION

Since the introduction of equipment capable of performing real-time digital subtraction, a large body of the literature has concentrated on the applications and techniques of intravenous contrast injection for digital subtraction angiography (IV-DSA). The digital subtraction technique as an adjunct to conventional intra-arterial catheter angiography has also been found quite useful in a number of situations. Our equipment consists of a Technicare DR-960 unit coupled to a General Electric Fluorocon 300 installed in the Neuro-Angiographic Suite at Vanderbilt.

In the course of slightly more than four months, a total of 53 patients have been evaluated in part or totally by the use of intra-arterial digital subtraction angiography (IA-DSA).

II. SPECIFIC CLINICAL APPLICATIONS

A. Angiography Planning Guide

Evaluation of vessel origins or carotid bifurcations for disease, before selective catheterization is attempted, can be easily accomplished using IA–DSA. This application is similar to the use of a 105 mm spot film device but with the advantages of real-time subtraction, i.e., improved images with smaller amounts of contrast material and no film-processing delay prior to viewing (Figs. 1–4).

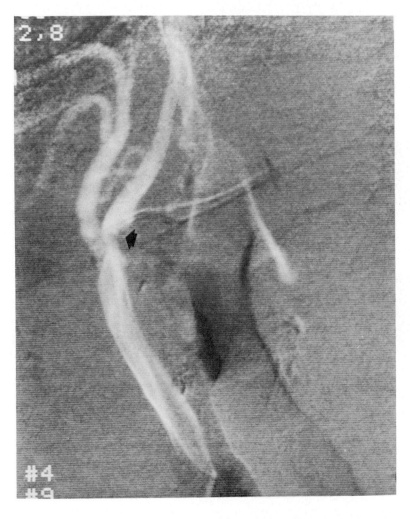

FIGURE 1. IA-DSA "spot film" of the right carotid bifurcation. This was obtained by injection of approximately 3 cc of Conray 60, diluted with an equal volume of Heparinized saline solution. The irregular narrowing of the internal carotid at its origin is readily seen (arrow).

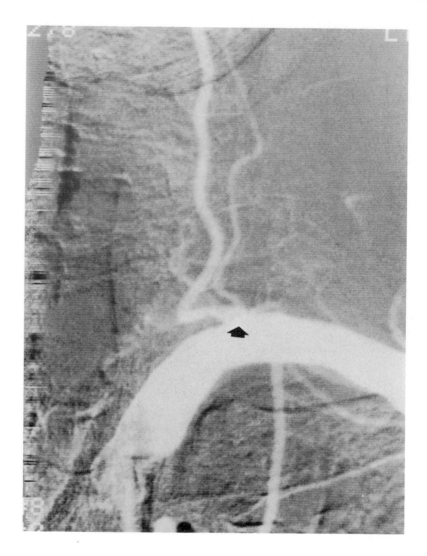

FIGURE 2. IA-DSA "spot film" of the left vertebral origin, showing it to be small but patent (arrow). Contrast utilized was approximately 3 cc of Conray 60 diluted with an equal volume of Heparinized saline.

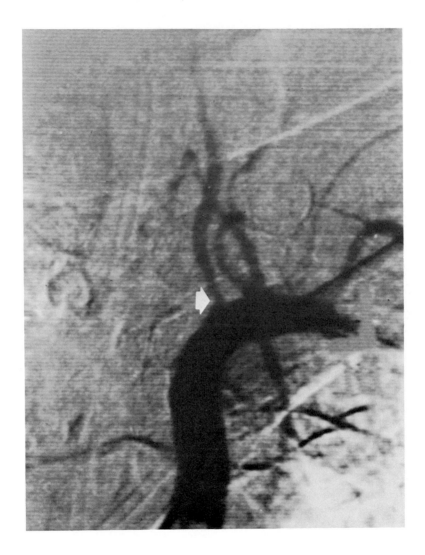

FIGURE 3. *Spot film of a left vertebral origin obtained in a manner similar to Fig. 2. This shows a minimal amount of stenosis at the origin (arrow).*

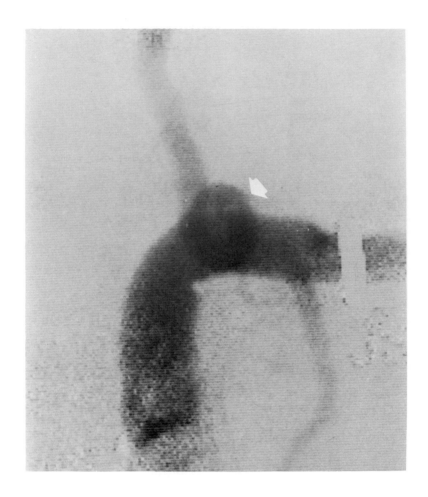

FIGURE 4A. IA-DSA "spot film" of the left vertebral origin showing its marked tortuosity (arrow).

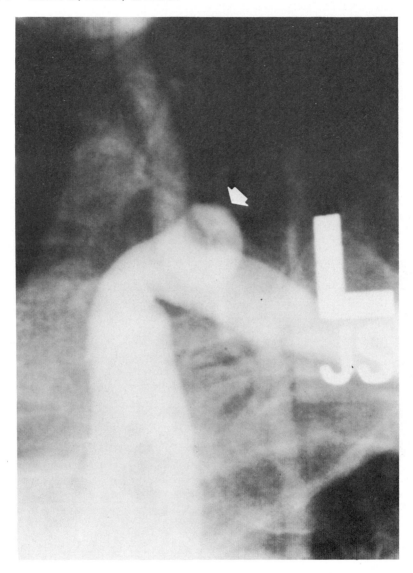

FIGURE 4B. *Same patient utilizing a "105 mm spot-film" camera with comparable resolution (arrow).*

B. Evaluation of Post-Subarachnoid Hemorrhage Spasm

Repeat angiography to evaluate spasm after definitive pan-angiography is occasionally necessary. If, however, only a single vessel requires angiography for a reason other than spasm, the presence or absence of spasm in other vessels can be readily evaluated by IA-DSA, utilizing a considerably smaller contrast dose than required by standard angiography (Figs. 5 and 6).

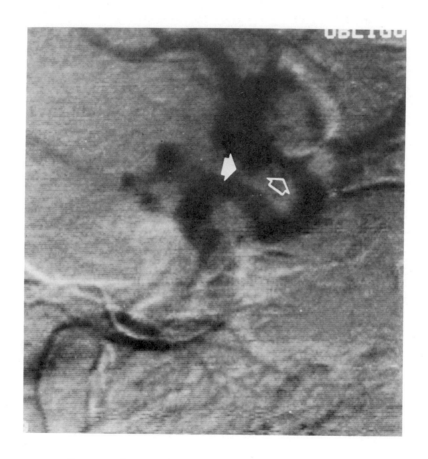

FIGURE 5. Patient with documented right carotid aneurysm at the posterior communicating artery level. Repeat angiography to reevaluate spasm. An IA-DSA view of the parasellar carotid shows clearly the presence of the aneurysm (closed arrow) as well as persistent residual spasm (open arrow).

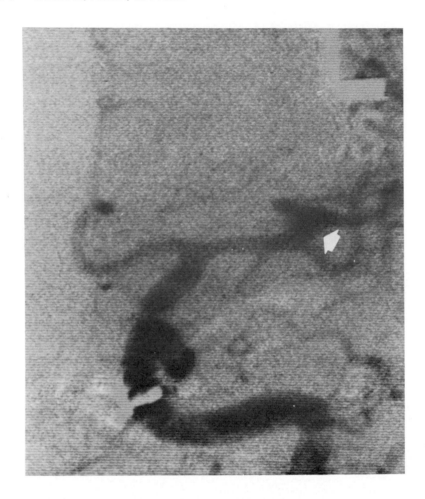

FIGURE 6. Patient with left middle cerebral artery aneurysm at the trifurcation. IA-DSA view of the left middle cerebral trifurcation clearly shows the aneurysm (arrow). No obvious spasm is identified.

C. EC-IC Bypass Patency Evaluation

For a patient who has undergone an extracranial-intracranial bypass procedure, evaluation of patency of the anastomosis can be accomplished by IA-DSA. This is particularly important if the parent vessel is difficult to catheterize and/or significantly diseased (Fig. 7). Selection of optimum patient position is also facilitated.

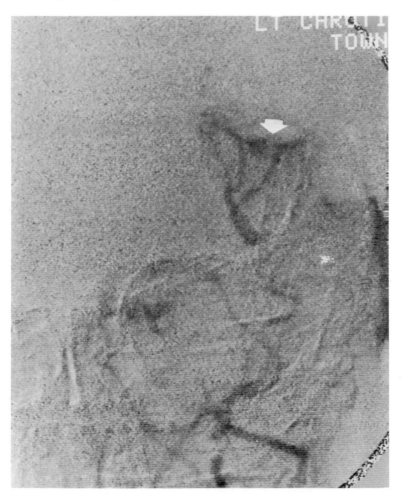

FIGURE 7. Patient with known internal carotid artery occlusion and s/p STA-MCA anastomosis. The IA-DSA view visualizes the flow into the middle cerebral distribution (arrow), although the exact anastomotic site is seen with difficulty on this film.

D. Vertebrobasilar System Evaluation

The vertebrobasilar system is readily evaluated for patency of vessels and flow direction without vertebral artery catheterization. Large aneurysms or significant arterosclerotic occlusive disease can be identified, although subtle detail is more difficult to detect. IA-DSA is particularly helpful in the face of significant vertebral origin disease, to determine if persistent attempts at catheterization or alternative routes are desirable to obtain more definitive information (Figs. 8-10).

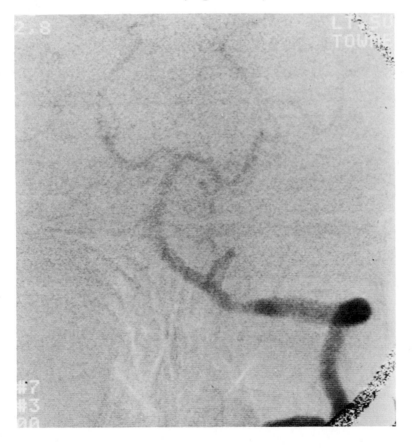

A

FIGURE 8. (A) AP and (B) lateral view of the vertebro-basilar circulation intracranially. Catheter tip was positioned in the left subclavian artery and hand injection of approximately 4 cc of Conray 60 with an equal volume of Heparinized saline. Gross patency and absence of focal stenoses or large aneurysms can be readily demonstrated by this technique.

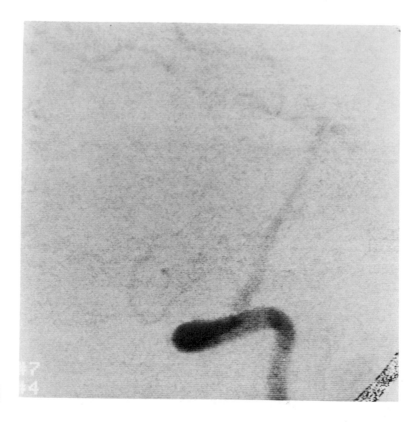

B

FIGURE 8 (continued).

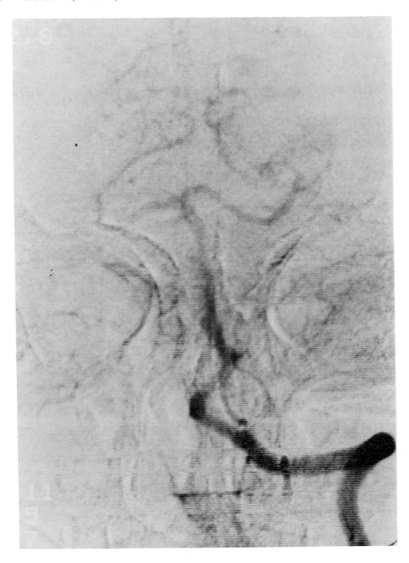

FIGURE 9. Similar catheter placement and injection technique used for Fig. 8 reveals (A) AP and (B) lateral views of the posterior circulation. Again, gross defects can be readily excluded.

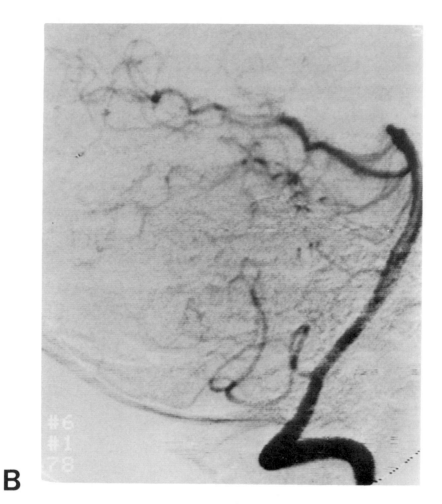

B

FIGURE 9 (continued).

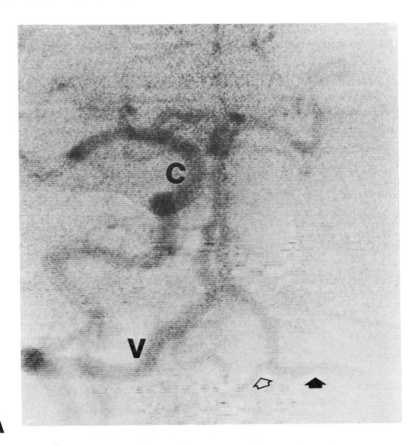

A

FIGURE 10. (A) AP and (B) lateral views were obtained by injection of approximately 5 cc of Conray 60 with equal solution of Heparinized saline in the inominate origin with subsequent filling of both the right carotid [C] and right vertebral [V] distribution. There is visualization of retrograde flow in the contralateral vertebral (closed arrow) distal to the origin of the contralateral PICA (open arrow).

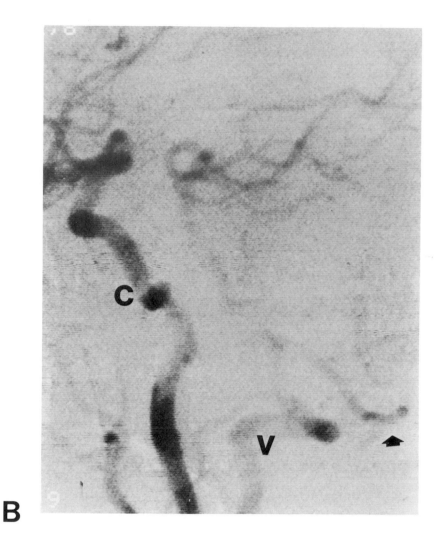

B

FIGURE 10 (continued).

E. Common Carotid Origin Evaluation

In a patient with documented "TIA's" but with a normal common carotid arteriogram, the common carotid origin can be readily evaluated using IA-DSA, without the additional hazard of performing an arch aortogram. This can be accomplished by either a hand injection into the origin of the vessel in question or by power injection in the ascending aorta, to obtain a digital subtraction "arch" (Figs. 11-13).

F. "Subclavian Steal"

Evaluation of the amount and direction of flow in the vertebrobasilar system can be readily accomplished without resorting to large volumes of contrast using IA-DSA. This can be particularly important in evaluating whether the basilar artery distribution distal to the vertebrobasilar junction fills from the vertebral distribution or is totally dependent on collateral flow from the anterior circulation (Fig. 14-16).

G. Evaluation of Carotid Artery "String Sign"

The utilization of real-time IA-DSA to determine the presence or absence of antegrade flow distal to a high grade carotid stenosis can be of paramount importance in surgical planning to determine whether carotid endarterectomy or a bypass operation would be the operation of choice.

H. Interventional Applications

The ability to evaluate vessels with real-time subtraction and with decreased contrast volumes would also seem to be a major contribution in multiple neuroradiologic interventional techniques. There has not been an opportunity to evaluate this as yet.

In the evaluation of intra-arterial digital subtraction angiography (IA-DSA), we have used from 4-10 cc of diluted Conray 60 [Iothalamate Meglumine Injection U.S.P. 60%, Mallinckrodt Pharmaceuticals, St. Louis, MO] (to an approximate concentration of 30%) for the hand injections and have mechanically injected from 8-15 cc over the course of 2-3 seconds of Conray 60 or Vascoray 76 [Iothalamate Meglumine 52% and Iothalamate Sodium 26% Injection U.S.P., Mallinckrodt Pharmaceuticals, St. Louis, MO] for the DSA-"Arch" injections.

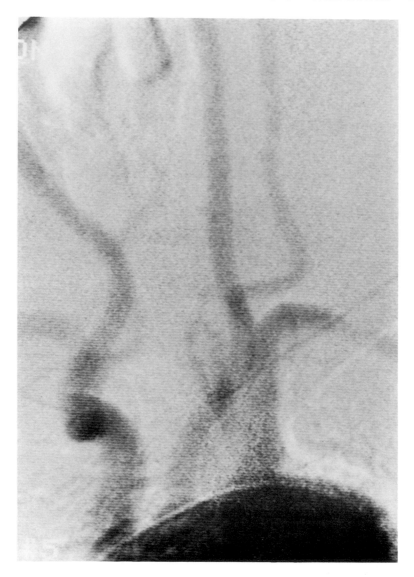

FIGURE 11. An RPO projection of an "arch aortogram," utilizing approximately 10 cc of undiluted Conray 60 and an IA-DSA technique. The origins of each of the four great vessels can clearly be seen to be patent.

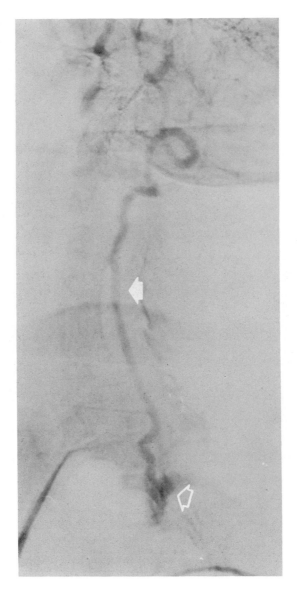

B

FIGURE 16 (continued).

III. <u>SUMMARY</u>

Utilization of digital subtraction techniques as an adjunct to intra-arterial catheter angiography can certainly provide adequate information to answer many questions with a significant reduction in constrast volumes, patient risk and patient discomfort. Spatial resolution is not comparable to standard cut film angiography but is certainly adequate in many instances.

20

SELECTED CLINICAL EXAMPLES FROM A GENERAL PURPOSE DIGITAL RADIOGRAPHY SYSTEM

Alvin N. Bird, Jr.

ADAC Laboratories
Sunnyvale, California

in collaboration with

Ronald R. Price
Alan C. Winfield
Jon J. Erickson
A. Everette James, Jr.

Department of Medical Imaging and Radiological Sciences
Vanderbilt University School of Medicine
Nashville, Tennessee

I. INTRODUCTION

Throughout this text, the emphasis has been upon the introductory aspects of the digital imaging process. This chapter serves mainly as an introduction to a particular typical commercially available system. The following studies are presented as typical clinical examples for the purpose of illustrating the image quality and flexibility of this present "state-of-the-art" digital radiography system. The images presented in this chapter were gathered from a number of medical centers who have recently acquired an ADAC DPS-4100 Digital Radiography system (ADAC Laboratories, 255 San Geronimo Way, Sunnyvale, California 94086). The software-based image processing system provides a facility for either continuous or pulsed digital fluoroscopy. In the continuous (cine) mode of operation, up to 30 frames per second real-time subtraction are possible, with the different images being recorded on an analog video storage device. When the system is operated in the pulsed (spot-film) mode, the digital images are recorded directly on a 40 Mbyte Winchester disk. The digital image storage rate with the disks that are used currently is approximately 1 per second for 512 X 512 images. The rate of storage of coarser images is increased in inverse proportion to the total number of picture elements in the image (see chapter by Price). The following examples were derived from systems in which the digital radiography components were "added on" to the existing x-ray equipment (see chapter by Freedman).

II. CEREBRAL ARTERIES

The images presented in Figs. 1A and 1B are the anteroposterior and lateral views of cerebral arteriograms and illustrate the typical normal vasculature. The images are the

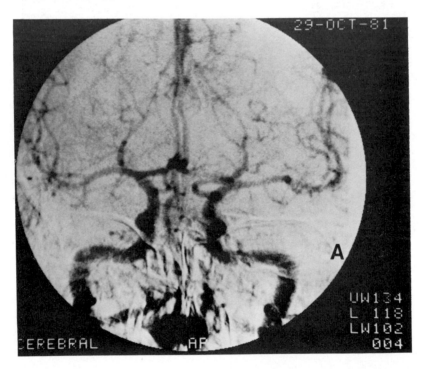

FIGURE 1A. *A normal intravenous digital subtraction AP cerebral angiogram (512 X 512 matrix using 45 ml injection of contrast media).*

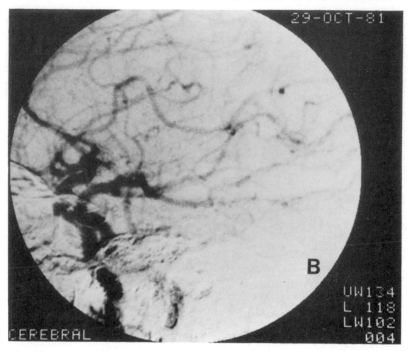

FIGURE 1B. Normal lateral cerebral IV angiogram (512 X 512 matrix following 45 ml injection of contrast media).

result of a methodology which used a 2 frame average acquisition with a 512 X 512 image matrix display. The radiographic technique was 800 mA, at 74 kVp. For the injection, a 5.0 French catheter was introduced into the right basilic vein and advanced to the superior vena cava, where 45-55 ml of Renografin 76 was injected at the rate of 15 ml/sec. The considerations of injection have been the subject of the chapter by Sackett and discussed by others. From these images, one can note the visualization of the intracranial vessels. As described elsewhere in this text, the ability to postprocess the digitally stored data improves our abilities to portray these vessels.

III. CAROTID ARTERIES

Throughout other chapters, the authors have described the necessity of evaluating the carotid circulation. Figs. 2A and 2B are LPO and RPO IV carotid arteriograms, respectively. These images clearly illustrate occlusion of the left external carotid. The images are the result of a 2 frame average acquisition and are both presented in a 512 X 512 matrix format. The radiographic technique was that of 360 mA, small focal spot (0.3mm) and exposed at 68 kVp. The injection was made through a 5.0 French catheter which had been positioned in the superior vena cava and a total of 45-55 ml of Renografin-76 was injected, at a rate of 15 ml/sec. Catheter placement and injection were performed by a physician (see chapter by Freedman).

Fig. 3 illustrates a magnification view of the carotid bifurcation and Fig. 4 is an example of an aortic arch study which was performed for the purpose of visualizing the origins of the carotid vessels.

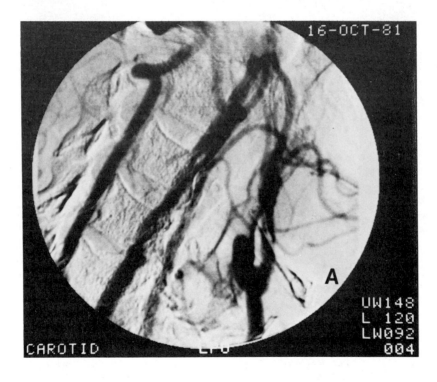

FIGURE 2A. LPO IV carotid angiogram with occluded left external artery (512 X 512 matrix with 45 ml injection of contrast media).

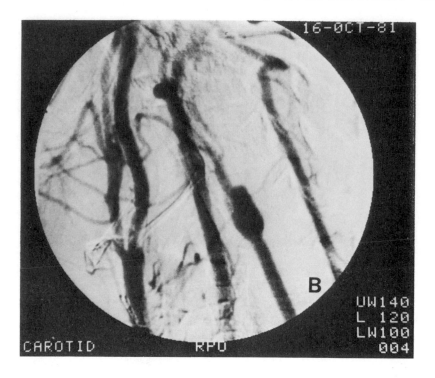

FIGURE 2B. RPO IV carotid angiogram (512 X 512 matrix with 45 ml injection of contrast media).

IV. <u>RENAL, ABDOMINAL AORTA AND ILIAC ARTERIES</u>

Figs. 5A and 5B illustrate an intravenous renal arteriogram in which the aorta and origins of the major renal arteries are clearly visualized. Fig. 5B demonstrates a magnified presentation of the same image.

Fig. 6 is an image of the abdominal aorta. The image is the result of a two frame average and is presented in a 512 X 512 matrix. The intravenous injection technique is the same as noted above, with a radiographic technique of 380 mA at 72 kVp. The tortuosity of the abdominal aorta and numerous plaques throughout the vessel are clearly evident. The origins of a number of vessels also demonstrate narrowing, irregularity and tortuosity.

Fig. 7 is an image of the common iliac bifurcation. The image illustrates tortuous and diseased iliac vessels with 30–40% stenosis on the right, with minimal stenosis on the left. This type of information would be most adequate as a

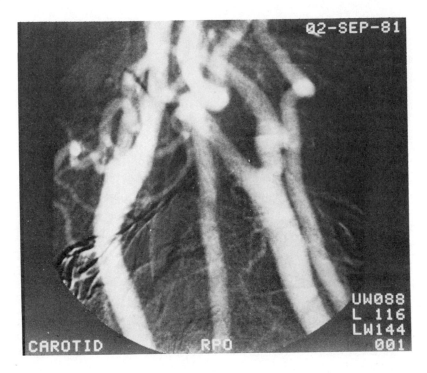

FIGURE 3. *Magnified carotid bifurcation IV digital subtraction angiogram (512 X 512 matrix).*

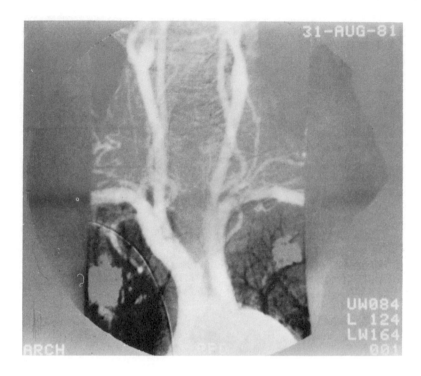

FIGURE 4. Intravenous digital subtraction aortic arch image (512 X 512 matrix).

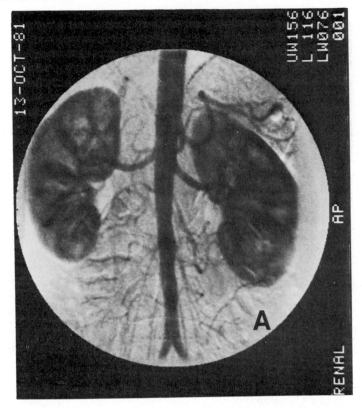

FIGURE 5A.   Intravenous renal arteriogram (512 X 512 matrix following injection of 45 ml of contrast media).

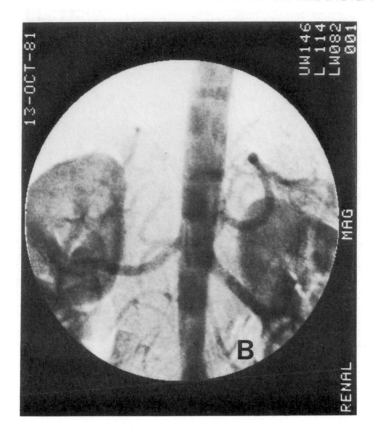

FIGURE 5B. Magnified view of Fig. 5A.

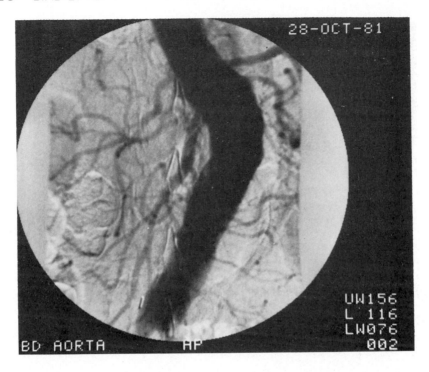

FIGURE 6. *Abnormal abdominal aorta image illustrating severe disease (512 X 512 matrix following 45 ml injection of contrast media).*

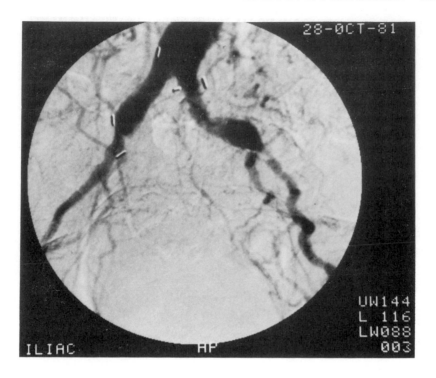

FIGURE 7. Abnormal iliac bifurcation image with significant stenoses (512 X 512 matrix with 45 ml of contrast media).

screening procedure and in many instances would be sufficient to plan whatever therapy anticipated.

V. INTRA-ARTERIAL INJECTIONS

As described in the chapter by Eggers, there are several advantages offered by digital subtraction in intra-arterial procedures. High quality images of the coronary arteries may be achieved using selective injections of smaller amounts of contrast media. Additionally, by postprocessing methods one may visualize smaller vessels more readily than with conventional methods. This may be especially relevant in areas where small arterial vascular systems may be covered by bone. The digital subtraction image of a coronary artery, shown in Fig. 8, was produced by a hand injection of only 0.5 ml of contrast media. At times, the images resulting from

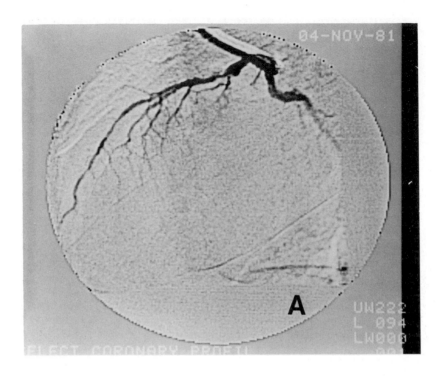

FIGURE 8A. *Digital subtraction image of a coronary artery following selective intra-arterial injections, 256 X 256 matrix (0.5 ml of contrast media).*

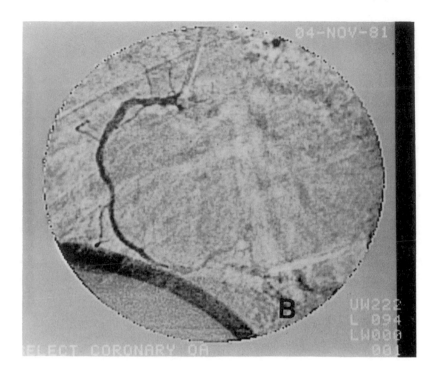

FIGURE 8B. Digital subtraction image of a coronary artery following a selective intra-arterial injection of 0.5 ml of contrast media.

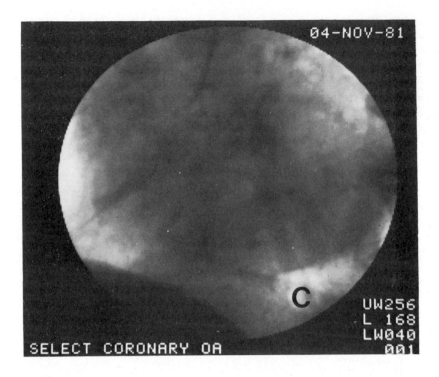

FIGURE 8C. Digital image of the same coronary artery as shown in Fig. 8B before subtraction of the mask image.

coronary angiography, as well as from intracranial cerebral angiography, may be improved by both subtraction and edge enhancement. The fine order branching of coronary vessels, anastomoses, and the presence of small collaterals can provide information of particular clinical significance. One might imagine the importance of the data one could achieve by visualization of these vessels in combination with an iodine density profile or a radionuclide myocardial perfusion study.

The image in Fig. 9 is an intra-arterial subtraction image of the hepatic arteries using only 1 ml of contrast media.

Fig. 10 represents a study of the parathyroid vasculature following a 0.5 ml arterial injection of Renografin-76. The technique factors were 64 kVp at 340 mA. There was no frame averaging and the image is displayed as a 512 X 512 matrix.

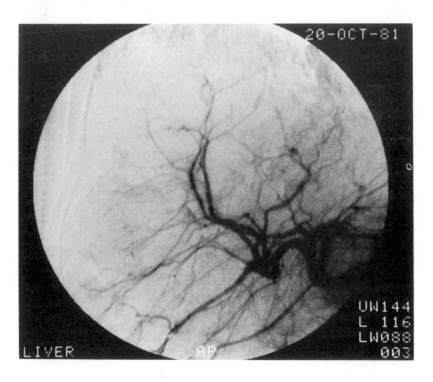

FIGURE 9. Digital subtraction image of hepatic arteries following an intra-arterial injection of 1 ml of contrast media.

VI. DISCUSSION

The digital imaging process offers significant clinical opportunities for improved information regarding vessel condition, blood flow, and regional perfusion. Many of these activities are discussed in this introductory text.

The two most common modes of operation, continuous digital fluoroscopy and pulsed fluoroscopy, are appropriately discussed in this text. In some ways, they are analogous to the conventional cine and "spot" radiographic modes of operation so familiar to medical imaging physicians. For these reasons, immediate applicaton of these techniques is predicted once the appropriate instrumentation is acquired. However, one should be circumspect in planning the addition of a system, as noted in the basic chapters by Mistretta and Price and specifically commented upon by Freedman and by Evens.

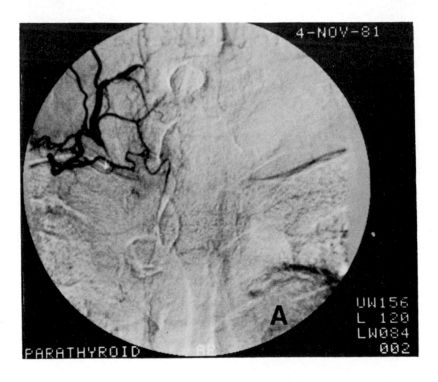

FIGURE 10A. Intra-arterial digital subtraction image of the parathyroid following 0.5 ml injection of contrast media.

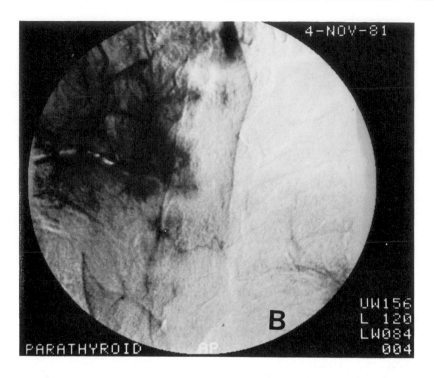

FIGURE 10B. Image of the parathyroid following the image shown in Fig. 10A, illustrating the parenchymal blush phase.

Most radiographic systems, if they have a high performance imaging chain, will conveniently and appropriately interface with a commercially available digital system. The imaging chain is a direct determinant of the quality of diagnostic output of any system; compromises in this area cannot be overcome by any fast acquisition. One should initially evaluate the characteristics of the existing system, compare these with the performance requirements for digital radiography, and upgrade the existing system before installation of the digital capability is initiated.

Applications of digital imaging outside the vascular system will be discussed in other chapters. However, in almost any area of organ or organ system imaging, significant clinical implications exist.

ACKNOWLEDGMENTS

The images in this chapter were provided courtesy of Drs. Harvey Eisenberg and Ben Arnold, South Bay Hospital, Redondo Beach, California.

The selective coronary artery images were from the Amboise Park, Paris, France.

21

ANALOG FILM–SCREEN SUBTRACTION INTRAVENOUS ANGIOGRAPHY

R. P. Schwenker
R. E. Wayrynen

E. I. DuPont DeNemours
Wilmington, Delaware

with the assistance of

S. J. Gibbs
O. M. Sloan
R. R. Price
A. E. James, Jr.

Department of Radiology and Radiological Sciences
Vanderbilt University Medical Center
Nashville, Tennessee

I. INTRODUCTION

The application of intravenous angiography to arteriography is currently and appropriately receiving a great deal of attention (1–4). This introductory text offers only an early insight into the implications of the process. With the fear of being repetitious, we might offer the following advantages of the intravenous approach as compared with conventional arteriography:

1. Intravenous angiography is substantially less invasive. This accepts the usual convention whereby it is common to refer to contrast injection into the venous system, either directly or via catheter, as noninvasive.

2. Patient trauma and discomfort are substantially reduced.
3. It is technically a simpler procedure to perform.
4. It may be performed as an outpatient procedure.
5. Cost to the patient should be reduced (See chapters by Evens and Freedman).
6. It is more readily applicable to the evaluation of high-risk patients and as a screening procedure for minimally symptomatic or asymptomatic patients.

While the advent of digital techniques has stimulated interest in intravenous subtraction angiography, it should be emphasized that this procedure can be accomplished using conventional film-screen imaging systems and existing automatic changers. These considerations will be the subject of this chapter.

II. ADVANTAGES OF ANALOG FILM-SCREEN SUBTRACTION

Intravenous angiography is made possible by subtraction techniques which remove unwanted anatomical information, thereby enhancing the perceptibility of images of contrast-containing vessels. In principle, the subtraction can be performed via either analog (photographic) or digital techniques (see chapters by Price and Mistretta). There may be certain advantages to utilizing the film-screen approach, including:

1. Excellent spatial resolution (response at 1 cycle/mm).
2. The ability to encompass a large field of view (up to 14 X 14 inches).
3. The acquisition of biplane data from a single contrast injection
4. The use of existing equipment.
5. The flexibility of registration of specific areas of interest.
6. Less contrast media generally required for a complete procedure.

Although this list is not exhaustive, and does not provide the overall considerations that each practitioner should have, it certainly provides a framework for discussion. The manual registration of the angiogram and mask permits x, y, and rotational alignment. This has not been greatly emphasized in this text or in the literature. Simple "pixel shifts" and other more direct means of misregistration correction may not properly account for all of the misalignment that occurs. For optimum results, registration can be adjusted for different areas of interest in the particular study. Using a film-based technique, this can be done by manual orientation during visual alignment.

Good photographic subtraction can easily be accomplished with little experience. Most darkroom technicians are quite familiar with the technique. This will obviate the requirements for additional personnel as discussed by Freedman and by Evens. Also, it might decrease the time involvement of the physician in the subtraction process, a cost-effective measure. Because of the larger field-of-view plus the possibility of bi-plane imaging, film-based procedures generally require fewer injections of contrast media. This not only benefits the patient by the reduced volume of contrast media but also reduces the cost of the procedure.

III. DISADVANTAGES OF ANALOG FILM-SCREEN SUBTRACTION

The inherent disadvantages of any film-based system include:

1. Film subtraction time. Typically, about ten minutes are required to obtain the subtracted results following completion of the radiographic procedure. Although the diagnostic quality of the results can often be predicted from visual evaluation of the angiograms, the patient should probably remain in position until completion of the photographic subtraction. This constraint might result in reduced patient throughput compared to a digital system, as discussed elsewhere in this text. In busy medical imaging departments, this factor could be substantial. However, in smaller departments, where intravenous angiography is only infrequently performed, the time element might well be offset by the cost implications of the two systems.

2. Manual technique. Photographic subtraction, while not technically difficult, requires manual handling, registering, and printing. In return for potential improved quality and flexibility, the simplicity of the digital approach is eliminated. Other considerations with regard to safety, and patient handling are common to both approaches.

3. Radiographic film cost. Typically, 25 to 30 sheets of film are used for an arch and carotid study with the film-screen technique. With a digital system, typically four to five sheets of film would be sufficient for display and archiving. Thus, there exists a trade-off of initial financing of digital system versus continuing costs of the film-based system.

IV. RADIOGRAPHIC PROCEDURE

Since this group of investigators initiated work in film-screen intravenous subtraction angiography, a number of radiology departments have begun performing these studies routinely. This text will describe a technique used by Holgate and Keller (5) in which the results have been clinically acceptable. One would not suggest that the procedure is necessarily optimum or that this is the only satisfactory method to perform film-based intravenous angiography. As in any radiographic procedure, the imaging physician should develop a method appropriate to the clinical needs and the available equipment.

A. Injection

For aortic arch and extracranial vessels in the neck, the usual injection is 60–80 cc of 75% Hypaque at 20–30 cc/sec, using a 7.2 French polyethylene "pigtail" catheter placed in the vena cava via a femoral or antecubital vein.

B. Radiographic Technique

Generally, Cronex 4 or 6-plus films with Cronex Quanta III screens are used. With this image system, AP exposures are performed at 33 mAs, 72–74 kVp, and lateral at 30 mAs, 78–80 kVp. In each plane, one pre-injection image is obtained, followed by 10–15 post-injection images at intervals of one second, beginning five seconds after injection.

It is important that the exposure technique is such that there is sufficient penetration in the densest areas of interest (including contrast-containing vessels) to produce a minimum density on the angiogram of at least 0.1 above base plus fog. One should avoid densities greater than 3.0 in any of the areas of interest.

C. Patient Positioning

From the supine position, the patient is moved to a 45° position with which the vertical (usually AP) tube-changer system will project a true lateral, and the horizontal (usually lateral) system, a true AP of the calvarium. The AP projection is then angled 15° caudally in an attempt to identify more clearly the origin of the vertebral artery.

Certain embellishments to the routine techniques have been found to be helpful in obtaining high success rates in film-screen intravenous angiography. Holgate and Keller suggest the use of:

1. A water bag, which provides greater uniform film exposure and permits greater flexibility in the radiographic technique.
2. A bite bar, to reduce swallowing artifacts, as discussed elsewhere in this text.
3. Instructions by the physician or attendant to the patient regarding breathing, especially first to hyperventilate, then hold breath on expiration, while simultaneously biting the bar.

Parenthetically, no sedation has been found necessary for this procedure.

Following angiography, photographic subtraction is accomplished using conventional methods. First, a subtraction mask is provided by making a contact print of the pre-injection (base) film on a negative type film with a contrast (γ) of 1.0, such as Cronex Subtraction Film. In cases of excessive patient motion, including swallowing, between the base and angiogram, an early (or late) angiogram can be used to make the subtraction mask. One should be certain that there is sufficient exposure of the mask film to produce some density in all areas of interest.

An angiogram image from the peak contrast period is selected visually and aligned with the subtraction mask (again visually) to provide registration in the primary area of interest. The two films are fastened together. (In some cases different alignment is required for the arch relative to the carotid bifurcation, but multiple alignment and printing can be obtained.)

A contact print is made through the angiogram-mask combination. The print can be made on a film of γ = 1.0,

such as Cronex Subtraction Film. For higher contrast, Cronex
Subtraction Print Film may be used. Again, one should assure
sufficient exposure to produce density in the print in all
areas of interest. Typical images of the aortic arch and
carotid arteries are shown in Figs. 1 and 2.

The DuPont Cronex Printer has been designed for the
printing steps required in this procedure. For further detail

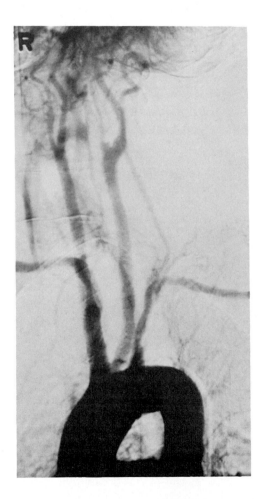

*FIGURE 1. Analog film-screen subtraction film following
intravenous injection of contrast media illustrating aortic
arch and carotid arteries. Note increased field-of-view
relative to digital video-fluoroscopic images allowing
visualization of aortic arch and carotid bifurcation
simultaneously.*

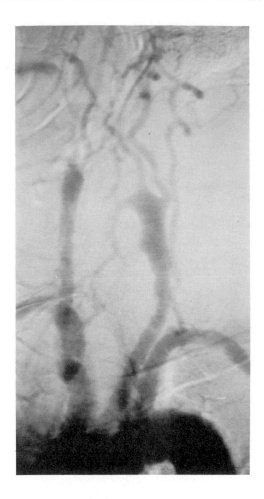

FIGURE 2. Analog film-screen subtraction following an intravenous injection of contrast media.

on photographic subtraction, one may refer to Principles of Subtraction in Radiology (6) or to any of the excellent articles in the radiology literature dealing with subtraction (7).

V. DISCUSSION

Intravenous angiography using a conventional film-screen system was reported as early as 1939 (1). However, early workers were not able to utilize the photographic subtraction techniques which have become available and are routinely used for subtraction angiography. Because of the poor visualization of the low concentrations of contrast media present in intravenous angiography, selective arteriography became the technique of choice for angiography. The recent developments in digital subtraction angiography has stimulated a re-evaluation of the film-screen approach utilizing photographic subtraction techniques (8).

Theoretical analysis and clinical results confirm that the film-screen approach provides contrast sensitivity comparable to that of the digital-electronic method. The dynamic range of the film-screen system is dependent on the film sensitometric properties. Therefore, with appropriate film choice, the dynamic range can significantly exceed that of the image intensifier.

Pure digital systems have certain inherent limitations and even some drawbacks. The dynamic range in these systems is a function of the slope (contrast) of the linear digitizing function and the luminance resolution (a function of the number of bits per pixel), as well as the dynamic range of the optical imaging system, generally intensifier-video. Clearly, contrast and dynamic range are antagonistic in these systems, as they are in film-based systems. Further, the linearity of these systems can be a disadvantage, particularly in the detection of a small amount of contrast above a high-level background. The logarithmic response of film is an advantage in these situations, since the signal:background ratio is independent of background level.

It may be argued that the capabilities of digital systems to provide processing other than simple subtraction cannot be matched by film-based systems. However, some manipulation of imaging parameters is possible with film. For example, it is possible to extend the dynamic range of the system by using low-γ films for the base and angiograms. Higher visual contrast can be obtained by using high γ films for the subtraction prints. The subtraction process, whether digital or photographic, cannot create information.

One of the major problems in digital angiography at present is the storage of images in real time. Film and conventional automatic changers remain a useful method of data acquisition and storage. Clearly, images stored on film may be digitized and processed exactly as would images that had been digitized directly from the intensifier.

VI. <u>CONCLUSIONS</u>

Excellent subtraction angiograms can be obtained with intravenous injections and either digital or film-screen techniques. It should be recognized, however, that the image quality will not equal that from selective arterial injections. Film-screen intravenous-injection subtraction angiography has been demonstrated as a useful, non-invasive diagnostic procedure for large vessel angiography. It is easily performed using existing equipment in most radiology departments. It has several advantages over digital techniques, which have been discussed. Film-based techniques, in certain situations, may be the method of choice, giving results equal or superior to digital systems.

<u>REFERENCES</u>

1. Robb, G.P., and Steinberg I., Visualization of the chambers of the heart, the pulmonary circulation and the great vessels in man: A practical method, <u>AJR</u> 41, 1 (1939).
2. Christenson, P.C., Ovitt, T.W., Fisher, D.H., et al., Intravenous angiography using digital video subtraction: intravenous cervicocerebrovascular angiography, <u>Amer. J. Neuroradiol.</u> 1, 379-390 (1980).
3. Mistretta, C.A., Crummy, A.B., and Strother, C.M., Digital angiography: a perspective, <u>Radiology</u> 139, 273-276 (1981).
4. Erickson, J.J., Price, R.R., Rollo, F.D., et al., A digital radiographic analysis system, <u>RadioGraphics</u> 1, 49-60 (1981).
5. Keller, M.A., Wortzman, G., and Holgate, R.C., Intravenous aortography, American Society of Neuororadiology, Los Angeles, California (March, 1980).
6. Pamphlet: Principles of Subtraction in Radiography, DuPont (A74787-1).
7. Horenstein, R., Lund, H., and Sjogren, S.E.., The subtraction method, <u>Acta Radiol.</u> (Diagn.) 2, 264-272 (1964).
8. Ducas de Lahitte, M., Marc-Vergues, J.P., Rascol, A., et al., Intravenous angiography of the extracranial cerebral arteries, <u>Radiology</u> 137, 705-711 (1980).

22

THE USE OF DIGITAL RADIOGRAPHIC TECHNIQUES
IN THE ANALYSIS OF WORKS OF ART
WITH AN EMPHASIS UPON PAINTING

A. Everette James, Jr.[1]
S. Julian Gibbs[1]
Joseph Diggs[1]
Thomas Brumbaugh[2]
Malcolm Sloan[1]
Kevin Grogan[3]
Ronald R. Price[1]
Jon J. Erickson[1]

[1]Department of Medical Imaging and Radiological Sciences
Vanderbilt University Medical School
Nashville, Tennessee

[2]Department of Fine Arts
Vanderbilt University
Nashville, Tennessee

[3]Cheekwood Fine Arts Museum
Nashville, Tennessee

This text is devoted to the digital imaging process and the emphasis is upon its implications to health care delivery. However, these technological advances may also be utilized in other areas to improve the quality of human life; we believe this is just such an application (1-4). Converting the values of density on x-ray images to discrete numbers and storing this data in computers allows evaluation of art objects especially paintings in a unique manner (5-7). The increase in availability of computers and microprocessor based data processing systems has made possible the implementation of several digital radiographic methods (8). These are readily adaptable to the analysis of art objects.

In this chapter, the term digital radiography is taken to mean any method of radiographic image production in which the silver halide based film is replaced by an electronic sensor for production of an image. For this purpose, there are three types of digital radiographic systems of interest to us. These techniques differ primarily in the method of image production and the rapidity with which images can be produced (9). The three methods discussed elsewhere in this text are: digital fluoroscopy, scanned projection radiography and the scanned point source radiography. Each has certain characteristics that, if properly utilized, will allow improved x-ray analysis of objects of art.

I. DIGITAL FLUOROSCOPY

Digital fluoroscopy, a major thrust of this text, is accomplished using a modified version of the standard imaging system in which depiction of density distribution is produced by causing x-rays to pass through a subject such as a painting and fall upon a receptor (Fig. 1). As noted elsewhere in this text, the receptor consists of a thin layer of material that will convert the x-ray energy into light (see chapter by Price). The receptor apparatus, as also noted previously, is mounted on an image intensifier tube. In most systems, the output of the image intensifier is viewed by a video camera for display or by a film/camera system for recording of a hard copy to share with art scholars, curators, collectors, and conservators. In many digital fluoroscopy systems, the normal video camera is replaced by a high-sensitivity, low-noise camera (usually around 500 to 1 signal-to-noise range). This entire system, especially the camera, is designed to minimize image distortion. The output of the video camera is converted from an analog signal to a digital format by a high speed analog to digital converter. This digital data is then available to be processed by computer hardware and is either processed in real-time for immediate display or stored on digital disks for replay and processing after completion of the study (Fig. 1). At this time, multiple characteristics of the work of art can be analyzed, especially such important assessments as support integrity, as well as pigment apposition, separation, cracking and crazing (10,11). Since most of these studies will be performed in a collaborative fashion, "post-processing" is quite important.

An advantage of a digital system for analysis of paintings is the ability to replay the data following completion of this study without the degradation involved in analog storage

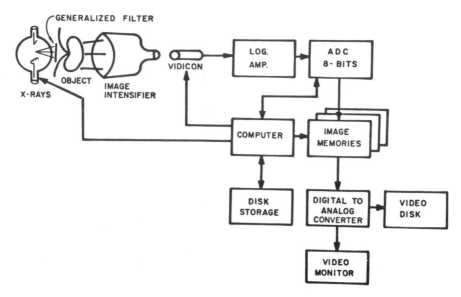

FIGURE 1. The digital radiology system consists of the standard x-ray image intensifier system with the digital processing hardware coupled to it. Digital data are stored on digital disk in order to be available for post-processing after collection.

techniques. Because of this facility, one then has the opportunity to manipulate the data to form subtraction images as well as to obtain quantitative values of density from certain parts of the images. In terms of analysis of paintings as noted, it is perhaps this post imaging capability which provides the most usefulness of this technique. One of the difficulties with obtaining adequate radiographs of paintings is that the attenuation characteristics of the structure and the pigment layer are usually unknown before several trial exposures have been made. This problem with conventional radiography makes it difficult to obtain an optimal radiograph for analysis. A digital fluoroscopy system allows manipulation of the image following collection of the density values in the computer system to produce a near optimum image for the intended analysis. Additionally, different areas of an individual work will often have dramatically different x-ray attenuation properties. Thus, post image processing will allow one to select and manipulate the image to optionally depict and analyze each area.

Because of the limited contrast ranges in conventional radiographs of paintings, as we have noted, it is often difficult to display the necessary range of densities with simple x-ray images. However, as has been discussed in this text, the attenuation properties of all materials that compose a work of art are a function of the energy of the incoming x-ray (12). Use of this principle has led to the ability to subtract the shadows produced by unwanted objects in the images of the art objects. Similarly, the ability to perform subtraction images using radiographs obtained at two different x-ray energy settings may provide additional information in the analysis of paintings. Two given pigments may have attenuation characteristics which are much the same at any particular x-ray energy, making it difficult to form a radiographic image with sufficient appreciable contrast to distinguish objects or specific materials in the work (2,3). However, it may be possible to perform subtraction images by combining individual radiographs taken at different x-ray energies, thereby enhancing the difference in the various pigment distributions (see discussion of dual energy subtraction by Jolles).

Dual energy techniques may take advantage of K edge absorption differences or different properties of compton scatter and photoelectric absorption. One can expose a painting in the scout mode of certain x-ray computed tomographic units at different energies (such as 85 kVp and 135 kVp) and combine these to form a "basis" image for later selective subtraction. Just as Brody and others have suggested that dual energy subtraction may form the basis of technology leading to tissue characterization, pigment and technique characterization may be similarly accomplished (5).

One of the advantages of using computers in image processing is the ability to perform mathematical manipulations. That is, one can perform statistical analysis on the distribution of the digital numbers or the distribution of intensity levels which reflect the image of the painting. This ability can be used to enhance the display of the image as shown in Fig. 2. Investigation of image processing and analysis techniques has made possible a large number of image manipulation procedures which may be used in the analysis of paintings (13). The Fourier transform is one such technique already discussed in this text. This concept is based upon the theory that any image is composed of a discrete number of spatial frequencies. Any combination of spatial frequencies can, therefore, be considered the "signature" of the image. By the use of these processing techniques, any image can be decomposed into the individual signature frequencies. These signature frequencies can be displayed upon a device for analysis. This technique might be considered as similar to that of voice prints in which the sounds are separated into

discrete temporal frequencies and displayed for analysis.   As
more is known about this technique, it may be possible to use
the Fourier transform analysis of images to achieve frequency
signatures which can be subsequently used to characterize
images and validate paintings of questionable origin or
authenticity.

One of the methods used by art scholars to validate
paintings is the analysis of the technique of a painting and
comparing these observations to the characteristic technique
that forms the "signature" of the painter in question.   Of
course, one recognizes that the usual concept of the signature
of an artist can be forged, embellished, or reinforced at some
later date.   It is much more difficult to copy the style of
any particular artist.   Using Fourier transform techniques on
digital images, it may be possible to simply take a radiograph
or a series of radiographs of a painting and compare the
technique "signature" of the painting with the frequency
signature of paintings of other artists that have previously
been stored in computer memory.   Obviously it would be quite
impossible to make an absolute identification by this
technique, but the weight of evidence might support the
evidence of a particular artist.

The spatial resolution of the digital fluoroscopy system
is on the order of two line pairs per millimeter, as has been
noted elsewhere.   However, the size of the image that can be
collected at present is relatively small when compared with
the size of some paintings.   Image intensifier fields-of-view
vary from approximately 4 inches to a maximum of 14 and soon
16 inches, which makes the use of digital fluoroscopy for the

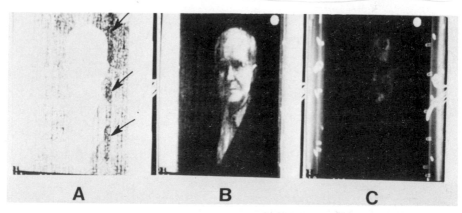

FIGURE 2. Digital data storage allows the image to be
manipulated to examine, in turn, (A) canvas defect (white
arrow), (B) pigment distribution, and (C) mechanical
mounting.

analysis of larger paintings rather restrictive if one is interested in imaging the entire painting. In the present format, multiple exposures may have to be taken with the composite images placed together in their proper orientation. This maneuver is not necessary with small paintings. However, the use of digital fluoroscopy is imperative if one is interested in performing high resolution or "signature" analysis because of the high resolution capabilities necessary.

Certain studies have shown that there is some decrease in observer performance for image analysis at a 512 X 512 CRT display but not with a 1024 X 1024 display. Also, the resolution (in line pairs/mm) is slightly reduced when one moves from a 10 X 10" format to a 14 X 14" format. This technique offers quite unique possibilities in being able in a non-destructive manner to evaluate a painting as well as compare the components, painting technique employed, and status of the condition of a series of works.

II. SCANNED PROJECTION RADIOGRAPHY

One of the outgrowths of modern computed tomographic (CT or CAT) scanning instrumentation is a method for performing digital radiography which has many of the features of an ordinary radiographic study but records each data point in a discrete, finite manner. This technique is often referred to as a "scout view" or a preview. At the present time, it is available in any radiology department with a "CAT" scanner and consists simply of placing the x-ray tube and detector assembly in such a position that the painting can be moved linearly through the x-ray beam to produce the view required (Fig. 3). As the painting is moved through the x-ray beam, data can be collected by the computer from the detector array. The image of the painting is thus stored in the computer memory for subsequent display and manipulation.

Following collection of the data and normalization for display, the image is depicted as a black and white representation on a television type monitor. In this image, the brightness of the individual image point or "pixel" is proportional to the density of the corresponding point in the painting. The resolution of this system is quite good and has a meaningful correspondence to the image in the painting. Spatial resolution on the order of 1.5 millimeters are possible in scan projection radiography of this type. Density differences of half a percent may be perceived by this

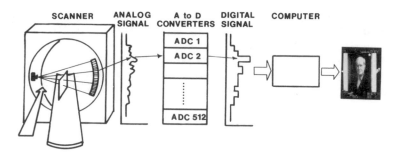

SCANNER · ANALOG SIGNAL · A to D CONVERTERS · DIGITAL SIGNAL · COMPUTER

ADC 1
ADC 2
ADC 512

FIGURE 3. Scanned projection radiography of paintings can be performed by use of a conventional computerized tomography scanner as shown here.

technique; better even than those with conventional radiography and xeroradiography (14).

An advantage of this method of digital imaging is that it is possible to change the energy of the x-rays over a relatively wide range and still produce an excellent image with manual manipulation. This is possible because the electronics of the detector array can be optimized by special calibration procedures for the particular x-ray energy being used. This calibration procedure is not possible either with a conventional x-ray system or with the usual form of digital fluoroscopy system previously discussed in this chapter. Larger paintings may be analyzed by this method since most scout view systems are able to accommodate a 16 x 16 inch field of view. The scout view technique also has the advantage of being able to image a much larger dynamic range of densities of material because of the electronic nature of the detector. This allows the user to display a much finer gradation in the densities. Because of the scatter removal or rejection properties of this type of system, very high contrast images can be achieved. Quite possibly, we may realize the promise that was initially enthusiastically offered when we first began to analyze the numerical expression of the x-ray attenuation properties (the so-called "Hounsfield numbers").

III. SCANNED POINT SOURCE SYSTEM

A third digital radiography method is the "flying spot" or scanned point source system (see chapter by Heller). In this system, the x-ray image is formed by scanning a fine pencil beam of x-rays over the part of the painting area being imaged (Fig.4). After passing through the object, the beam is detected by a large scintillation crystal whose output is measured by light detectors and then stored in computer memory. The formation of the pencil beam of x-rays is accomplished by a mechanical system of collimators which block the beam and move in such a manner that the beam is scanned over the imaged area in a rectilinear raster. The time required for a radiograph of a painting (16 x 24 or 20 x 24 inches) is of the order of 5 seconds.

This technique has not been widely used in clinical medicine because until recently the imaging time was in the order of 15 seconds. Additionally, the spatial resolution is not as great as with the other digital methods, placing this technique in the framework of a screening method. Although the image is of relatively high quality, the low resolution and extended imaging time make it useful in only a very limited number of clinical medical problems. However, neither of these represents formidable obstacles in the analysis of art. At the present time, it is possible to form images with a resolution on the order of 2 line pairs per millimeter. Images can be stored in computer memory and one can perform

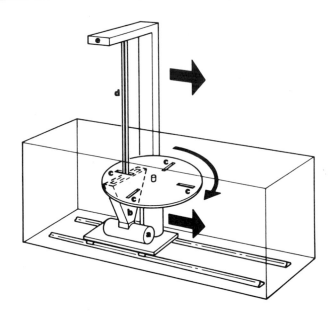

FIGURE 4. In the scanned point source system, the image is constructed one point at a time by moving the x-ray beam over the area to be imaged in a predetermined path by means of a collimation system.

several scans of the same area, sum the images to form a higher quality picture, and manipulate the data to optimize the display. This technique has not received sufficient use that our experience allows us to evaluate and compare it with the other more widely accepted digital methods. For the moment this is a potential method to study works of art and does not appear to have the promise of fluoroscopic radiology or "scout film" x-ray computed tomography.

IV. SUMMARY

The recent advances in computer processing of images and the development of electronic detectors have made possible the development of digital radiographic techniques. These processes which replace the ordinary silver halide film with electronic detectors have great potential in the analysis of objects of art especially paintings. The ability to distinguish very small differences in attenuation characteristics provides the possibility of quantitative analysis of pigment. The very sophisticated image processing techniques that have been developed for the space industry and medicine also may be applied to the analysis of paintings through the use of the digital radiographic images.

ACKNOWLEDGMENTS

We are most appreciative of the advice of conservators Caroline Keck of Cooperstown, and Cynthia Stow and Shelly Reisman of Nashville. The encouragement of the late Joshua Taylor, Robert C. Vose, Jr., and Dr. Robert Coggins was most helpful.

REFERENCES

1. James, A.E., Freedman, J., Robertson, J., Brumbaugh, T., and James, J., The Ahls, Vanderbilt Press (1980).
2. James, A.E., Gibbs, S.J., Diggs, J., et al., The use of x-rays to evaluate paintings, (in press).
3. James, A.E., Gibbs, S.J., Price, R.R., et al., Uncovering works of art, Diagnostic Imaging (June, 1981).
4. Minton, L., and James, A.E., The Cowan Collection, Antiques Magazine (November, 1980).

5. Brody, W.R., Macowski, A., Lehmann, L., et al., Intravenous angiography using scanned projection radiography: Preliminary investigation of a new method, Invest. Radiol. 15, 220–223 (1980).

6. Mistretta, C.A., Ort, M.G., Cameron, J.R., et al., A multiple image subtraction technique for enhancing low contrast, periodic objects, Invest. Radiol. 8, 43–49 (1973).

7. Roehrig, H., Nudelman, S., Fisher, A.D., Frost M., and Capp, M.P., Photoelectric imaging for radiology, IEEE Transactions on Nuclear Science, NS-28(1), 190–204 (1981).

8. Coulam, C.M., Erickson, J.J., Rollo, F.D., and James, A.E., Jr., eds., "The Physical Basis of Medical Imaging," Appleton–Century–Crofts, New York, (1981).

9. Erickson, J.J., Price, R.R., Rollo, F.D., et al., A digital radiographic analysis system, RadioGraphics 1(2), 49–60 (1981).

10. Keck, C.K., "The Care of Paintings," Watson–Guptill, New York, (1967).

11. Bridgeman, C., and Keck, S., The Radiography of Paintings. Eastman Kodak Co., Rochester, New York, (1961).

12. Rao, G.U.V., Fatouros, P., and James, A.E., Physical characteristics of modern radiographic screen-film systems, Invest. Radiol. 13, 460–469 (1978).

13. Partain, C.L., Price, R.R., Patton, J.A., Erickson, J.J. Pickens, D.R., and James, A.E., Jr., The potential impact of digital radiography (DR) on the specialty of nuclear medicine, Clin. Nucl. Med. 6(108), P2–P5 (1981).

14. James, A.E., Montali, R.J., Novak, G.R., and Bush, R.M., The use of xeroradiographic imaging to evaluate fracture repairs in avian species, Skeletal. Radiol. 2, 161–168 (1978).

23

NEW TECHNIQUES IN MEDICAL IMAGING
WITH SPECIAL EMPHASIS UPON DIGITAL RADIOLOGY

M. Paul Capp[1]

A. Everette James, Jr.[2]

with the assistance of

Sol Nudelman[1]
H. Don Fisher[1]
Theron W. Ovitt[1]
Gerald D. Pond[1]
Bruce J. Hillman[1]
Joachim Seeger[1]
Jon Erickson[2]
Don Baker[3]
C. Leon Partain[2]
W. Hoyt Stephens[2]
James A. Patton[2]
Ronald R. Price[2]
Arthur C. Fleischer[2]
Alan C. Winfield[2]

[1]University of Arizona
Tucson, Arizona

[2]Vanderbilt University School of Medicine
Nashville, Tennessee

[3]University of Washington
Seattle, Washington

The developments in physics, engineering, computer sciences and other basic disciplines are being increasingly applied to medical imaging in recent years. These advances provide exciting new opportunities for improved diagnosis and more specific therapeutic regimens.

When Wilhelm Roentgen produced the first medical radiographic image on December 22, 1895, he initiated a revolution that continues until this day. In the first fifty years after this monumental discovery, radiologic technology developed with advances in x-ray tubes, film, intensifying screens, and image intensifiers. The ensuing thirty years have seen major advances in special procedure technology, nuclear medicine, ultrasonography, microwave and computed tomography.

At present, we are either in early clinical trials or at the threshold of clinical introduction with the "new" imaging modalities of real-time and pulsed Doppler diagnostic sonography, positron emission tomography (PET), "dynamic" computed tomography, digital radiographic techniques, and nuclear magnetic resonance (NMR). This communication will consider many of these topics and relate these to the subject of this text—digital radiography.

I. MICROWAVE IMAGING

Bragg et al. (1) have developed a technique by which they can use microwaves to accurately monitor changes in lung-water. For this measurement, a transmitter is placed across the chest of the patient. Phase and magnitude signals from the microwave interrogating pulse are measured and clearly demonstrate their direct relationships to increasing concentrations of pulmonary water. This technique, one of the most sophisticated indicators of lung-water detection to date, can perceive and record changes in lung-water of 2% to 3%. Lung-water must be doubled to be determined on chest radiographs. The double indicator radionuclide technique to measure extravascular pulmonary water is accurate but complex to perform (2).

Human trials are beginning in the development of this simple, inexpensive, low-dose method which measures an important finding in the lungs. This technology could influence therapy, particularly for patients in intensive care areas, to detect early forms of pulmonary edema. Videodensitometry and digital radiography offer viable alternatives to microwave imaging.

II. NUCLEAR MAGNETIC RESONANCE (NMR)

For several decades, NMR has been a recognized method of analysis of specimens and samples. Some half-dozen years ago, investigators began to explore the possibility that this technique could be employed to produce clinical images representing proton distribution as well as other parameters. Recently, this imaging modality has improved to the point that it is of sufficient anatomical resolution to provide images comparable to those achieved by radiography, sonography, nuclear medicine, and, at present, even x-ray computed tomography (3-6). The signals utilized to produce NMR images contain unique chemical and structural information which other techniques do not provide. NMR appears to represent a technology of greater imaging potential than many others. In the past year, data acquisition time requirements and spatial resolution have quite favorably improved (7-9). The basic principles of this imaging technique are sufficiently unfamiliar to the potential users that this characteristic may initially prove to be a limitation.

A. NMR: Basic Concepts

Nuclei of atoms possess a positive charge. Some nuclei also possess an intrinsic spin which results in the creation of a magnetic field. Intrinsic spin resembles the motion of a spinning top rotating about an axis. These nuclei when placed in an external magnetic field will experience a torque (Fig. 1). These nuclei will then attempt to line up either parallel or antiparallel to the external magnetic field and will move in a pattern called "precession" around the magnetic field. The precessional frequency for each nucleus is determined by the external magnetic field strength and a characteristic property of the nucleus, the "gyromagnetic ratio." The characteristic (precessional) frequency for a particular nucleus is known as the "Larmor frequency".

After being placed in a homogenous static magnetic field, the nuclei under study are irradiated with a radiofrequency electromagnetic pulse equal to the Larmor frequency. A resonant effect will be created (Nuclear Magnetic Resonance—NMR). In this resonant condition, the nuclei to be studied will absorb energy from the RF pulse and change their alignment relative to the applied magnetic field. Following the RF pulse, the nuclei will "relax" to their original

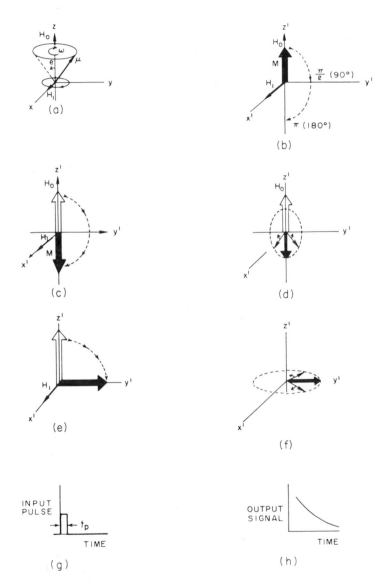

FIGURE 1. *(a) Precessing nucleus (proton) with magnetic moment, μ; at an angle, Θ, with respect to the magnetic field H_0; at an angular velocity, ω, with superimposed radiofrequency field, H_1.*

(b) Net magnetic vector M, prior to π pulse in T_1 experiment.

(c) M after π pulse.

(d) Return to equilibrium after removal of H_1 radiofrequency field.

(e) M after $\frac{\pi}{2}$ pulse.

(f) Return to equilibrium after $\frac{\pi}{2}$ pulse.

(g) Width of π pulse, t_p.

(h) Decay in time of output signal.

alignment and will reradiate the absorbed energy to the surroundings. The re-emitted energy provides the NMR signal which can be detected and measured. If the information in this signal is spatially resolved, it can be employed to form an image.

The length of time ("relaxation time") necessary for the nuclear rearrangement is in general terms related to the general nuclear environment. Short relaxation times imply a greater facility to pass energy to the neighboring nuclei and promptly return to the original energy state. Two different relaxation times have been identified, the spin-lattice or longitudinal relaxation time (T_1) and spin-spin or transverse relaxation time (T_2). T_1 is the exponential time constant corresponding to the decay of that component of magnetization parallel to the external field. T_2 is the exponential time constant corresponding to the decay of the component of magnetization perpendicular to the external field (Fig. 2). The other important NMR parameter is the nuclear density (ρ) which represents the concentration of the nuclei of interest in the area of the body under study.

The parameters, ρ (nuclear density), T_1 and T_2, describe or reflect both the characteristics of the nuclei to be analyzed and the environment in which these nuclei exist. The NMR signal (free induction decay, FID) generally provides information which is a combination of ρ, T_1 and T_2, depending upon the NMR experiment chosen by the investigator. Thus, the information derived can be controlled by the election of the experimental design (10).

B. Imaging By The NMR Method

If all areas of the sample are subjected to the same static magnetic field and have the same resonant frequency,

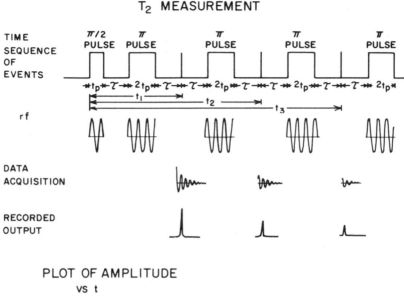

FIGURE 2. Typical T_2 pulse sequence.

one cannot derive spatial data. Spatial information has been achieved with NMR techniques by a number of different approaches. If a known field gradient (usually linear) is applied in addition to the static magnetic field, then different areas of the sample will be in slightly different fields. Thus, the nuclei in each area will resonate at slightly different frequencies. The resonant frequency can then be directly related to the spatial location.

A pulsed NMR experiment is a broadband experiment and the duration and shape of the pulse can be tailored to excite uniformly a precisely known band of frequencies corresponding to a specific area of the sample. The excitation bandwidth is chosen to match the range of resonant frequencies imposed upon the sample by the application of the linear field gradient. The transient time domain response (FID) following the resonant RF pulse in the presence of a field gradient is then

the summation of decays of all frequency components present in
the sample. By the mathematical process of Fourier
transformation the spatial distribution of spectral components
can be obtained. This frequency domain spectrum in this
instance represents a one-dimensional projection of NMR
response along the particular field gradient direction. A set
of angular projections can be obtained by rotating the field
gradient, and at each gradient angle position, performing the
pulsed NMR experiment, collecting the transient NMR response,
and then performing the Fourier transform. The field gradient
rotation can be achieved by producing a single field gradient
which is the vector sum of fields produced by two separately
driven, mutually orthogonal field gradient coil sets.

The above described methodology has a number of parallels
in imaging techniques in clinical use. The rotation of a
field gradient to form angular projections is analogous to the
rotation of the x-ray tube and/or detectors in x-ray computed
tomographic scanning. The projection data can be processed
mathematically to provide a two-dimensional image by using the
filtered backprojections algorithm. Reconstruction of an
image from a set of projections was among the first NMR
imaging techniques developed (5). The requirement of sample
rotation to obtain projections may be obviated by rotating a
static linear field gradient, an advantageous process which
may not require mechanical motion.

Plane definition is a prerequisite for medical imaging
since the body does not possess cylindrical symmetry; in x-ray
computed tomography, beam collimation determines "slice"
thickness. In the process of NMR imaging, frequency, not
wavelength, determines spatial resolution. Two complementary
slice definition techniques presently predominate and have
been successfully used to produce high quality thin section
images of human structures. These techniques are described as
selective irradiation and the use of time-dependent gradients.
In the selective irradiation technique, a long, spectrally
tailored RF pulse with a narrow excitation bandwidth is used
to excite the spin system. This is performed in the presence
of a relatively strong field gradient in a particular
direction and the signal collected in the presence of a
gradient placed in another plane to provide a projection.

In the time-dependent gradient technique, data acquisition
takes place continuously in the presence of two field
gradients: 1) the x-y gradient forming the projection and 2)
an oscillating z gradient to define the slice. The
oscillating gradient makes the signal from all parts of the
sample time-dependent except for a thin slice situated at the
gradient null plane (6). In the selective irradiation
technique, the length and shape of excitation pulse and field

gradient strength determine slice thickness. In the time-dependent gradient technique, frequency of gradient oscillation and strength of gradient determine slice thickness. The time-dependent gradient technique has a particular advantage because coordinate axes can be reassigned so that the defined imaging plane can be spatially located in any direction. The capability has been used to produce direct coronal and sagittal NMR sections of the brain and thorax (7,11,12). The acquisition of images from oblique planes is also feasible with this technique and may overcome any spatial resolution differences when compared with x-ray computed tomography.

To present projection reconstruction as the only method of NMR image formation would not be correct. Other methods are sensitive point "line scanning" and methods of collecting data from two-dimensional sets of points or an entire three-dimensional array [projection reconstruction, 2-D FT (e.g., "spin-warp"), "echo planar", 3-D reconstruction]. NMR imaging is intrinsically a low sensitivity, noise limited modality. Even with the most elegant experimental and technological designs, the relaxation times (T_1 and T_2) of biological tissue and the thermal noise of the body ultimately determine the signal-to-noise ratio in the image. Within limits, using the most sensitive NMR techniques, higher spatial resolution can only be achieved by increasing the acquisition time with reduced image signal-to-noise ratio and/or spatial resolution. Compared to x-ray computed tomography, NMR sensitive point and line scanning can be compared with a single beam/single detector and fan beam computed technology, respectively.

Computed tomography using x-ray energy will very likely be the "gold standard" by which we are to judge NMR imaging. Although with improved understanding of NMR images with higher spatial resolution, more favorable signal-to-noise ratios will be produced, they do not necessarily have to compete in these particular terms with the images produced by the current generation of computed tomographic scanners. The major advantage that NMR imaging may offer medicine is the ability to provide contrast in a unique manner, one not due to the attenuation of x-rays.

The type of NMR system which will offer the greatest clinical cost/benefit and risk/benefit advantages remains to be determined. At present, it appears that a common choice of design will employ either an air-core, water-cooled type or a superconducting magnet. No general agreement exists as to what should be or is being displayed in any particular nuclear magnetic resonance image. NMR images often do not represent a two-dimensional map of a single parameter in a defined area of the objects. The image is often a function of the relaxation times (T_1 and T_2) and the proton density at each point in the body section studied. Thus, the image formed by an NMR experiment is usually a spatial representation of what corresponds to a composite NMR signal. For this reason, we predict a rather long lag time between the physical understanding of these parameters and understanding of their implications for physiological assessment and the determination of health and disease.

Clinical trials will be necessary to determine the particular NMR experiments that record the parameters (ρ, T_1, T_2) or the combinations and ratios of parameters that are significant in pathophysiological terms. Although one can observe differences in various tissues, expressing this discrimination in clinical terms awaits correlation. The theoretical utility of the NMR form of tissue characterization has profound clinical implications--probably greater than ultrasound and x-ray computed tomography.

The fundamental difference in relaxation times can be advantageously employed in the NMR imaging of biological materials. The time differences of pulsing and data accumulation can be utilized to create different appearances of body areas much as attenuation is employed to create image differences in x-ray computed tomography.

The NMR imaging technique of reconstruction by projections has been utilized by many laboratories (7,11,13-17). Alternative designs involving movement of the patient or the machine would pose certain definite constraints regarding data acquisition time. Because of these constraints, NMR imaging techniques have been devised and employed which appear to utilize modifications of the applied magnetic fields. Since the spatial definition of the magnetic field is coupled to the RF electromagnetic field by the nuclei of the tissue or organ studied, the technique has been termed zeugmatography, to express "joining together to form a picture" (18). As we have noted in this summary discussion, NMR is a rather complex technique with multiple potential areas of clinical applications to medicine. Several of the more promising areas will be considered--recognizing that this communication is not complete and the omission of certain important investigations is accepted.

C. Certain Clinical Uses of NMR

Certain proponents of NMR have advocated the concept that disease has traditionally been regarded in patho-anatomical terms. However, analysis by NMR techniques will allow investigation of health and disease in chemical/physiological terms (19-21). Biochemical differences in human structures may serve as the basis for contrast resolution in NMR images. As an example, white and gray matter can be distinguished on the basis of lipid and water content.

The finding that the relaxation times of malignant tissues differ from those in normal tissues of the same histologic type was greeted with enthusiasm and has led to a number of investigations of these phenomena (22-26). Results have indicated that malignant tissues generally have longer relaxation times than their normal tissue equivalent. There is overlap in the relaxation time parameters which have been produced by studies to date. Female breast tumors and liver metastases have been demonstrated to have an increased T_1 relaxation when compared to adjacent normal tissue (21). Some preliminary results have also shown that tissue adjacent to inflammation, local immunological reactions, and neoplasia show increased T_1 relaxation times even before there are detectable abnormal histologic changes.

An NMR experiment can be designed to measure the number of nuclei at specific phase angles, thereby accurately determining the motion of these nuclei. Because of this property, blood flow can be accurately measured by NMR techniques (27-29). The magnetization direction of the protons in blood retain their direction for almost a second. This has been referred to as the "memory". The temporal relation of signal and proton motion can be used as a "tracer" to monitor blood flow and to rather accurately calculate the blood flow velocity.

In measurement of complex blood flow systems, NMR technology provides a method to determine the exact characteristics of flow, providing an analysis of distribution functions and irregularities of flow in specific areas. Because of the short time required by NMR to determine blood flow, pulsatile blood can be measured and blood flow as a function of the cardiac cycle can be studied. How this will evolve in relation to digital radiography and pulsed Doppler ultrasound has not yet been determined. The simplicity of the digital procedures and their familiarity to the medical imaging specialist may prove significant. NMR and pulsed Doppler will require the user (medical imaging physician) to understand and employ basic principles not directly transferrable from conventional radiographic techniques. This may, indeed, become a limiting factor in the introduction and widespread application of these techniques. Conversely, the lack of x-radiation and its biological implications has significant appeal.

The combination of NMR proton density imaging with blood
flow measurement promises to be of great clinical utility.
Singer and his colleagues are presently attempting to develop
a system by which the NMR anatomical image will be portrayed
by cross-sectional view of the body displayed in shades of
gray (28). Color, representing the blood flow measurements in
the same area will be superimposed on the gray level image
providing a physiological "picture" with an anatomical
orientation. Other groups are approaching this exciting area
utilizing similar methodologies.

Realizing the potential of creating images with nuclei
other than the proton ^1H has been attempted by several
groups of investigators. The difficulties imposed by the
constraints of nuclear abundance and signal strength have, in
the past and at present, proven formidable. If we are able to
correlate pathophysiology with metabolic information, this
would appear to be particularly important for conditions
involving compromised blood flow and oxygenation, such as
myocardial and cerebrovascular ischemia and infarction. A
number of groups have oriented their major activities in these
areas.

NMR studies using ^{31}P could allow documentation of the
location and extent of tissue injury in any human structure or
organ (30-34). We may also develop techniques to determine
the efficacy of therapy or to document the presence of
irreversible damage in cardiac and cerebrovasular disease
using NMR technology. Hollis, et al. have reported studies of
myocardial ischemia in which they did not attempt spatial
localization (31), whereas Nunnally and his group have applied
surface coils to study the regional metabolism in myocardial
muscle by ^{31}P NMR (30). Recent investigations have
demonstrated that in vivo determinations of heart metabolism
by ^{31}P NMR can be made and appear to be an area of future
promise. Will coronary angiography and organ perfusion
techniques as emphasized by the Vanderbilt and several other
groups using digital methodology offer a more cost effective
diagnostic procedure? The answer is obviously not available
at the time of this publication. Intravenous coronary
angiography has not been clinically achieved but we are of the
opinion that it will.

"Topical magnetic resonance" is a newly developed in vivo
method to acquire ^{31}P NMR spectra from an area of tissue.
The NMR studies require constructing a combination of static
field (B) gradients in which homogenous and non-homogenous
regions are identified. In the homogenous volume of known
dimensions, tissues placed within the gradient volume will
produce high resolution NMR spectra distinguishable from the
broadened spectra produced from the non-homogenous volume. In

the muscle of the human forearm, spectra from adenosine triphosphate (ATP), phosphocreatine (PCr) and inorganic phosphate (P_i) have been obtained and changes in these spectra, due to reduced blood supply, have been determined (34). We are aware of the value of the information, but at present the clinical implications are not fully appreciated. A classification scheme has been developed to evaluate damaged human tissue by measuring the ^{31}P spectrum as well as by determining the ability to maintain low sodium content relative to the perfusing blood.

Some investigators believe that ^{31}P NMR has a potential advantage over the measurements of ^1H because the body contains only a few types of phosphorus compounds. However, the ^{31}P ratio to ^1H in human organs in tissues is approximately 10^{-3} to 10^{-5}. Although these differences between these nuclei are compelling, the severe signal-to-noise constraints of ^{31}P measurements must be overcome before NMR images comparable to those achieved by protons are achieved. Other nuclei of interest have significantly lower NMR sensitivity than protons and are much less abundant in human tissues.

To overcome these inherent limitations, various laboratories have been investigating the use of paramagnetic agents such as manganese or oxygen by infusion or injection; a method analogous to "contrast media" in conventional radiography to alter the parameters of nuclear density, relaxation times, or to change the time course of the spectra of the nuclei themselves (35). Others have infused ^{19}F intravenously in normal canine hearts and canine hearts with an experimentally produced myocardial infarction (36). ^{19}F "washes out" of ischemic tissue to the extent that this parameter might allow differentiation of ischemic myocardium from normal. Clinical trials and prototype instrument developments are being initiated to improve this technology and determine its value in the health care system.

Appropriate attention must be directed to the issue of the biological implications from NMR. One may assume that NMR machines are free of hazard just so long as the exposure parameters remain within certain rather broadly defined limits (37–41). The National Radiological Protection Board (NRPB) in England has concluded that the hazards of using static (B) magnetic fields of several kiloGauss are not biologically significant. In high strength fields, however, flow potentials in major blood vessels or cardiac chambers might present a hazard. An upper limit of 20,000 Gauss has been recommended in response to this concern. With regard to RF power levels, at frequencies below 15 MHz, one should not employ levels corresponding to 70 watts average absorbed power, which would cause a rise of over 1°C in average body temperature.

The National Council of Radiation Protection (NCRP) has organized a committee to produce a document regarding the possible biological effects of electromagnetic energy. Some believe that the most serious biological hazard may result from the rapidly changing magnetic fields which could induce currents in the human body or cause acute deleterious physiological responses. Certain groups have recommended that the maximum rate of change for any part of the exposed body should be less than 20 Tesla/second for pulses of 10 milliseconds or longer. There is specific concern for patients with surgical implants, cardiac pacemakers and certain prosthetic devices. The various compositional materials should be tested for their reaction to the radiofrequency fluxes and magnetic field intensities to be employed.

The rigorous investigation that has accompanied concerns regarding ionizing radiation is yet to occur in NMR. We do not have the body of data in the literature that can be applied as it is in the case of digital radiography. One would anticipate that these studies will be stimulated by the marked increase in the application of NMR techniques to clinical circumstances. Other parameters of biological inquiry may have to be developed to fully evaluate this effect of NMR upon human tissues—as is also true of ultrasound.

Nuclear magnetic resonance, digital radiography and other modalities herein discussed are techniques of analysis and imaging that have the potential to significantly change the practice of medicine. If the potentials of these techniques can be realized, they will offer considerable improvement in our capabilities of diagnosis and evaluation of human disease processes.

III. EMISSION TOMOGRAPHY

Radionuclide emission tomography has received renewed emphasis due to the success of high resolution x-ray transmission computerized tomography (CT) systems. Emission tomography is utilized in a manner similar to CT to obtain images of planes or sections of radionuclide distributions within the body. Conventional radionuclide imaging devices provide images that represent projections of three-dimensional distributions onto two-dimensional displays. Scintillation cameras and most rectilinear scanners have this as an inherent limitation. Depth, the third dimension, can be obtained by complementary views at different angles. The difficulty in this approach is that with these imaging devices, underlying or overlying radioactivity often prevents the imaging device from obtaining an accurate representation of the plane of interest.

Emission tomography systems can be classified into two general types based on the image plane that is visualized (Fig. 3) (42). Emission tomography permits the separation of organs into either longitudinal or transverse sectional maps of radioactivity distributions. The two major advantages of emission tomography are that depth information is provided and the effects of underlying and overlying activity distributions eliminated.

Certain requirements must be imposed on emission tomography systems in order to obtain diagnostic quality images (43). Uniform resolution and sensitivity versus depth characteristics for the detector system are essential since variations in detector response with depth cause unacceptable image distortions. Also, accurate corrections for photon attenuation should be made in order to compare activity concentrations at various tissue depths. Adequate discrimination against scattered radiation is important in all radioisotope image procedures but is even more essential in emission tomography in order to preserve image contrast. Accurate detector positioning and sampling are also necessary because most tomography techniques require geometric reconstruction.

A computer is required for emission tomography imaging because of the complexities of most of these techniques, resulting from the quantity of data processed. High spatial resolution systems are necessary in order to accurately reconstruct the radioactivity distributions under study. Detectors with high sensitivity are required to provide adequate statistics for reconstruction algorithms. It is also necessary that the reconstruction algorithms provide images that compare quantitatively with the actual radionuclide distributions in the human body.

Another fundamental division in emission tomography is made on the basis of the type of radiations emitted from the radionuclide being imaged. Emission tomography systems are classified as either single-photon counting systems (SPC), which make use of routine gamma emitters such as Tc-99m, I-131, I-123, Ga-67, etc. and annihilation coincidence detection systems (ACD), which detect the 511 keV annihilation radiation from positron emitters such as C-11, N-13, O-15, F1-18, Ga-68, etc. (44). Both SPC and ACD tomographic systems have been used to produce both longitudinal and transverse section images.

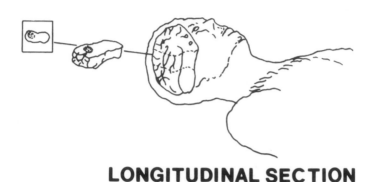

LONGITUDINAL SECTION

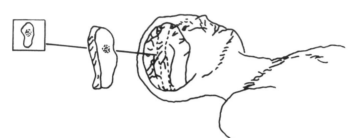

TRANSVERSE SECTION

FIGURE 3.   Illustration of the concepts of longitudinal and transverse section tomography.

Single-photon counting systems are generally designed to collect data from as large a solid angle as possible. This is accomplished either through the use of large, position-sensitive detectors or by measurements at multiple angles; in addition, there exist techniques which combine both forms of data acquisition. Images of the radioactivity distribution are reconstructed by projecting as accurately as possible each detected photon back to its point of origin.

The detectors which employed focused collimators in common use in the rectilinear scanners of the late 1960's did provide longitudinal section images of tissue planes. These tissue planes or "slices" were 1-4 cm thick because of the large solid angle and limited depth of response that were characteristic of the crystal and detector arrangements available in these instruments. An extension of this concept employs multiple detectors with focused collimators utilizing a common focal point.

An instrument using this concept and consisting of an array of nine high purity germanium detectors is undergoing evaluation (Fig. 4). The system remains stationary while the patient is moved in a rectilinear raster beneath the system with a computer-controlled scanning bed (45). Data in this instrument are maintained separately for each detector. Nine arrays of data are stored in a PDP-11 computer and images are reconstructed after the study has been completed. The images correspond to the arrays collected by the system when imaging a distribution consisting of a radioactive letter "+" 1-1/2 inches above the focal plane (F) in plane A and a radioactive letter "0" 1-1/2 inches below the focal plane in plane B. The data illustrated in Fig. 5 from the central detector is analogous to a standard frontal plane image acquired by conventional instrumentation.

The simplest form of image reconstruction of a plane with this technique is produced by backprojection reconstruction.

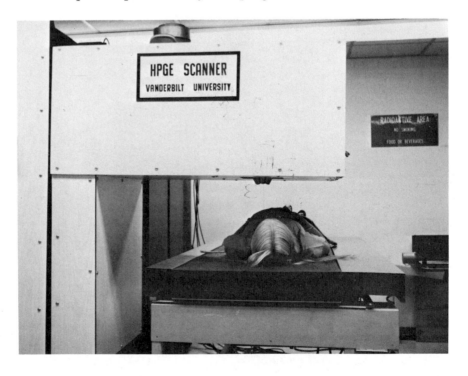

FIGURE 4. An array of nine high purity germanium detectors with tomography collimators for longitudinal section tomography.

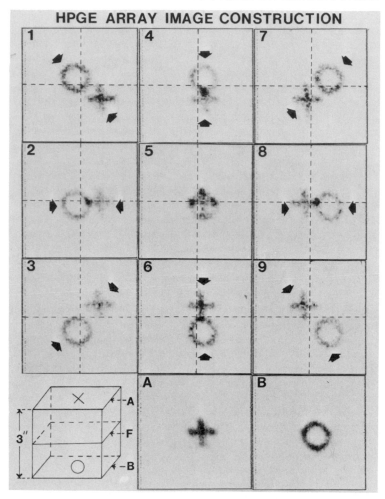

FIGURE 5. An example of image reconstruction by linear superposition of backprojections from a nine detector array.

This method of image formation involves projection of each radionuclide emission event back through the image space along the line from which the radioactivity was initially detected. Activity in a plane is then reinforced by superposition of the data points, whereas contributions from activity in other planes are blurred and thus deemphasized. The superimposition of back projections is accomplished by translating the data arrays in the X and Y directions. This translation distance is determined from the distance from the plane of interest to the common focal point of the system. The directions of the translations are determined by the relation of the plane of interest to the focal plane. Almost any type of multidetector arrangement can be used to produce longitudinal section images using backprojection reconstruction.

The multi-detector arrangement described is only a special use of the generalized theory of longitudinal section tomography or focal plane tomography. These techniques were also developed for position-sensitive detectors (46) and have been applied to a multiplane tomographic scanner which is currently being marketed by Siemens Gammasonics, Inc. The newest system (Pho/Con Model 192) consists of two 9.3 inch diameter scintillation cameras (each with 19 photomultiplier tubes and an intrinsic resolution of 6.5 mm) which scan in a rectilinear raster for simultaneous anterior and posterior imaging (Fig. 6). By electronically determining the coordinates of the geometrical center at the time a radioactive event occurs, as well as the coordinates of the event within the scintillation camera itself, it is possible by means of analog circuitry to use the backprojection technique to reconstruct multiple planes from a single scan.

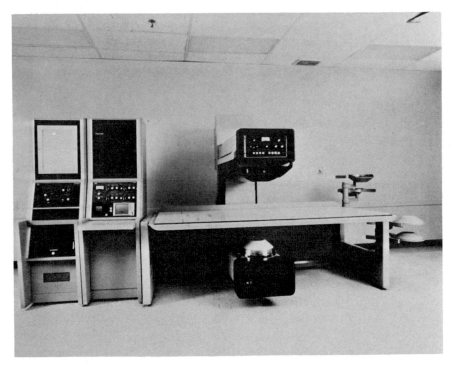

FIGURE 6. The Pho/Con tomographic scanner manufactured by Siemens Gammasonics, Inc.

The instrument employs 12 longitudinal section planes, 6 from each detector. All 12 planes are produced for each scan with the separation between planes pre-selected by the operator.

Several attempts have previously been made to develop tomographic techniques using the scintillation camera. The development of the tomographic capability as an accessory to a conventional scintillation camera would represent a significant economic advantage. A rotating, slant-hole collimator has been used with a moving bed to provide such a longitudinal section imaging device (47). This system was not widely accepted due to circular artifacts inherent in the type of data collection process. Another technique, based on the use of a seven pinhole collimator coupled to a large-field scintillation camera and optimized for longitudinal section imaging of the myocardium, has also been developed (Fig. 7) (48). Data are acquired and stored in a computer from images projected onto seven independent areas of the camera crystal. Images of a point at a standard distance from the center of the collimator and of a uniform plane source are used to establish the imaging characteristics of the system. Images of multiple planes are then reconstructed by a translation and addition-multiplication algorithm.

A. Transverse Section Imaging

Transverse section images with single photon counting are generally obtained by one of two techniques. Multiple sets of data about the region of interest can be obtained with a single detector, or multiple detectors can be used. An

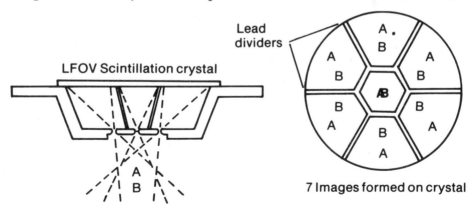

FIGURE 7. Diagram of the seven pinhole collimator used with the scintillation camera for longitudinal tomography.

example of such a system is shown in Fig. 8 (49). Each detector rotates about its support axis (A) to collect counts as a function of angle (B) for each detector. The image is reconstructed by projecting each detected event along the line of origin (backprojection), as shown in (C) for a single detector, (D) for four detectors and (E) for all eight detectors.

The addition of background subtraction results in image (F). This image represents the simplest of transverse section image reconstructions. However, the images acquired in this manner are relatively low in contrast, may contain artifacts due to summing effects, and are therefore not quantitatively accurate. Other techniques for image reconstruction can be used to obtain higher quality images (50), such as the iterative (repetitive) reconstruction procedure in which an initial image is generated (such as a simple backprojection image). Corrections are applied successively in order to force the image into better agreement with the true distribution. The iterative process continues until the image converges to a point such that further corrections do not cause a significant change in the image.

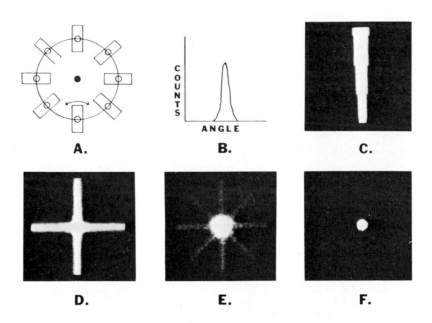

A. B. C.

D. E. F.

FIGURE 8. Image reconstruction of a point source by linear superposition of backprojections from data obtained with the Vanderbilt University Tomographic Scanner.

Analytical reconstruction techniques may be employed for image formation in which exact equations are solved to provide the final image. Filtered backprojection algorithms (computerized mathematical techniques similar to but slightly different from those used in transmission computed tomography) may be used. These algorithms alter the individual projections by applying mathematical correction factors before projecting them back into the image array. In the projection array, those projections are summed together. Two-dimensional Fourier reconstruction algorithms may be implemented by taking the one-dimensional transform of each projection and plotting this in the Fourier plane. Interpolation is used to provide a two-dimensional array of Fourier coefficients. The final image can be produced by taking the inverse two-dimensional transform of the array.

To make reconstructed images quantitatively accurate, one must correct for photon attenuation due to tissue interposed between the radioactive nuclei and the detector. In single photon imaging, this correction has been approached in several ways. A successful technique has utilized a phantom which simulates the area under study. This phantom can be scanned to obtain a correction matrix to be applied to the reconstructed images (51). Conjugate views and transmission scans have also been used to develop correction factors which are then applied to the original projection data. Transverse section radionuclide tomography by single photon counting was accomplished early by Kuhl and Edwards (51). Their machine was optimized for brain scanning, utilizing detectors that were structurally fixed (Fig. 9). Different projections can

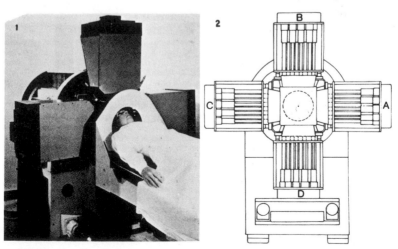

FIGURE 9. The Mark IV Transverse Section Tomographic Scanner optimized for imaging of the brain.

be obtained by rotating the entire frame so that the fields of view of the detectors are interlaced. Images are reconstructed by an iterative technique which Kuhl has termed the Cumulative Additive Tangent Correction (CATV), which is an additive correction process by which corrections are based on pairs of orthogonal projections (Fig. 10). Non-uniformities in count rates experienced by different detectors are corrected by data obtained from a plane source placed immediately in front of each detector. Attenuation corrections are obtained daily by scanning an 18 cm diameter plastic cylinder of activity as a reference. Clinical results with this system indicate that section scanning, as compared to rectilinear scanning, is quite helpful in the basal regions of the brain, by virtue of improved image separation and statistics.

Another transverse section imaging device for single photon counting that was commercially available for a time consisted of twelve 8" X 5" X 1" NaI(T1) detectors with focused collimators (6" focal length). The instrument of this type designed for body imaging consists of ten detectors with focused collimators positioned symmetrically in a gantry about the scan field (52). Data collected by axial movement of the detectors was then coupled with a rotational movement of the gantry. Tomographic images were produced by optimizing the focal point response of each detector which repeatedly moved from the center to the outer edge of the scan field during the scanning interval. Another system of this general design consisted of two opposed detectors mounted in a gantry with rotational movement permitted for data collection. Data could

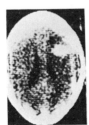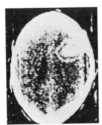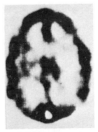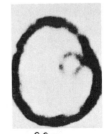

XCT   XCT (contrast) ^{99m}Tc-RBC ^{99m}TcO$_4$

FIGURE 10. Images obtained by x-ray computed tomography and emission computed tomography of a patient with a dense intracerebral hematoma.

be summed from the two detectors providing a cylindrical response of 15 cm in diameter (53).

Transverse section imaging has also been accomplished using the parallel hole collimator of a scintillation camera coupled with a computer (54–57). This technique employs the various reconstruction methods that have been previously described. Static images are collected at multiple angles about the patient. These data are used to reconstruct multiple sections through the patient. This technique employs the various reconstruction-by-projection methods that have been previously described. Advantages of the scintillation camera based system are its ability to record simultaneously images from multiple planes and the capability of using an imaging device which can be employed in routine imaging. A disadvantage with this configuration is loss of spatial resolution and sensitivity with depth.

Yet another system with improved capabilities of the camera-type arrangement has recently been developed (58). This system consists of two opposed large-field-of-view scintillation cameras which can be used with either conventional parallel hole collimators or specially designed one-dimensional converging collimators. The system makes use of filtered backprojection reconstruction algorithms and attenuation correction techniques. These provide excellent resolution uniformity with variation in sensitivity of approximately 10% throughout a 30 X 21 cm elliptical scan field. Most of the major manufacturers are now offering versions of the single or dual rotating camera design as commercial products. Our clinical experience at present is not sufficient to completely evaluate the clinical applicability of these systems.

B. Annihilation Coincidence Detection (ACD): Basic Principles

The use of positron emitters is well suited to applications in emission computed tomography. The positron (a positively charged electron) has a short lifetime and, when emitted from a nucleus, travels only a short distance before losing kinetic energy and uniting with an electron. At that point, the masses of the two particles are then converted into energy in the form of two 511 keV gamma rays which move from the site of their production in opposite directions (180°). If these photons are detected simultaneously in two detectors located directly opposite each other, the origin of the positron annihilation would then lie at a point along a straight line between the two detectors. This annihilation phenomena can be used for longitudinal and transverse section imaging. Locating each recorded pair of 511 keV gamma rays is immediately reduced to a one-dimensional problem. This is to determine the point at which these positrons were produced and in this manner locate the origin of the decay event. The origin of the detected emissions is determined by the physical characteristics of the annihilation process. This circumstance eliminates the need for conventional radionuclide collimators and only "electronic collimation" is necessary.

C. Longitudinal Section Imaging

Camera-type devices have been used for longitudinal and transverse section tomography utilizing ACD (Fig. 11). The two detectors located opposite each other record the coordinates of the two 511 keV photons that arrive in coincidence. These coordinates are then employed to project a line back through the image space. The linear superimposition of these backprojections will allow one to create an image of a longitudinal plane while deemphasizing blurred off-plane information. Using the filtered backprojection technique, it is possible to obtain an improved rendition of the three-dimensional distribution of a radionuclide within the organ or structure of interest. A positron camera device for this purpose is characterized by: 1) lack of collimators to be used in the imaging process, 2) more than one detector, and 3) sophisticated electronics to perform the coincidence detection. Several camera-type imaging devices are being developed as positron tomography systems. One of these positron cameras consists of two opposed detector arrays, each containing 144 small NaI(T1) detectors which are arranged in a

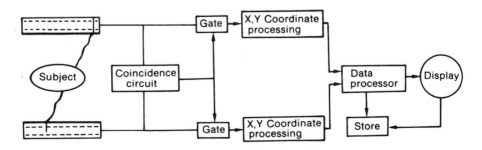

FIGURE 11. A conceptual diagram of camera-type systems used for longitudinal and transverse section tomography with positron emitters.

square array (59). This was developed at the Massachusetts General Hospital, PCII, Boston, Mass. In this system, each crystal is wired in coincidence with 25 crystals in the opposite array. As a stationary imaging system, the detector arrays can produce images of longitudinal sections. Sampling problems are reduced by scanning in the vertical and horizontal direction.

A multiwire proportional-chamber (MWPC) camera has been built that consists of two detectors, each with a sensitive area of 48 cm X 48 cm and with a single converter for each chamber (60). The multiwire proportional-chamber detectors with lead converters are suitable for a large area positron camera because of relatively low cost for large area detectors, adequate spatial resolution, and acceptable uniformity of response. The disadvantages encountered with present types are low detection efficiency and long resolving times.

A scintillation camera can be modified to be used as a detector for positron tomography (61). One such system consists of two large-field-of-view (LFOV) cameras with 1.0 inch thick sodium iodide crystals. Detector electronics can be modified to allow each camera to record a higher count rate than in the usual mode of operation. Coincidence circuitry has been designed such that each position in one crystal has the potential to determine coincidence with the entire crystal of the opposed detector. This type of device is currently undergoing initial clinical trials.

D. Transverse Section Imaging

Transverse section images of positron-emitting distributions can be fashioned using scintillation camera-type devices. The ability to do this is achieved by rotating the detection systems about the object of interest (the patient). Specialized devices making use of multiple detectors have been constructed for transverse-section imaging. One such system employs 32 stationary detectors, arranged in a circle, with corresponding coincidence circuitry (62). Another slightly different instrument has been developed utilizing a ring of 64 detectors with rotational capability (63). Each detector is coupled in coincidence with 23 opposed detectors creating a fan beam geometry with a central cross-sectional field of 25 cm (64,65).

One system which is commercially available is the ECAT which is manufactured by the Ortec Corporation of Oak Ridge, Tennessee. The ECAT represents an improvement of the prototype system (PETT III) of Phelps, Hoffman, Ter-Pogossian and co-workers (66) of the Mallinkrodt Institute of Radiology in St. Louis, Missouri. This device (Figs. 12 and 13) consists of 66 detectors arranged in a hexagonal array with 11 detectors in each of 6 detector banks. Each of the 11 detectors in a bank is separately wired to an equivalent detector in the opposite bank. Therefore, a total of 363 lines for response are present in this system. The resolution of the system is improved by collecting data as the detector banks are moved synchronously to perform linear scans over a distance of 3.5 cm. The entire system is then rotated 5° and the linear scan repeated. This process is continued until the entire system has been rotated 60° and an image is reconstructed using the Fourier techniques of linearly superimposing filtered backprojections. The only collimation employed in this device are slit shields to reduce the coincidence count rate from scattered radiation and single event count rate that can produce random coincidences. Photon attenuation corrections are performed by using geometrical factors determined for the head or abdomen or one may actually measure the attenuation with an external ring source containing a positron emitter. The image acquisition times are variable from 10 seconds to several minutes per view and resolution ranges from 9 mm to 1.8 cm under the operator selection method. This system can perform rectilinear scans which provide three simultaneous views (anterior, 60° LAO, and 60° RAO). An improvement of this system utilizes elongated sodium iodide crystals with two photomultiplier tubes per crystal and "position logic" to provide 4 simultaneous images, each approximately 8 mm thick.

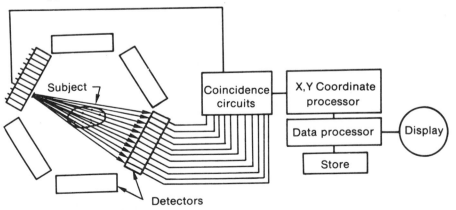

FIGURE 12. *A schematic of the ECAT system marketed by Ortec, Inc.*

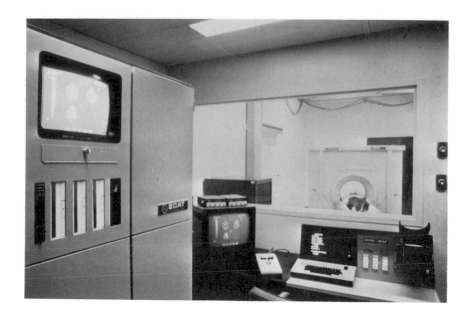

FIGURE 13.   The ECAT system for positron emission
tomography.

Another system of this type consists of a circular array
of 280 detectors with a 31 cm diameter field of view (62).
This instrument does not move and has 14,000 coincidence lines
of response. Because of the geometry of the sampling
procedure, the resolution of this system is circular at the
center of the image field (8 mm FWHM) and becomes elliptical
at a significant distance from the center (8 X 13 mm at 10 cm)
(Fig. 4) (67).

A distinct advantage of these types of systems is the
ability to use isotopes C-11, N-13, O-15, F-18, and Ga-68 as
radiotracers in labeling a wide variety of metabolically
active compounds. However, with the exception of F-18, these
isotopes have short half-lives and therefore must be obtained
from an on-site cyclotron or isotope generator (Ga-68).
Conversely, single photon counting systems use
radiopharmaceuticals that are more generally available, do not
require a cyclotron and are in common use for other
radionuclide studies. The radiopharmaceuticals currently
available for clinical use do not provide the physiological
information that is as fundamentally important as that
provided by the radionuclides of positron emitters (68,69).

Many opportunities will be created with the development of new and improved radiopharmaceuticals.

Since x-ray transmission tomography images are superior in anatomical resolution to radionuclide emission tomography, are there characteristics that might favor the continued development of emission tomography? Transmission tomography provides excellent anatomical information, but emission tomography provides information regarding the functional status of the organ or region under study, making the information different and sometimes complementary. Radionuclide emission tomography, although a well-established concept, has not achieved widespread application. This is due in part to the equipment complexity and cost, the sophistication of personnel needed and requirements of space. The "market" currently appears to be limited although there are some half dozen tomographic systems that are commercially available (Table I). Future developments in radiopharmaceuticals and the outcome of detailed current clinical trials should provide valuable information to determine the cost-benefit ratio for radionuclide tomography as a routine diagnostic procedure.

Emission tomography and digital radiography appear to be only peripherally related. Information provided by these modalities does not appear to be competitive. Limited resource allocation might limit the availability of both of these techniques but digital radiography does not appear to have a great deal of potential as an alternative to emission tomography.

IV. REAL-TIME SONOGRAPHY

Many of the recent technical advances in diagnostic ultrasound instrumentation have been made in the area of real-time imaging. There are currently four basic types of real-time scanners available; these are: 1) linear sequenced arrays, 2) linear phased arrays, 3) annular phased arrays, and 4) mechanical sector scan types. Each of these designs has very definite advantages and each possesses certain limitations. Differences between these instrument types are a result of differences in the transducer design.

To be utilized for cardiac imaging, a transducer should be physically small enough to fit between the ribs or to be angled under the rib cage. Equipment capabilities to record at least 25 frames/sec are also required for cardiac studies. In general, these scanners employ either the linear phased array or the mechanical sector scan transducer. Real-time

TABLE I. Commercially Available Systems

System	Image type	Isotope	Detector description	Spatial resolution
Siemens Pho/Con	Longitudinal	Single Photon	Two scanning cameras with focused collimators	6.5 mm Intrinsic
Union Carbide[a]	Transverse	Single Photon	Circular array of 12 detectors with rotational and axial movement	7–8 mm
Tomogscanner[a]	Transverse	Single Photon	Two opposed detectors with rotational movement	15 mm
Siemens, Picker, GE, Technicare, Toshiba	Longitudinal & Transverse	Single Photon	Scintillation camera mounted on rotational gantry	15–20 mm
Cycoltron Corp. PC-II (MGH)	Longitudinal & Transverse	Positron	Two opposed detector arrays with rotational movement	15 mm
Ortec, Inc. ECAT	Transverse (also recti- linear mode)	Positron	Six banks of 11 detectors each with translational and rotational movement	9–18 mm

[a]No longer available.

imaging can also be applied to much of the rest of the body, especially to the abdomen and neck. One of the advantages of real-time imaging is that this methodology permits a large region to be studied in an expeditious manner and allows a rapid determination of optimum scan planes. This is particularly important, for example, in fetal scanning where one must determine the correct plane through the fetal abdomen for diameter measurements. This also obtains for biparietal diameter measurements.

Because the image is viewed continuously and instantaneously, linear structures such as blood vessels can be followed with real-time systems and their three-dimensional nature reconstructed. With real-time imaging there is less need for the patient to remain immobile or to suspend respiration during the scan. Thus, infants, children, and patients whose physical conditions render them uncooperative or otherwise present obstacles to static imaging, may be studied with less difficulty than with conventional static B-mode scanners. Because study and viewing angles are rapidly achieved, structures can be evaluated, and their size, shape and internal consistency determined quickly. There is less dependence upon the skill and experience of the ultrasonographer. Thus, unlike studies done in static B-mode scanning, these avoid such artifacts as those produced by image overwriting. Within limits, the image quality is independent of the speed at which the transducer is moved over the body. The transducer can be more variable in size and shape for real-time abdominal and pelvic scanning in adults, than for cardiac scanning. However, there is a need to produce as large a field-of-view as possible to permit easy identification of anatomical landmarks and to simplify image orientation for interpretation. Skill of the ultrasonographer is still necessary to obtain the proper image plane necessary to insure an appropriate study.

Real-time instrumentation has introduced the practice of using the water enema to determine relative anatomical orientation and sometimes fixation of structure (Fig. 14). In addition, air bubbles in a liquid may be used to provide a sonographic "contrast media," not unlike that obtained in radiographic fluoroscopy or digital radiography. Another technique of real-time "contrast" study involves the patient ingesting decanted or water mixed with methyl cellulose to create an "acoustic window" through the stomach and duodenum. This latter technique is illustrated in Fig. 15.

The two types of real-time tranducers which have been designed specifically for body scanning are physically large. They are the linear sequenced array transducer (Fig. 16) and the annular phased array transducer. Linear phased array and mechanical sector scan transducers give rise to sector shaped images with an apex angle typically between 60 and 90 degrees (Fig. 17). While this format presents no significant physical constraints in cardiac imaging, the restricted field-of-view in the apex of the sector is inconvenient for imaging superficial structures and organs during body scanning. In comparison, linear sequence array and annular phased array instruments yield rectangular and trapezoidal image formats, configurations which are much more suited to body imaging (Fig. 18).

One of the important determinants of real-time scan quality is the echo dynamic range that can be discerned on the display (70). For x-y oscilloscopes, which are usually employed in analog based real-time scanners, the echo dynamic range is significantly restricted. Clinically, such analog scanners can display only a limited amount of echo amplitude

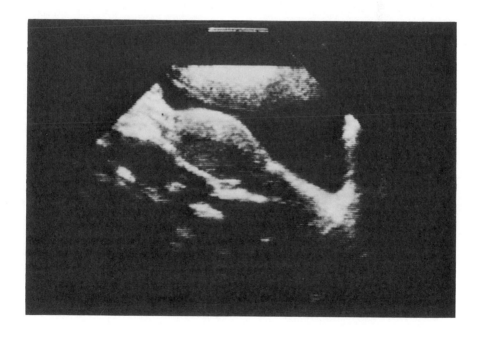

FIGURE 14. Water distension of the rectosigmoid colon utilizing real-time sonography (sector real-time scan taken during water distension of the rectosigmoid colon). Although a rectouterine mass was suspected on the pre-water enema sonogram, distension of the rectum and rectosigmoid colon utilizing real-time sonography failed to demonstrate any rectouterine abnormality.

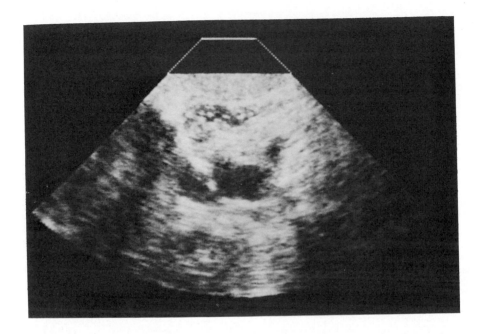

FIGURE 15. Water distension of the duodenum allowing for detailed delineation of the pancreatic head (sector real-time image taken through a transverse plane in the upper abdomen after ingestion). The pancreatic head is clearly outlined when the duodenum is distended with water.

information. Usually the display will only include the stronger echoes which originate from specular reflections at gross tissue interfaces and does not record the smaller and less definite interfaces which record "tissue texture". Digital based real-time instruments may provide a much wider echo dynamic range so that gross tissue interfaces as well as fine parenchymal details can be depicted. This equipment promises the potential to display the echoes from the parenchymal structures which make up the internal composition of organs such as the liver, spleen, and placenta. The ability to "tissue characterize" is a goal in ultrasound which many believe is gradually being achieved. However, at present, certain changes in texture of specific organs are sufficiently characteristic to suggest certain diagnoses.

Real-time instrumentation appears to be a very important direction for progress in ultrasound development. At present, there exists some controversy regarding the wisdom of having a real-time or a static B-mode instrument as the only ultrasound

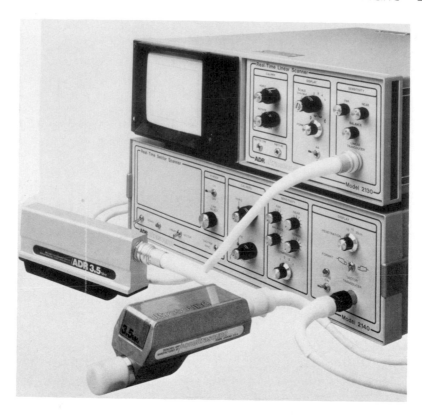

FIGURE 16. Linear array transducer configuration. The linear array transducer is shaped like a bar and contains numerous smaller transducer elements which are activated in a sequential manner. This type of transducer configuration produces a rectangular depiction of a region of interest. Elements are not, however, activated individually but rather in groups in order to form beams that move perpendicular to the transducer plane, unlike the field from a single small transducer which has extremely poor directional properties. The large rectangular field-of-view of the multi-element linear array is best suited for abdominal and obstetrical applications because of the relatively unlimited contact area and need for additional landmark information. (Courtesy of ADR Ultrasound, Tempe, Arizona.)

imaging device in a single department. We believe that these types of imaging instruments offer such different capabilities that in many clinics both may be necessary. There is a compelling need in ultrasound for physiological evaluation and monitoring; this can only be achieved by real-time imaging. There is also the need to record images that have the same resolution as those created during the actual performance of the studies. Many observers believe that only articulated arm B-mode instruments offer this capability at present. Improvements in static recording from real-time studies will be an accomplishment in the near future. We are most certainly approaching a time in which the majority of real-time devices will not be "add on" units.

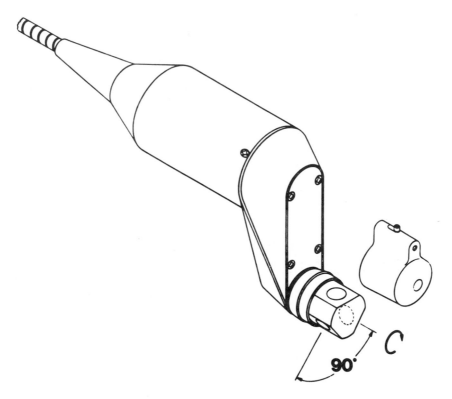

FIGURE 17. Rotating wheel mechanical sector transducer configuration. Within the scanning head of this transducer are three small transducer elements which are rotated. This allows a high frame rate as well as an increase in density. (Courtesy ATL, Bellevue, Washington.)

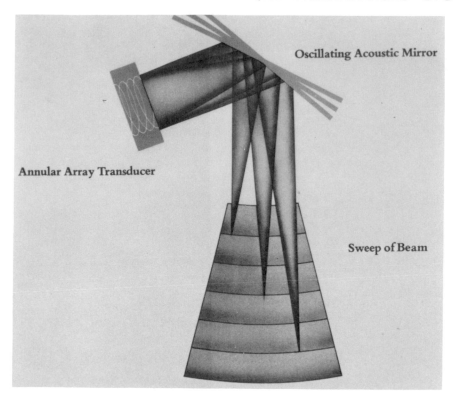

FIGURE 18. *Annular array with oscillating mirror configuration. Annular array transducer configurations allow for the best type of focusing, usually with the use of a water path. The oscillating acoustic mirror focuses the acoustic beam on different areas within the body. (Courtesy Smith Kline Instruments, Philadelphia, Pennsylvania.)*

V. DOPPLER TECHNIQUES

Until recently, no practical or entirely satisfactory ultrasonic method had been developed for the noninvasive determination of volumetric blood flow (71). Even now, availability of this instrumentation is limited. To appreciate the difficulty of this measurement, one needs to understand the concept of volumetric blood flow and measurements which are required to derive it. No directly calibrated "one step" measurement of volumetric blood flow using noninvasive methods seems possible with our present technologies, including digital radiography. Volumetric blood flow (Q), while having the units of liters/minute, actually is derived from two independent measurements when determined ultrasonically. These include the vessel lumen cross-sectional area (Acm^2) and the average flow velocity (Vcm/sec) over that determined and measured area. Determining the average velocity requires a dual measurement since the angle between the sound beam and the blood flow direction or axis (θ) must also be determined. This can be expressed as:

$$Q = VA$$

where   Q = volumetric flow rate in liters/min. or cubic centimeters/sec.

V = average velocity in centimeters/sec., moving along the vessel axis at 90° to the plane of the cross-sectional area. V is a vector having both direction and magnitude.

A = blood vessel lumen area in square centimeters.

Medical ultrasonic Doppler techniques have concentrated almost entirely on only one aspect of this problem; the detection and measurement of flow velocity. Vessel area (A) and sound beam angle (θ) are potentially measureable using recent developments in instrumentation. Before discussing these, blood flow variables as clinical parameters should be considered in detail. Since volumetric flow measurement is technically difficult, other more readily derived parameters, resulting from velocity measurements, have evolved and are being evaluated. These include (72):

1.   Average velocity over the vessel lumen presented as an analog waveform. This method is commonly used in peripheral vascular disease diagnosis.

2.   Velocity distribution within a small sample volume or point located within the vessel or heart and displayed as a frequency spectrum. This is the primary detection and display mode used in cardiac and certain vascular applications.

3.   Velocity at a point within the vessel or intracardiac structure presented as an analog waveform. This particular technique has been employed by some in analysis of certain aspects of cardiac vascular disease.

4. Velocity distribution summed across the lumen of a blood vessel and displayed as a frequency spectrum.

5. Two-dimensional flow images of the blood vessel lumen either in the long axis or in the cross section, depending upon the type of Doppler instrument employed, especially whether it is pulsed or continuous wave. This technique is utilized almost exclusively in peripheral vascular disease evaluation.

We would now like to consider this technology on its own merits and later infer some of the comparisons and correlations which will probably occur in relation to digital radiography. At present, none of these parameters is routinely calibrated to give the true flow velocity or spectra. Blood flow images are "semi-calibrated" but most often appear larger than actual size due to sound beam distortion and resolution effects. Since calibration for quantitation is difficult to accomplish clinically at the present time, most of the Doppler blood flow applications are qualitative and subjective. Physician observation currently serves as a competitive processing system to evaluate normal and abnormal blood flow signals. Clinical experience will determine whether digital radiography will make this statement incorrect.

Accurate use of Doppler blood flow detection techniques requires a thorough understanding of fluid dynamics in a biological setting. In addition, the observer must have appropriate knowledge and appreciation of the Doppler principals and some "feel" for the interaction of ultrasound with moving blood (73). The simplest Doppler instrument transmits a continuous beam of ultrasound into the tissue and vessels of interest at frequencies in the range of 3 to 10 MHz. The ultrasound intensities will vary from 10's of milliwatts per square centimeter (mw/cm^2) to several $100mw/cm^2$ on some of the present commercial units. The ultrasound beam dimensions, including lateral width and position of the focal zone, will depend on the size of the transducer element and whether a lens is fixed to the crystal face. Beam widths which are as narrow as 1 mm or less can be achieved at a frequency of 10 MHz with a sharply focused transducer. In a continuous wave Doppler, the appropriate resolution specifications of interest clinically depend on the lateral width of the ultrasound beam.

We would now consider some of the more general actions of sound in matter. When the sound wave leaves the transducer face and propagates through the tissue, it will undergo

several effects. First, it will be absorbed to reduce the
sound intensity at each point along the beam--a decrease of
approximately 1 dB/cm/MHz. For a 4 MHz wave traveling 10 cm
through the tissue, the loss would thus be 40 decibels or a
factor of 100. Twenty decibels would be the equivalent of a
loss factor of 10, and 60 decibels would correspond to a loss
factor of 1000. Ultrasound would be reflected in this system
at each point along the beam that the acoustical impedence
changes, according to the relation as expressed in $Z = PC$,
where P = tissue density and C = velocity of sound in tissue,
which is about 1540 meters/second. If the structure is
stationary, the frequency of the reflected wave will be
identical to the impinging wave. A moving structure will
cause the backscattered signal frequency to be shifted up or
down by an amount proportional to the interface velocity
acting along the sound beam axis. This shift is given by the
following equation (72):

$$\pm \Delta f_o = \frac{2Vf_o}{c} \cos \theta$$

where Δf = Doppler shift in Hertz (Hz)
          V = vector velocity of interface cm/sec.

          f_o = frequency of impinging sound beam Hz

          c = velocity of sound in tissue media cm/sec.

          θ = angle in degrees between sound beam axis and
             velocity vector

the actual received frequency (f_r) from a moving structure
would thus be:
$$f_r = f_o \pm \Delta f$$

therefore, $\pm \Delta f = f_o - f_r$

When the impinging ultrasound beam passes through a blood
vessel, scattering of the sound wave occurs. In this process,
small amounts of sound energy are absorbed by each red cell
and re-radiated in all directions. If the red blood cell is
moving with respect to the source, the backscattered energy
returning to the receiving transducer will be shifted in
frequency; the magnitude and direction of this shift is
proportional to the velocity of the respective cell. If the
ultrasound beam is considered to fill the entire lumen of a
blood vessel, then the backscattered signal will consist of
all the Doppler shifts produced by the red cells moving
through the ultrasonic beam. Since there will always be a

range of velocities present, from zero at the vessel wall to a peak value near the center of the vessel lumen, a spectrum of Doppler shift frequencies will always be present. This spectrum can become quite complex with pulsating blood flow and vessel wall motion.

Blood flow disturbances due to anatomical defects, i.e., vessel wall irregularity or ulcerated plaques, narrowed or partially occluded vessels, or other abnormalities such as stenotic heart valves, can be readily detected by noting differences in the frequency spectrum of the Doppler signal. Usually, these can be determined by having the observer listen to the Doppler difference frequency, Δf. For ultrasound frequencies in the range of 3 to 10 MHz, Δf will vary from zero to approximately 10 KHz for velocities from zero to 100 cm/sec. A partial occlusion would therefore cause a region of high flow velocity to exist in the narrowed area. This velocity can be readily detected from the Doppler signal by recording the high pitched frequencies which will be present. Another effect which also assists in detection of the abnormality occurs as a result of the vessel narrowing. The moving blood will gain kinetic energy as it accelerates through the narrowed vessel or valve opening. However, as the blood passes the narrowed point into a region of larger caliber, the velocity will then decrease. In this region, the stored kinetic energy will be given up in the form of blood flow disturbances or turbulence.

Although "true engineering turbulence" may not exist, the blood flow will be sufficiently disturbed to produce eddies and vortices. The flow velocity vectors in this circumstance will rotate like a ball or vane in all directions not unlike the motion of an oscillating string. Doppler instruments are quite sensitive to this kind of flow. The output will contain a wide spectrum of Doppler shift frequencies due to the rapidly changing wide range of velocities present in disturbed flow. Clinical auscultation has its utility because disturbed blood flow has a characteristic harsh sound compared to smooth blood flow, which has a definite harmonous tonal quality.

A variety of simple, continuous wave Doppler flow detectors is available to evaluate the peripheral circulation by detecting sites of high velocity or disturbed flow due to partially occluded vessels. These flow detection devices are useful if one is familiar with the method and interpretation of the signals. Both arterial and venous flow in the lower extremities can be assessed by these devices and methods.

With the use of continuous wave (CW) Doppler instruments, the transmitted and received signals are continuously being mixed or compared by the receiving transducer. Because ultrasound is constantly being radiated into the tissue in this circumstance, there is an abundance of non-Doppler shifted signals present from the many stationary interfaces occurring along the sound beam. These large amplitude, overriding, non-shifted signals mix with the very low amplitude Doppler return from moving blood in vessels within the same beam. Following this inherent mixing process, the Doppler difference frequency Δf can be determined by using the amplitude modulation (AM) detection methods employed in radio communications.

For many clinicians, the complexity of the Doppler blood flow signal has been an obstacle, as may also be true in nuclear magnetic resonance. There have previously been no images to view; flow waveforms and frequency spectrum plots seem remote from the disease process, even when the user has a thorough understanding of the physics. A number of imaging schemes have been devised to give the user some orientation to the vessel anatomy and to indicate the site of blood flow detection. These are undergoing clinical trials. The simplest of these uses a continuous wave (CW) Doppler transducer fixed to a mechanical arm. As the transducer moves back and forth over a vessel of interest, an image is produced on a storage oscilloscope corresponding to each site of inquiry. The various deficiencies of the simple continuous wave (CW) Doppler instruments cause them to fall far short of providing a basis for quantitative blood flow measurement. More sophisticated methods and devices will be developed to achieve the goals of calibration of the blood flow through specific vessels. The combination of pulsed Doppler and digital techniques may offer great promise.

The most practical means to add depth resolution to a Doppler instrument is to pulse the source and add a range gate to the receiver. The entire pulsed Doppler methodology being tested in many laboratories is an implementation of this idea. These devices are similar to a pulse echo instrument in that bursts of ultrasound are emitted at a regular repetition rate into the body tissue. A new pulse will not be transmitted until echoes from the previous pulse have ceased or significantly diminished. The depth of a pulse can be determined by noting the time of its flight to an interface and return. Relatively short bursts of approximately 0.5 to 1.0 μ sec duration can be used to give high axial resolution for detection of the location and separation of interfaces to within 1 mm or less. This type of resolution appears to satisfy most clinical needs.

With the caveat that both employ ultrasound energy, the principal of the pulsed Doppler is quite different from that employed with a pulse echo instrument. To determine the Doppler shift of an echo at a particular depth or at many

depths simultaneously requires determination of the precise
frequency of the original transmitted sound burst from the
transducer. This measurement is best accomplished by exciting
the transmitting transducer at a precise and known frequency.
When the echoes return, the observer must have the capacity to
compare their frequency with the original transmitted sound
impulse to determine the difference or Doppler shift. Each
transmitted burst excitation is derived from a master
oscillator (MO) which operates in a continuous mode at a
frequency of something in the range of 5 MHz.

   Initially, this technique will divide the continuous
frequency of 5 MHz into a frequency of approximately 12.5 KHz.
This low frequency is precisely related to the 5 MHz and
becomes the pulse repetition frequency (PRF) of the
transmitted bursts. This PRF signal is used to sample or time
gate the 1.0 μsec long burst (5 cycles at 5 MHz) from the
5 MHz MO which are precisely spaced 80 μsec apart. When
oriented in this manner, each transmitted burst will be
exactly in step with the master oscillator frequency. This
signal can then be amplified and applied to the transmitting
transducer crystal. The fact that there is an 80 μsec space
or time between each transmitted burst means that, for this
example, it will be possible to ultimately detect flow signals
from vessels as deep as 6 cm, based on a calibration of 13
μseconds of transmission time from the tissue for each
centimeter of depth. If the pulse repetition frequency can be
lowered, evaluation at greater depth is possible. Conversely,
if the pulse repetition frequency is increased, the
examination is limited to more superficial depths in soft
tissue. It is believed that pulse Doppler techniques will
provide a future avenue of tremendous clinical growth of
ultrasound use. We will defer the in-depth discussion of this
in relation to digital radiography until the concluding
remarks.

VI. ANALOG TOMOGRAPHY

   "Poor man's CT", or analog tomography, was described by
Barrett and Swindell (74). Film is used as a detector, and
reconstruction is optical rather than digital. During an
exposure, a patient is rotated, and the film is moved
vertically. Consequently, points in the patient appear on the
radiograph as sine waves with varying amplitudes and
frequencies. The radiograph is then placed in a light-box,
and sine waves of known, varying amplitudes are matched to the
sine waves generated by the points. The result of this

matching is filtered optically with a convolutional algorithm, and the signal is transmitted to a photomultiplier tube and displayed on a TV monitor. The results compare favorably to results from CT. Kujoory and others (75) are using this new imaging method to differentiate cortical and medullary excretion in rats (Fig. 19).

One big advantage of analog tomography is that it allows geometric magnification, and cross-section resolution that is impossible with CT. A potential advantage is low cost. At the University of Arizona, scientists anticipated designing a system that would cost approximately $50,000 and could be included in any radiographic room. Rotation of the patient is a definite disadvantage, but all ambulatory patients could be imaged.

This analog method contradicts the prediction that "All images will be stored electronically." However, predicting the state of radiologic imaging in 2000 A.D., even with 90% accuracy, would be a major accomplishment.

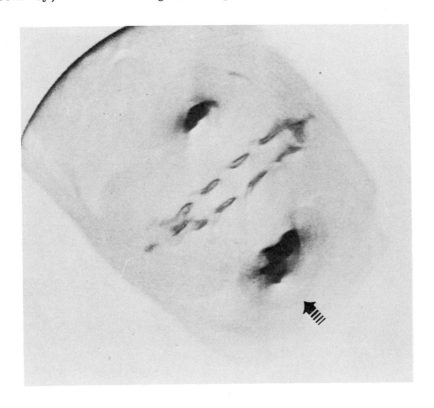

FIGURE 19. Analog tomography differentiating cortical and medullary activity in a kidney of a rat.

VII. <u>PHOTOELECTRONIC RADIOLOGY (DIGITAL)</u>

In 1973, at the University of Arizona, an investigation of the role of photoelectronic radiology in clinical medicine was begun. The goal was to explore the possibility of replacing all x-ray film. At that time, there was data that sophisticated television images were approaching detail found on x-ray films. However, the system for replacement was not ready and there was a question as to whether there was any component of it that could be clinically applicable. The problem of imaging the vascular system was addressed in this way: the conventional technique of film subtraction was used and applied digitally (76). Bernstein, et al. (77) and Steinberg, et al. (78) described digital angiography as early as 1958 and 1959, respectively.

Fig. 20 demonstrates the first successful computerized subtracted image of carotid arteries in a dog (1976). At about the same time, the University of Wisconsin, under Mistretta, et al. (79,80), working independently, also were successful in developing a system to do intravenous video

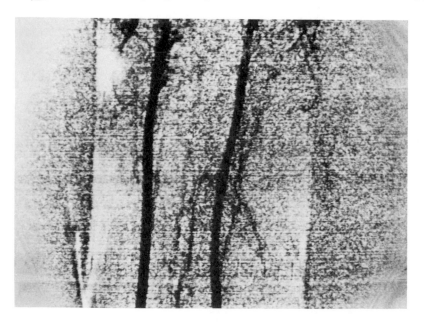

FIGURE 20. This is the subtracted digital image with contrast enhancement of a dog done in 1976. The excellent visualization of the carotid artery led to applying this to humans.

subtraction. The Arizona intravenous video subtraction images in patients started in the research laboratory in 1977 and in March of 1980 a biplane special procedures room was dedicated to photoelectronic imaging (no film) (81,82). This was quite successful and clinical examples will be given later. Current efforts toward total replacement of film are underway. This is an immense problem, one that will require a much greater sophistication of computers, storage devices, systems analysis, and great cooperation from both the radiologist and the clinician (83). The University of Arizona Department of Radiology theoretically converted its 70,000 procedures per year to complete photoelectronic imaging (no film). It was estimated that this would save approximately five million dollars over ten years (84). Extrapolating this to the entire United States would result in a conservative estimate of savings of one billion dollars per year. Not included in these mathematics are the cost-effective savings of all physicians' time and effort.

A. Methods

Approximately 600 patients have been done at the University of Arizona. These are virtually all performed on an outpatient basis. A number 16 angiocath is inserted into the antecubital vein and, using Seldinger technique, a 7 French catheter is advanced into the Superior Vena Cava. Approximately 40 cc of Renografin 76 is injected over two seconds and exposures are made at the rate of one per second for about 15 seconds.
Fig. 21 demonstrates the system block diagram of our current system. The input dose to the image intensifier is about 1 to 1-1/2 milliroentgens per frame or about 150 milliroentgens per exposure skin dose to the patient. Image intensifiers of 9 inch, 6 inch, and, rarely, 4 inch diameter have been used. These will be replaced by a special 16 inch and a 9 inch CGR intensifier, to better handle the high exposure levels and to give a larger area of exposure. The output of the intensifier is coupled to the video camera. The analog signal is then put through an A-D converter. The digitized video signal is fed in real time to a 512 X 512 X 8 bit memory and from there, very quickly, to the VAX 11-780 processing facility. A minimum of two pictures is necessary for intravenous angiography, one before the injection and one after the injection. The computer then performs a linear or logarithmic subtraction of the two images. The differential image is then enhanced in contrast, using a digital "density window", and is displayed on the high resolution CRT. For

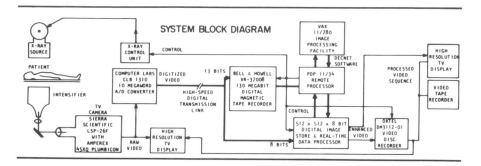

FIGURE 21. This is a system block diagram representing the photoelectronic department of radiology at the University of Arizona. This system is quite sophisticated and obviously very expensive. From this system was devised a more simple, inexpensive one seen in Figure 22.

dynamic imaging such as is necessary for blood flow or cardiac pulsations, the digitized video goes to a high density, digital tape recorder which can record up to 21,600 frames of 512 X 512 X 13 bit video in real time.

It is important to point out that this is a rather complex system which is designed to do research on photoelectronic imaging devices in order to find optimum system components. Fig. 22 demonstrates the phototype model of the CGR (DIVAS) system which is operational in several x-ray departments. This system has the capability of stopping motion with one mr exposure at the intensifier, delivered in 10 milliseconds. The output of the intensifier is optically coupled to a high resolution TV camera using the Ampex 45 X Plumbion. The camera provides both interlaced and noninterlaced video formats with a signal-to- noise ratio of 1,000. The camera's output signal is digitized to 10 bits and fed to the freeze frame digital memory in 1/30 of a second. Simultaneously, the digital data is transferred to a 300 megabyte disk at rates of up to three frames per second. Raw data can be viewed instantly; it can also be recalled at the completion of the procedure for analysis in the image processor. Most image analysis functions are performed in 1/30 of a second, including subtraction, filtering, contrast stretching, averaging and magnification. More complicated algorithms such as geometric correction for patient motion require more time, depending upon complexity.

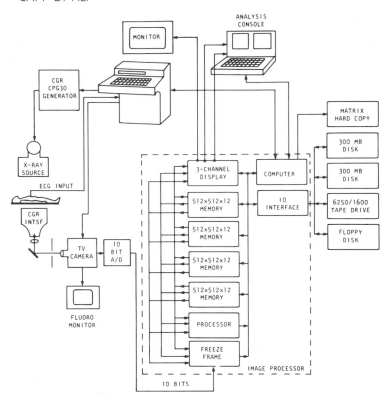

FIGURE 22. This is a simplified, inexpensive, commercially available digital intravenous angiographic system (CGR-DIVAS) developed at the University of Arizona.

The image processor has a configuration with three independent display channels. The user has complete control over the processing environment. Routine functions are initiated through predefined function keys on either of the consoles. More sophisticated processing can be done through commands entered at the keyboard.

The acquisition console provides the interface for control of the x-ray image acquisition system. This includes programmable acquisition patterns to reduce patient dose and data storage. It accepts an EKG gate to reduce patient motion or to synchronize for cardiac studies. The analysis console has the same keyboard, knobs, joystick, interface as the acquisition console, with the exception that the data acquisition function keys are not present. A "reading room" remote from the examination room would be a likely location for the analysis console. This console contains two independent image displays to allow for comparison of different views taken at different studies, different times in the same study, pre and follow-up studies and/or the output of different processing algorithms.

Space required for all this system sophistication is quite reasonable. It will fit comfortably in the hospital environment. For example, the only additional space required for the controls at the examination room fits comfortably in the housing provided for the CGR generator control desk. The analysis console is the size of a standard office desk. The image processor with all of its peripherals can be placed in a room of 10 X 10 ft.^{2} area, located within a coupling electrical cable length of 300 feet from the two consoles.

B. RESULTS

1. Neurological Disease. The University of Arizona has done 300 intracranial neck studies and 200 intracerebral studies using digital angiography (85). Initially, the success rate for intracranial studies was 80% and neck studies 87%. More recently, after the development of a head holder, this has risen to 95% for neck studies and 90% for intracranial studies (86).

Fig. 23 demonstrates a normal digital carotid angiogram in a patient with TIA. Noise in the system has beem reduced to a minimum.

Fig. 24 is an intracranial study in the same patient which demonstrates a normal cerebral angiogram. Detail down to 1 and 2 mm vessels has now been obtained. The exact role of digital subtraction angiography (intracranially) versus conventional cerebral angiography remains to be evaluated. Digital cerebral angiography eliminates the risk of stroke which is always present with arterial catheterization. Digital cerebral angiography seems to be a reliable screening procedure to evaluate certain intracranial abnormalities suspected at CT brain scanning, such as aneurysm, arteriovenous malformations, or vascular tumor. However, the greater spatial resolution and selectivity of conventional angiography make it still the preferred examination for obtaining precise angioarchitectural information, especially preoperatively. The importance of a negative intravenous study of good technical quality should also be emphasized. In many instances, this has obviated the need for conventional angiography. Digital subtraction angiography can replace cerebral angiography in most cases of postoperative evaluation of aneurysm clipping, AV malformation obliteration and various carotid bypass procedures.

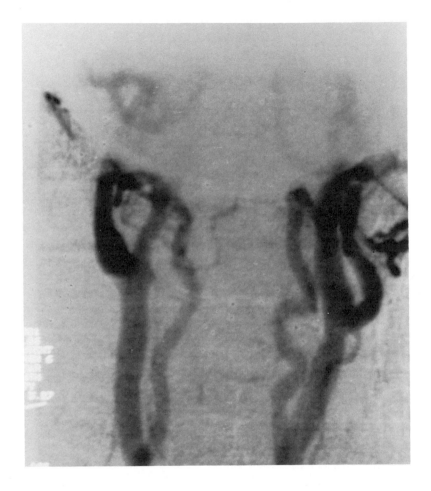

FIGURE 23. This patient's digital subtraction carotid angiogram appears normal. Note the relatively small amount of noise.

2. Abdominal Disease. Most of the intravenous subtraction angiography of the abdomen has been limited to evaluation of the renal vessels and kidneys. Of the first 100 renal cases of the University of Arizona, fifty-three have been of hypertension, twenty-one renal allografts, twelve characterization of renal masses, ten potential renal donors and four were "others". Seventy-six studies resulted in image quality and diagnostic information comparable to that which would be expected by conventional catheter aortography (87,88). Eighteen were judged suboptimal because of poor

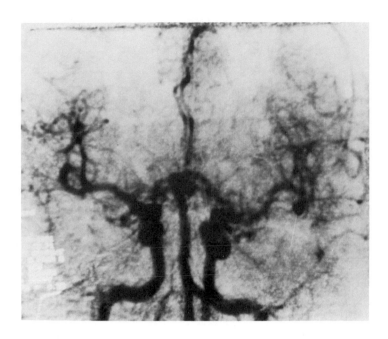

FIGURE 24. This is the intracerebral study of the same patient as noted in Figure 23, demonstrating the normal cerebral arterial circulation.

cardiac output, patient obesity, or nondisplaceable, peristalsing bowel gas; in all of these cases, however, sufficient diagnostic information was generated to permit diagnosis. In six cases, no diagnostic information was obtained. Details of these studies have been reported by Hillman, et al. (89,90). Fig. 25 demonstrates stenosis of the right renal artery.

3. <u>Pulmonary Intravenous Angiography</u>. The University of Arizona has a total of 25 patients where there was a suspicion of pulmonary thromboembolism. Where this is suspected, intravenous angiography is done following a nuclear medicine pulmonary scan. This is felt to be considerably safer than a routine pulmonary angiogram. Success from a technical standpoint was achieved in approximately 75% of the patients from a technical standpoint. No cases were seen in which a negative pulmonary intravenous angiogram was not negative when followed by a routine pulmonary angiogram (91).

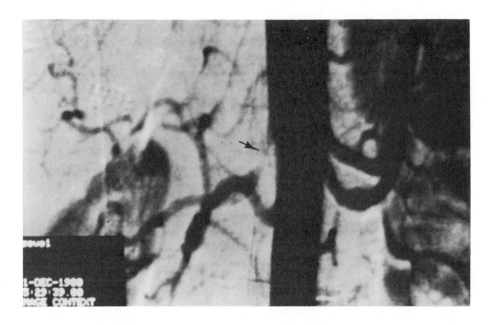

*FIGURE 25. This patient, with hypertension, demonstrates
a stenosis of the right renal artery, small right kidney,
normal left renal artery and a large hyperplastic left
kidney.*

Fig. 26 demonstrates a digital subtraction pulmonary
angiogram, which appears to be normal, in a patient suspected
of having a pulmonary embolism.

4. Cardiac Angiography.   Fig. 27 demonstrates an
intravenous subtraction angiogram in a dog, demonstrating the
left atrium, left ventricle and part of the aortic valve and
aorta. Comparable visualization has been defined in humans.
We have recorded both at 30 and 60 frames per second. The
original system block diagram shows a Bell and Howell digital
magnetic tape recorder for this function. However, this unit
is difficult to work with and already obsolete. Faster
digital recorders that are easier to work with are currently
commercially available. Evaluation of ejection fraction and
areas of dyskinesis is easily done in real-time. The long
term goal is to be able to screen high risk patients for
coronary artery disease. This will probably require the
biplane mode and sophisticated digital tape recording in
real-time.

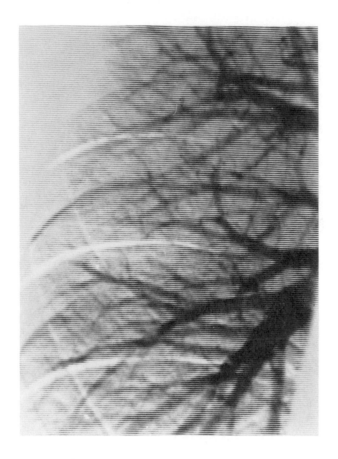

FIGURE 26. Normal digital subtraction pulmonary angiogram in a patient suspected of pulmonary embolus.

5. Miscellaneous. Vessels in upper and lower extremities have been sucessfully evaluated. Fifty studies have been done at the University of Arizona, all of which have been diagnostic. These are patients with aneurysms, vascular bypass grafts, thromboendarterectomy sites and suspected arterial occlusions. Intra-operative or postoperative routine angiograms are used as comparison, if available. A limitation in the procedure is the size of the image intensifier (9 inches). This precludes comprehensive evaluation of the entire lower extremity and aorta in patients with diffuse atherosclerotic disease. Further information will be gained

from using the 16-inch intensifier which is currently being installed. In addition, using some of the experimental contrast media with a much longer half-life within the blood volume will also improve peripheral angiography.

C. The Future Photoelectronic Radiology Department

Long term goals at Arizona are a photoelectronic department with total film replacement for all imaging modalities (92). This will happen but only with improved technology. This transition will occur because of improved physician efficiency, cost effectiveness and some modest improvement in diagnosis. The most important of these three is the cost effectiveness. A theoretical cost effective study was done converting the University of Arizona's Diagnostic Radiology Department from film to a photoelectronic system. This study was done by converting each of the 13 conventional diagnostic rooms to image intensifier sensors and included anticipated hardware requirements for the storage and imaging processing facility. Included in the hardware were digital

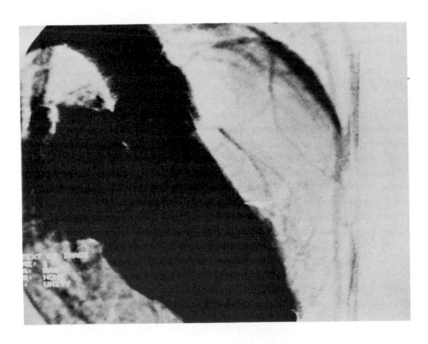

FIGURE 27. This is a levogram phase of a subtracted cardiac demonstrating the left atrium, left ventricle, aortic valve and aorta.

laser beam recorders for archival storage, large capacity high speed disks for intermediate storage and sufficient memory to drive 96 displays. On the basis of 65,000 diagnostic examinations per year, it is estimated that five million dollars would be saved over a ten-year period. Obviously, the front-end costs would be considerable, but this would be more than made up over the ten years. Extrapolating this figure in converting all radiology departments in the United States demonstrates a savings to the health care industry of one billion dollars per year. Many assumptions must be made in this calculation but the figures are probably on the conservative side.

One of the earliest studies done at the University of Arizona included a psychophysical evaluation of the effect of TV scanning lines on diagnostic accuracy, and a judgment of the information content in the radiological image (93,94). A set of radiographs, using a 3-M phantom and sponge soaked in renographin to mimic lung tissue (Fig. 28), were developed (95). In some of the radiographs was simulated a small (1 cm in diameter) pulmonary nodule. Radiologists were asked to detect the pulmonary nodule, comparing various TV scan line display monitors to these same radiographs observed on a view

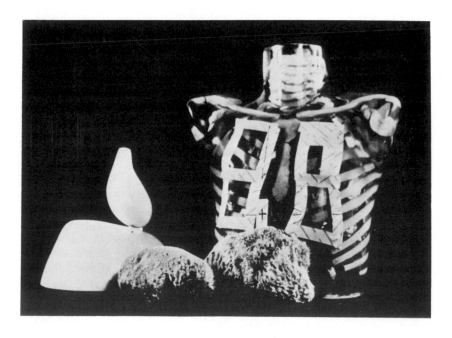

FIGURE 28. This is a 3-M phantom with sponges soaked in diluted contrast material simulating lungs.

box (Fig. 29). Fig. 30 demonstrates that the radiologists performed significantly better in evaluating these nodules from the film on the view box, as compared to both TV systems, 525 X 525 and 525 X 1,000. Fig. 31 demonstrates the detection rate when comparing film to much higher scan line systems. Two different types of film were used and compared to a 1,023 X 1,000 TV line system. There was no significant difference in detecting the pulmonary nodules in terms of percentage correct. Further details of this experiment are found in a publication by Seeley, et al. (94).

A photoelectronic radiology system is currently functional in the Department of Radiology, University of Arizona (Fig. 32). The core of the network consists of a DEC VAX 11-780 computer. The computer system is 350 million bytes of disc storage, 1600-800 BPI magnetic tape system, 256,000 bytes of core memory and a floating point processor (Fig. 33). The VAX 11-780 system will function as a "network scheduler",

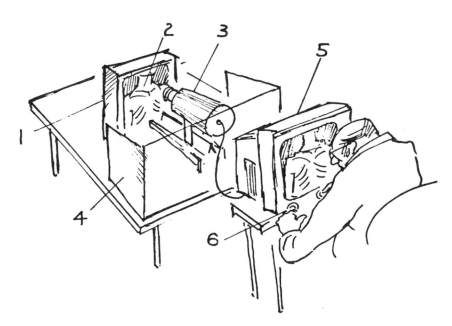

FIGURE 29. Experiment set up for video studies. 1) standard light box, 2) film image of phantom, 3) video camera, 4) opaque curtain, 5) monitor, 6) contrast-brightness controls.

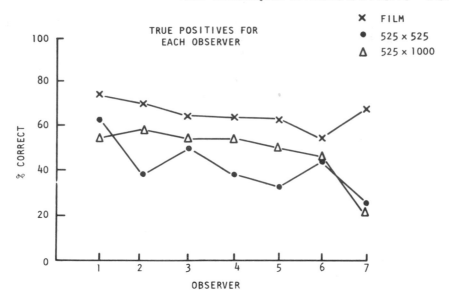

FIGURE 30. This shows that seven radiologists performed better detecting the pulmonary nodule on film compared to the 525 X 525 and 525 X 10000 TV monitors.

queuing tasks for the array processor, providing a time-shared environment for general image analysis, and providing mass storage capability and hence a common data base for the acquisition modes in the network. Further details of this system can be found in the article by Nudelman, et al. (95).

The greatest limitation at the present time is determining which type of x-ray sensor will be the most efficient. Fig. 34 demonstrates four possible x-ray sensors, showing each in combination with some video capability. Each has very significant limitations varying from low spatial resolution to limitation in field size. Technical developments will emerge in the next few years determining which of these four, or possibly other sensors, will be most acceptable.

Another interesting experiment was done to further test the effect of TV camera degradation. Seven sets of pediatric cases (on film) were photographed from a view box as well as from a 1024-line TV monitor. These were shown via slides to several groups of radiologists, who were asked to detect the differences in the slides taken from the 1024-line TV monitor versus the slides from the view box. On a subjective basis, they were unable to detect any difference. The technical sophistication where the quality of the digitized image approaches that of film is closer. For pulmonary structures, however, digitized images are not yet developed. Improvements in technology and more comparative testing need to be done.

Fig. 35 is a schematic diagram demonstrating the functions involved in a photoelectronic radiology department. Three sensing devices are offered. The x-ray screen optically coupled to a video camera should be emphasized. This type of sensing device may well be the most cost effective. Each room contains a display supported by memory. This assures the technologist in that room of quality control. Images would be retrievable seconds after the exposure has been made. Since diagnosis is not carried out here, the display need only be of a conventional quality. The image acquisition, archival storage and imaging processing have been combined together in Fig. 35. Image acquisition involves a video camera at the front end whose signal is immediately digitized and then must be sent to some device where the image is captured and held for as long a time as image manipulation requires. High speed

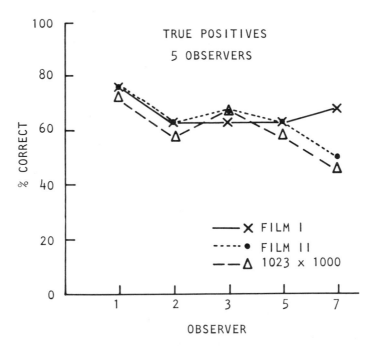

FIGURE 31. This figure demonstrates that five observers performed equally well in detecting the pulmonary nodule comparing two types of film versus the 1023 X 1000 TV monitor.

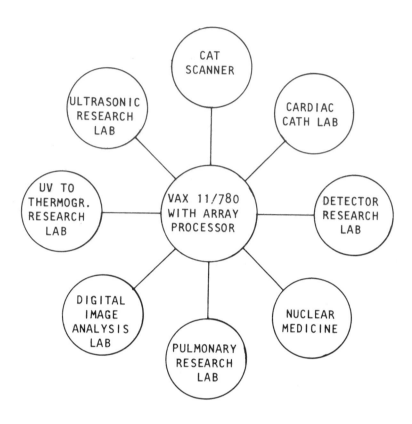

FIGURE 32. This figure demonstrates the photoelectronic
radiology system as currently exists, strictly experimentally,
at the University of Arizona.

digital tapes are available for archival storage and will
serve an anticipated short term need. It is expected that the
long term device for storage will be the laser beam digital
disk recorder, which is able to store more than 10^{86} bytes
per disk side.

A group of digital memory units is also included here to
acquire images for retention and transmission of images to
designated displays (offices, clinics, conference rooms,
etc.).

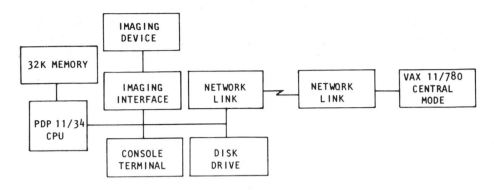

FIGURE 33. Typical satellite.

The reading room requirement is for six stations each with eight displays. This is probably an "overkill". It remains to be seen what the ideal display requirements will be. For example, for most diagnostic applications, 1024 X 1024 pixels will suffice. However, displays at 2048 X 2048 pixels will probably be necessary for greater spatial resolution. Experimentation will have to be done to determine whether or not 4096 X 4096 pixels are necessary.

All radiographic information would be stored on a laser digital disk recorder. From there, using various memory

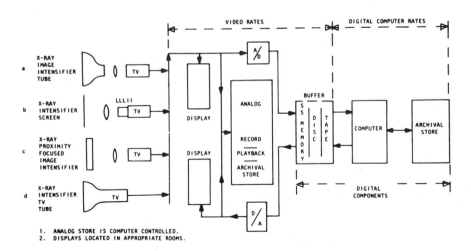

1. ANALOG STORE IS COMPUTER CONTROLLED.
2. DISPLAYS LOCATED IN APPROPRIATE ROOMS.

FIGURE 34. This figure demonstrates four types of x-ray sensors as the imaging receptor. This is by no means conclusive.

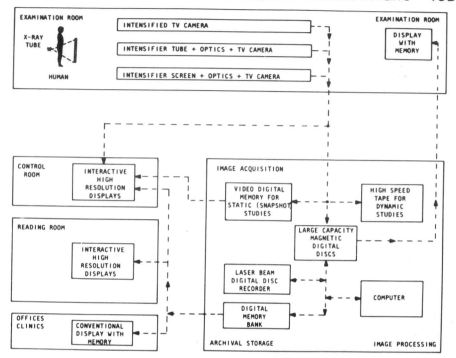

FIGURE 35. This figure demonstrates the functional components of a potential photoelectronic radiology department.

banks, it could be transmitted to the reading room, clinics, offices, etc. Doctors in their own offices would have access at all times to the image as well as to the video report from the radiologist. The educational and service functions of the wards and clinics would be served the same way, eliminating the inefficiency of clinicians coming down from the various parts of the hospital during the day or night seeking films. How long it will take to totally convert to a photoelectronic radiology department depends on the technlogy of x-ray sensors and the technology of archival storage. Dr. Capp's original prediction was by the year 2000, but he now suspects it will be closer to 1990.

VIII. <u>CONCLUSION</u>

Unfortunately, the U.S. Government has invested relatively little into the research and development of new medical-imaging technology. Ten or fifteen years ago we ought to have been where we are today. The National Institutes of Health must redirect some of its funding, possibly by defining a new institute of radiologic sciences. Funds from such an institute could then be channeled into research for the new technologies. This would accelerate the solutions to the problems of clinical medicine and help to achieve the primary goal--better care for patients.

<u>REFERENCES</u>

1. Bragg, D.G., Durney, C.H., Johnson, C.C., and Pederson, P.C., Monitoring and diagnosis of pulmonary edema by microwaves: A preliminary report, <u>Invest. Radiol.</u> 12, 289-91 (1977).

2. Strauss, H.W., Pitt, B., and James, A.E., "Cardiovascular Nuclear Medicine," Mosby, St. Louis, (1974).

3. Damadian, R., Field focussing nuclear magnetic resonance (FONAR) and the formation of chemical scans in man. <u>Philos. Trans. R. Soc. Lond.</u> (1980).

4. Hinshaw, G.N., Image formation by nuclear magnetic resonance: The sensitive point method, <u>J. Appl. Phys.</u> 47, 3709-3721 (1976).

5. Lauterbur, P.C., Image formation by induced local interactions: Examples of employing nuclear magnetic resonance, <u>Nature</u> 242, 190-191 (1973).

6. James, A.E., and Partain, C.L., Proceedings, Vanderbilt Nuclear Magnetic Resonance (NMR) Imaging Symposium. <u>J. Comput. Assist. Tomogr.</u> 5, 285-305 (1981).

7. James, A.E., Jr., Partain, C.L., Holland, G.N., Gore, J.C., Rollo, F.D., Harms, S.E., and Price, R.R., Nuclear magnetic resonance imaging: The current state, <u>AJR</u> 138, 201-210 (1981).

8. James, A.E., Jr., Partain, C.L., Rollo, F.D., Erickson, J.J., Patton, J.A., Coulam, C.M., and Price, R.R.: Nuclear magnetic resonance (NMR) imaging: The potentials and the technic, <u>Southern Medical Journal</u> 74, 12 (1981).

9. Holland, G.N., Moore, W.S., and Hawkes, R.C., Nuclear magnetic resonance tomography of the brain, <u>J. Comput. Assist. Tomogr.</u> 4, 1-3 (1980).

10. Hawkes, RC., Holland, G.N., Moore, W.S., and Worthington, B.S., Nuclear magnetic resonance tomography of the brain: A preliminary clinical assessment with demonstrations of pathology, J. Comput. Assist. Tomogr. 4, 577–586 (1980).

11. Partain, C.L., James, A.E., Watson, J.T., Price, R.R., Coulam, C.M., and Rollo, F.D., Nuclear magnetic resonance and computed tomography, Radiology 136, 767–770 (1980).

12. James, A.E., Jr., Price, R.R., Rollo, F.D., et al., Nuclear magnetic resonance imaging: A promising technique, JAMA 247(9), 1331–1334 (1982).

13. Partain, C.L., Price, R.R., Patton, J.A., and James, A.E., Jr., Nuclear magnetic resonance (NMR) imaging: potential impact on medical diagnosis and digital data communications, SPIE 318 (1981).

14. Partain, C.L., Price, R.R., Rollo, F.D., and James, A.E., Jr., "Nuclear Magnetic Resonance (NMR) Imaging," W.B. Saunders Company (1982).

15. Moore, W.S., and Holland, G.N., Experimental considerations in implementing a whole body multiple sensitive point nuclear magnetic resonance imaging system, Philol. Trans. R. Soc. Lond. 289, 511–518 (1980).

16. Moore, W.S., and Holland, G.N., The NMR CAT scanner--a new look at the brain, J. Comput. Assist. Tomogr. 4, 1–7 (1980).

17. Holland, G.N., Hawkes, R.C., and Moore, W.S., Nuclear magnetic resonance tomography of the brain: coronal and sagittal sections, J. Comput. Assist. Tomogr. 4, 429–433 (1980).

18. Lauterbur, P.C., and Lai, C.M., Zeugmatography reconstruction from projections, IEE. Trans. Nucl. Sci. 27, 1227–1231 (1980).

19. Hinshaw, W.S., Andrew, E.R., Bottomley, P.A., et al., Display of cross-section anatomy by nuclear magnetic resonance imaging, Br. J. Radiol. 51, 273–280 (1978).

20. Shepp, L.A., Computed tomography and nuclear magnetic resonance, J. Comput. Assist. Tomogr. 4, 194–197 (1980).

21. Damadian, R., Tumor detection by nuclear magnetic resonance, Science 171, 1151–1153 (1971).

22. Hollis, D.P., Economou, J.S., Parks, J.C., et al., Nuclear magnetic resonance studies of several experimental and human malignant tumors, Cancer Res. 33, 2156–2160 (1973).

23. McLachlan, L.A., Cancer-induced decreases in human plasma proton NMR relaxation rates, Phys. Med. Biol. 25, 309–315 (1980).

24. Goldsmith, M., Koutcher, J.A., and Damadian, R., NMR in cancer XIII: Application of the NMR malignancy index to human mammary tumors, Br. J. Cancer 38, 547–554 (1978).
25. Eggleston, J.C., Saryan, L.A., and Hollis, D.P., Nuclear magnetic resonance investigations of human neoplastic and abnormal tissues, Cancer Res. 35, 1326–1337 (1975).
26. Mansfield, P., Morris, P.G., and Ordidge, R., Carcinoma of the breast imaged by nuclear magnetic resonance (NMR), Br. J. Radiol. 52, 242–243 (1979).
27. Kolin, A., Improved apparatus and techniques for electromagnetic determinator of blood flow, Rev. Sci. Instrum. 23, 235–242 (1952).
28. Singer, J.R., Blood flow measurements by NMR of the intact body, IEEE Trans. Nucl. Sci. 27, 1245–1249 (1980).
29. Garroway, A.N., Velocity measurements in flowing liquids by NMR, J. Physics D. (Applied Physics) 7, 159–163 (1974).
30. Nunnally, R., and Bottomley, P.A., ^{31}P NMR studies of myocardial ischemia and its response to drug therapies. J. Comput. Assist. Tomogr. 5, 296 (1981).
31. Hollis, D.P., Bulkley, B.H., Nunnally, R.L., Jacobus, W.E., and Weisfeldt, M.L., Effect of the manganese ion on the phosphorous nuclear magnetic resonance spectra of perfused rabbit heart: a possible new membrane probe. Clinical Research 26, 240 (1978).
32. Nunnally, R.L., and Hollis, D.P., Adenosine triphosphate compartmentation in living hearts: a phosphorous nuclear magnetic resonance saturation transfer study, Biochemistry 18, 36–42 (1979).
33. Hollis, D.P., Nunnally, R.L., Taylor, G.J., et al., Phosphorous nuclear magnetic resonance studies of heart physiology, J. Mag. Res. 29, 319–330 (1978).
34. Fossel, E.T., DeLayre, J., and Ingwall, J.S, Potential of nuclei other than protons in NMR imaging, J. Comput. Assist. Tomogr. 5, 301 (1981).
35. Doyle, F.H., Gore, J.C., and Pennock, J.M., Relaxation rate enhancements observed in vivo by NMR imaging, J. Compt. Assist. Tomogr. 5, 295 (1981).
36. Goldman, M.R., Fossel, E.T., Ingwall, J.S., and Pohost, G.M., Use of ^{19}F NMR in evaluation of ischemia and infarcted myocardium, J. Comput. Assist. Tomogr. 5, 304 (1981).
37. National Radiological Protection Board, "Exposure to Nuclear Magnetic Resonance Clinical Imaging," (1980) (Available from the Secretary, NRPB, Harwell, Oxon. OX11 ORQ, United Kingdom).

38. Budinger, T.F., Thresholds for physiological effects due to RF and magnetic fields used in NMR imaging, IEEE Trans. Nucl. Sci. 26, 2821-2825 (1975).

39. Barnothy, M.F., ed., "Biological Effects of Magnetic Fields," Plenum Press, New York, (1964).

40. Bottomley, P.A., and Andrew, E.R., RF Magnetic field penetration, phase shift and power dissipation in biological tissue-implications for NMR imaging. Phys. Med. Biol. 23, 630-643 (1978).

41. Saunders, R.D., and Stewart, J., Biological Effects of NMR, in "Nuclear Magnetic Resonance (NMR) Imaging" (C.L. Partain, R.R. Price, F.D. Rollo, and A.E. James, eds.), W.B. Saunders, Philadelphia (in press)

42. Patton, J.A., Emission Tomography, in "The Physical Basis of Medical Imaging" (C.M. Coulam, J.J. Erickson, F.D. Rollo, and A.E. James, eds.), pp. 253-263. Appleton-Century- Crofts, New York, (1981).

43. Kuhl, D.E., and Edwards, R.O., Image separation radioisotope scanning, Radiology 80, 653-661 (1963).

44. Phelps, M.E., Hoffman, E.H., and Kuhe, D.E., Physiologic tomography (PT) in medical radionuclide imaging, IAEA-SM 210/303, 233-253 (1977).

45. Patton, J.A., Price, R.R., and Brill, A.B., A mosaic germanium radioisotope scanning device with longitudinal section scanning capability. IAEA-SM 210/165, (1977).

46. Anger, H.O., Tomographic Gamma-Ray Scanner with Simultaneous Readout of Several Planes, in "Fundamental Problems in Scanning," pp. 195-211. Thomas, Springfield, IL, (1971).

47. Muehllehner, G., A tomographic scintillation camera, Phys. Med. Biol. 16, 87-96 (1971).

48. Vogel, R.A., Kirch, D., LeFree, M., et al., A new method of multiplanar emission tomography using a seven pinhole collimator and an Anger scintillation camera, J. Nucl. Med. 19, 648-654 (1978).

49. Patton, J.A., Brill, A.B., and King, P.H., Transverse Section Brain Scanning with a Multicrystal Cylindrical Imaging Device, in "Tomographic Imaging in Nuclear Medicine," pp. 28-43. Society of Nuclear Medicine, New York, (1972).

50. Brooks, R,A., and DiChiro, G., Principles of computer assisted tomography (CAT) in radiographic and radioisotopic imaging, Phys. Med. Biol. 21, 689-732 (1976).

51. Kuhl, D.H., Edwards, R.I., Ricci, A.B., et al., The Mark IV system for radionuclide computed tomography of the brain, Radiology 121, 401-413 (1976).

52. Advertising brochure, Union Carbide Imaging Systems, Inc., Norwood, MA (1978).

53. Wooley, J.L., Williams, B., and Penilatesh, S., Cranial isotopic section scanning, Clin. Radiol. 28, 519-528 (1977).

54. Freedman, G., Tomography with gamma camera, J. Nucl. Med. 11, 602-606 (1970).

55. Jaszczak, R., Huard, D., Murphy, P., et al., Radionuclide emission computer tomography with a scintillation camera, J. Nucl. Med. 17, 551 (1976).

56. Keyes, J.W., Orlander, N., Heetderks, W.J., et al., The humogotron--a gamma camera transaxial tomography, J. Nucl. Med. 17, 552 (1976).

57. Budinger, T.F., Gullberg, C.T., McRae, J., et al., Isotope distribution reconstruction from multiple gamma camera views, J. Nucl. Med. 15, 480 (1974).

58. Murphy, P., Bordine, J., Moore, M., et al., Single photon emission computed tomography (ECT) of the body, J. Nucl. Med. 19, 683 (1978).

59. Burnham, C.A., Brownell, G.L., A multicrystal positron camera, IEEE Trans. Nucl. Sci. 19, 201-205 (1972).

60. Kaplan, S.N., Kaufman, L., Perez-Mendez, V., et al., Multi-line proportional chambers for biomedical applications, Nucl. Inst. Methods. 106, 397-406 (1973).

61. Muehllehner, G., Buchin, M.P., and Duder, J.H., Performance parameters of a positron imaging camera, IEEE Trans. Nucl. Sci. 23, 528 (1976).

62. Robertson, J.S., Marr, R.B., Rosenblum, M., et al., 32 Crystal Positron Transverse Section Detector, in "Tomographic Imaging in Nuclear Medicine," pp. 142-153, Society of Nuclear Medicine, New York, (1973).

63. Cho, T.H., Chan, J., and Erickson, L., Circular ring transaxial positron camera for 3-D reconstruction of radionuclide distribution, IEEE Trans. Nucl. Sci. 23, 613-622 (1976).

64. Hoffman, E.J., Phelps, M.E., Mullani, N.A., et al., Design and performance characteristics of a whole body transaxial tomography, J. Nucl. Med. 17, 493-502 (1976).

65. Phelps, M.E., Hoffman, E.J., Coble, C.S., et al., Some performance and design characteristics for the PETT III, in: Reconstruction Tomography in "Diagnostic Radiology and Nuclear Medicine," University Park Press, Baltimore, (1977).

66. Ter-Pogossian, M.M., Basic principles of computed axial tomography, Semin. Nucl. Med. 7, 109-128 (1977).

67. Derenzo, S.E., Budinger, T.F., Cahoon, J.L., et al., High resolution computed tomography of positron emitters. IEEE Nucl. Sci. 24, 554-558 (1977).

68. Advertising brochure. Ortec, Inc., Oak Ridge, TN.
69. Phelps, M.E., Emission computed tomography, Semin. Nucl. Med. 7, 337–365 (1977).
70. Carson, P.L., Gray-scale ultrasound: Understanding and innovation in imaging to speed realization of its potential, Appl. Radiol. 6, 185–189 (1977).
71. Baker, D.W., Personal communication.
72. Baker, D.W., Application of pulsed Doppler techniques. RCNA 18, 79–104 (1980).
73. Wells, P.N.T., Halliwell, M., Mountford, R.A., et al., Tumor detection by ultrasonic doppler blood-flow signals, NBS Special Publications 525, 173–176 (1979).
74. Barrett, H.H., and Swindell, W., Analog reconstruction methods for transaxial tomography, Proc. IEEE 65, 89–107 (1977.)
75. Kujoory, M.A., Hillman, B.J., and Barrett, H.H., High-resolution computed tomography of the normal rat nephrogram, Invest. Radiol. 15, 148–154, (1980).
76. Roehrig, H., Frost, M., Baker, R., et al., High-resolution low-light level video systems for diagnostic radiology, SPIE 78, 102 (1976).
77. Bernstein, E.F., Greenspan, R.H., and Loken, M.K., Intravenous abdominal aortography, a preliminary report, Surgery 44, 529–535 (1958).
78. Steinberg, I., Finby, N., and Evans, J.A., A safe and practical intravenous method for abdominal aortography, peripheral arteriography fand cerebral angiography, AJR 82, 758–772 (1959).
79. Kruger, R.A., Mistretta, C.A., Lancaster, J., et al., A digital video image processor for real-time x-ray subtraction imaging, Optic Eng. 17, 652 (1978).
80. Kruger, R.A., Mistretta, C.A., Houk, T.L., et al., Computerized fluoroscopy in real time for noninvasive visualization of the cardiovascular system: preliminary studies, Radiology 130, 49–57 (1979).
81. Christenson, P.C., Ovitt, T.W., Fisher, H.D., et al., Intravenour angiography using digital video subtraction: Intravenous cervicocerebrovascular angiography, AJNR 1, 379–386 (1980).
82. Ovitt, T.W, Christenson, P.C., Fisher, H.D, et al., Intravenous angiography using digital video subtraction: X-ray imaging system, AJNR 1, 387–390 (1980).
83. Roehrig, H., Nudelman, S., Fisher, H.D., Frost, M., and Capp, M.P., Photoelectronic imaging for radiology, IEEE Transactions on Nuclear Science NS-28(1) (Feb. 1981).

84. Nudelman, S., Fisher, D., Frost, M., Capp, M.P., and Ovitt, T., A study of photoelectronic--Digital Radiology (Part I) The Photoelectronic--Digital Radiology Department, (to be published in IEEE, 1982).

85. Seeger, J.F., Smith, J.R.L., and Carmody, R.F., A head immobilizer for digital video subtraction angiography, (to be published in Jan./Feb. issue of AJNR).

86. Hillman, B.J., Zukoski, C.F., Ovitt, T.W., Ogden, D.A., and Capp, M.P., Digital video subtraction angiography in the evaluation of potential renal donors and renal allograft recipients, (to be published).

87. Hillman, B.J., Ovitt, T.W., Capp, M.P., Fisher, H.D., Frost, M.M., and Nudelman, S., Renal digital video subtraction angiography: 100 Cases, (to be published).

88. Hillman, B.J., Ovitt, T.W., Capp, M.P., Fisher, H.D., Frost, M.M., and Nudelman, S., Renal digital videosubtraction angiography: 100 cases, (to be published).

89. Hillman, B.J., Ovitt, T.W., Capp, M.P., et al., The potential impact of digital video subtraction angiography (DVSA) on screening for renovascular hypertension, (to be published).

90. Pond, G.D., Smith, J.R.L., Hillman, B.J., Ovitt, T.W., and Capp, M.P., Current clinical applications of digital video subtraction angiography, Vasc. Diag. Ther. (Nov. 1981).

91. Capp, M.P., Radiological imaging--2000 A.D, Radiology 138, 541-550 (1981).

92. Gray, J.E., Seeley, G.W., and Capp, M.P., Psychophysics: A tool for evaluation of radiographic systems, Presented at the Tutorial Seminar in Optics in Diagnostic Medicine. Tucson, AZ, Jan. 9-11, 1974.

93. Seeley, G.W., Roehrig, H., Nudelman, S., et al., Psychophysical evaluation of video systems compared to film, J. App. Photo. Eng. 4 (1978).

94. Seeley, G.W., Roehrig, H., Nudelman, S., and Capp, M.P., Psychophysical evaluation of radiology performance from a high-resolution video system compared to film, "Image analysis and Evaluation", SPSE Conf. Pro., July 19-23, 1976. pp. 495-502, 1977.

95. Nudelman, S., Capp, M.P., Fisher, H.D., Frost, M.M., and Roehrig, H., Photoelectronic imaging for diagnostic radiology and the digital computer, SPIE 164, 138 (1978).

A GLOSSARY OF DIGITAL RADIOGRAPHY TERMS

Algorithm - A specific set of well-defined steps for the solution of a problem.

Analog - A physical quantity whose measurable magnitude may take on a continuum of values as opposed to digital quantities which can have only discrete values. In DR, the light output from the image intensifier or the output voltage signal from the video camera which views the output phosphor of the image intensifier are analog quantities. (See digital.)

Analog-to-digital converter (ADC) - A device which converts analog quantities to digital quantities. In DR, the analog video signal is converted (digitized) to digital values (numbers) and stored in a digital memory.

Aperture - An opening in an optical lens system. In DR, the aperture opening is varied (f-stop setting) to control the amount of light from the output phosphor of the image intensifier which reaches the video camera.

Area detector - In photoelectronic imaging, a video-image intensifier is an area x-ray detector. (See point scan radiography and line scan radiography.)

Array Processor - Special hardware which is designed for high speed processing of large volumes of digital information. Some systems have fixed (hard wired) programs while others can be reprogrammed as needed.

Bandwidth - The range of frequencies (lowest to highest) which a system can transmit. High spatial frequency objects (small objects or objects with sharp edges) within x-ray images require large bandwidths. Electronic noise in video systems, however, increases with increased bandwidth.

Binary - The base two (2) number system as opposed to the more common decimal or base ten (10) number system. The binary system uses only two digits, 0 and 1. All modern digital computers are based on the binary number system. (Compare decimal and binary numbers: 1=1; 2=10; 3=11; 4=100; 5=101; etc.).

Bit - A single binary digit can have a value of 0 or 1.

411

Byte — A group of bits (binary digits). In most computer systems, a byte is taken equal to 8 bits. A byte can be used to represent a number from 0-255. In DR, the brightness at a point in the x-ray image is usually represented by a byte; i.e., the brightness can be one of 256 (including 0) values.

Central processing unit (CPU) — That part of the computer which controls the execution of commands specified by the software program.

Compiler — A special computer program, usually provided by the manufacturer, which can convert a program written by a user in a high-level language into a form which can be used directly by the computer.

Composite video — A video signal which contains image video as well as all control pulses and signals for blanking and synchronization.

Conspicuity — The ability of a structure to stand out from its surroundings. In DR structured noise in the form of bones and other anatomy is removed so that the opacified vessels can be made more conspicuous.

Continuous digital subtraction radiography — Images from a video image intensifier system operated in the continuous fluoroscopic mode are digitized and subtracted at video imaging rates. Subtracted images are generally stored as analog video since digital storage devices are generally not fast enough.

Contrast — The difference between two regions divided by the average of the two regions. Subject contrast measured in terms of transmitted photons, image contrast measured in terms of optical density, DR numbers or CT numbers.

Contrast sensitivity — (See contrast) — The ability to detect small contrast differences.

Conversion time — The time it takes for the analog-to-digital converter to convert the analog signals to the digital numbers.

Core — A special type of digital memory consisting of arrays of ferrite rings (cores) which are magnetized to represent either a binary digit (bit) of value 0 or 1.

CRT display - A special display device, usually a video monitor, used to either display images or for operator communications.

Digital - The representation of the magnitude of a measurable physical quantity which can take on only discrete values. The number of discrete values which can be assigned depends upon the number of binary bits used in the digitizing process; e.g., 8 bits = 256 levels, 9 bits = 512 levels and 10 bits = 1024 levels.

Digital Radiography (DR) - Acquisition or display of radiographic images using digital techniques includes digital video-fluoroscopy and scan-projection radiography (SPR). Also includes digital subtraction angiography (DSA), digital intra-venous angiography (DIVA) and computed tomography (CT).

Digital Subtraction Angiography (DSA) - (See Digital Radiography.)

Digital-to-Analog Converter (DAC) - A device used to convert digital quantities to analog quantities. In DR, a DAC is used to convert image data stored in digital memory to analog video for viewing on a video monitor.

Direct Memory Access (DMA) - A channel for data transfer to or from the main storage memory of the central processing unit.

Disk - An electro-mechanical device used to store digital data. Disks are circular shaped magnetic surfaces (platters) and may be either rigid or flexible (floppy). Disk speed and capacity are determined by rotation speed, writing density and the number of surfaces. The size of a disk is usually expressed in terms of Mega bytes or Mega words of storage capacity.

Disk-operating-system (DOS) - An executive software system or set of programs which utilize a disk for temporary storage resulting in faster and more efficient operations.

Dual-energy subtraction - An imaging technique which uses images produced at two different kVp settings along with the measured attenuation coefficients to produce images in which either the bone or soft tissue is removed.

Dynamic range — Refers to the range of values over which image information is stored or displayed. In traditional radiographic imaging, it refers to the maximum minus minimum detectable radiation exposure. For a digital system, the range of radiation exposures that may be recorded is limited by the number of bits used to store the information.

Field — In standard video systems, a scene is scanned from top to bottom using 262-1/2 horizontal scan lines. This scan sequence is called a video field and is performed in 1/60 sec. A videoframe is composed of two interlaced video fields.

Floppy disk — A special type of magnetic disk which is flexible in structure. Floppy disks are usually slower in data transfer rates and smaller in storage capacity than rigid disks.

FORTRAN (FORmula TRANslator) — A high level user programming language. A language similar to English text which is particularly useful for mathematical expressions and calculations.

Frame — In standard video systems, a complete video image (frame) consists of two interlaced fields. A video frame is formed in 1/30 sec.

Frame grab — To digitize and store a video image in digital form as it is created; i.e., one complete frame in 1/30 sec. or one field in 1/60 sec.

Hardware — The electronic components and mechanical devices which physically make up the computer system.

Hertz (Hz) — A unit of frequency, 1 Hertz is 1 cycle/sec.

Image repetition rate — The rate at which images can be repeated. This rate is usually dictated by the rate of the digital storage device (disk).

Instruction — A set of characters (letters and numbers) which specifies a particular operation to be performed by the central processor.

Interface — A device between two components of a computer system which ensures compatible data flow.

Interlaced video — Standard 525 line video frames are formed from two independent video fields which are displaced vertically with respect to one-another (interlaced). Positive interlace implies accurate positioning of the two fields and random interlace implies no precise positioning.

K-edge subtraction — The same technique as employed in dual-energy subtraction with the added requirement that the energies are selected to be just below and just above the K-edge of iodine (33 keV).

Kilo — Commonly a prefix meaning 1000. However, because computers are binary systems (base 2) kilo refers to 1024 which is the power of 2 closest to 1000. For example, 64K bytes actually refers to 65536 bytes of memory.

Line pairs (lp) — Used to specify the spatial resolution of imaging systems. The largest number of observable alternating opaque and transparent lines in a given distance is a measure of the system resolution; e.g., DR is about 1 lp/mm while film may be 4-8 lp/mm.

Line scanning radiography — An imaging system which uses a linear array of detectors and an x-ray fan-beam which is scanned over the patient to produce an image. Detector arrays may be scintillator/photo-diodes or high pressure xenon detector arrays.

Log amplifier — An amplifier which amplifies input signals according to a logarithmic function rather than linearly; i.e., small signals are amplified while large signals are compressed. In DR, log amplification of the video signals prior to digitization provides more quantitative estimates of iodine content.

Machine language — A language that is used directly by the computer.

Mask mode subtraction — Sometimes called time-mode subtraction where a "mask" image acquired before the appearance of iodinated contrast media is stored and subtracted from each subsequent image.

Matrix — The number of picture elements (pixels) into which an image is divided in both horizontal and vertical directions. Typical matrix sizes are 256 X 256 and 512 X 512.

Memory size – The number of words or bytes of memory that can be used to store either programs or images. For example, a 512 X 512 image requires 262,144 memory locations.

Misregistration artifacts – Subtraction image artifacts resulting from relative motion between the two images being subtracted. In DSA, common motion artifacts are caused by swallowing, bowel gas motion and patient movement.

Modulation-Transfer-Function (MTF) – A parameter of the fidelity with which an imaging device reproduces the spatial information contained within an object. MTF generally decreases with increasing spatial frequencies.

Noise – Everything within an image not part of the structures of interest. Noise can consist of other anatomical structures, electronic, digitization and x-ray quantum noise.

Non-interlaced readout – A special video scanning method in which the video camera viewing the output phosphor of the image intensifier is scanned only once vertically from top to bottom. As opposed to a standard interlaced frame which consists of 2 fields of 262-1/2 lines, each a non-interlaced frame consists of 525 lines from a single scan. Both type frames are created in 1/30 sec. (See progressive readout.)

Off-line – Usually refers to devices not in direct communication with the CPU.

On-line – Refers to devices in direct communication with the CPU.

Pixel (picture element) – Digital images are divided into a matrix of picture elements. Each pixel consists of a memory location which has an established one-to-one correspondence with a location within the x-ray image.

Point scanned radiography – A radiographic system in which the image is created by scanning a pencil beam of x-rays over the patient.

Post-processing – Digital manipulation of stored images; e.g., different mask selection or edge enhancement.

Program – A set of instructions arranged in a specific order to cause the computer to perform a particular process or the development and creation of such a set of instructions.

Progressive readout - A method of reading a video camera image phosphor in which the phosphor is scanned only once vertically during a 1/30 sec. period, unlike standard video scanning in which the phosphor is scanned twice and interlaced. Progressive readout is used in pulsed mode DR.

Pulsed mode - Digital fluoroscopic images created using short pulses of x-rays at high currents. Video readout of the image is synchronized to follow the x-ray pulse. Short pulses help eliminate patient motion.

RAM (Random Access Memory) - Information stored in ram memory may be modified and accessed at will with all locations equally accessible.

Real-time subtraction - Digital subtraction of images as they are generated; i.e., no delay between image production and the display of the subtracted image.

Remasking - Choosing a different mask for subtraction following data storage. Usually a post-processing function.

ROM (Read Only Memory) - Memories of this type are used to store programs which are used frequently and which should not be modified or erased.

Scan projection radiography (SPR) - a general category of digital radiography including line scanning and point scanning systems.

Signal-to-noise ratio (SNR) - The ratio of the signal magnitude to the uncertainty (fluctuations) in the signal.

Slit radiography - A special case of scan projection radiography using a slit to create a collimated beam of x-rays which is scanned over the patient.

Software - The collections of programs associated with the operation of the computer.

Spatial resolution - The ability of an imaging system to depict structure within an object. Measured in terms of line pairs/mm. (see line pairs).

Synchronizing pulses - Timing pulses used to assure that x-ray production, video scanning, digitization and digital data storage are coordinated.

Temporal resolution - Relates to the speed of image formation and the image repetition rate. The higher the imaging rate, the higher the temporal resolution.

Time-interval difference (TID) - A real-time digital difference imaging in which temporally adjacent video images are subtracted and displayed in real-time. This mode of imaging presents a continuous display of the difference between adjacent video frames.

Time-mode subtraction - Same as mask mode subtraction where an image acquired and stored prior to the apperance of the contrast media is subtracted from all subsequent images.

Timeshare - The use of a device by several other devices or human users.

Video disk - An analog storage device used to store video frames or fields in real-time. Images stored on video disk or video tape must be redigitized for post-processing operations such as remasking.

Veiling glare - Non-zero light levels detected under radioopaque objects with an image intensifier due to lateral transmission of light from bright areas of the field into the dark areas. Veiling glare makes quantitative imaging difficult in digital radiography.

Winchester disk - A special high speed, large capacity fixed disk used in most DR system for digital image storage.

Word - A combination of binary bits. A word in most DR computer systems is either 16 or 32 bits or alternatively 2 or 4 bytes.

Xenon detector array - A type of detector array used in SPR systems.

INDEX

A

Abdominal vessels, 252, 311, 392
Acute tubular necrosis, 237
ADC. *See* Analog-to-digital converter
Addressing, computer, 32
Adenosine triphosphate, 356
Agency law, 127
Algorithm, 75
Aliasing. *See* Digital images
Allograft, 225
Amipaque, 152
Analog, 9, 27, 29, 35, 64, 308, 375, 385
Analog-to-digital converter, 35
    characteristics for DSA, 54
    contrast resolution, 8, 35
    conversion time, 35, 36
    DSA system component, 7, 83, 388
    sampling, 10
    spatial resolution, 35
Analog disk, 59, 60
Analog film-screen, 325
Analog images, 27
Anastomosis, 162
Aneurysm, 189, 286, 391
Angiocardiography, 63
Angiocatheter, 156, 245
Annihilation radiation, 367
Annular array. *See* Ultrasound
Aorta, 170, 189, 296, 316, 395
Aortic arch, 44, 193, 248, 250, 313, 330
Aortic valve ring, 260
Aperture, 65
Archival (digital) storage, 34, 60
Array. *See* Digital images
Array processor, 399
Arrhythmia, 153

B

Art, 335
Arterial imaging, 253
Arterial catheterization, 98
Arteriogram, 201
Arteriosclerosis, 224, 395
Arteriovenous malformation, 164
Artifacts, in digital subtraction
    angiography, 45, 364. *See also*
    Motion artifacts
Attenuation factor, 13
Averaging, of digital images, 82, 83

B-mode ultrasound. *See* Ultrasound
Backprojection, 351, 364
Bandwidth (video), 24, 25
Billing, methods of, 118
Binary numbers, 9, 30
Biological effects of electromagnetic
    energy, 357
Bi-plane fluoroscopy, 206
Bit, 31
Bits per inch, 34
Blanked (video), 21, 26
Blood flow, 232, 379
Blue Cross/Blue Shield, 104, 105
Bolus, 216
Bowel gas motion. *See* Motion artifacts
Brain, 165, 366
Break-even analysis, 99, 117
Broadcast video, 20
Bruit, 158
Bypass graft, 157, 177, 180, 254
Byte, 29, 31

a
2 b
3 c
4 d
5 e
6 f
7 g
8 h
9 i
8 0 j